METHODS IN MOLECULAR BIOLOGY

Series Editor
John M. Walker
School of Life and Medical Sciences
University of Hertfordshire
Hatfield, Hertfordshire, AL10 9AB, UK

For further volumes:
http://www.springer.com/series/7651

Non-Viral Gene Delivery Vectors

Methods and Protocols

Edited by

Gabriele Candiani

Polytechnic University of Milan, Milan, Italy

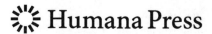 Humana Press

Editor
Gabriele Candiani
Polytechnic University of Milan
Milan, Italy

ISSN 1064-3745   ISSN 1940-6029   (electronic)
Methods in Molecular Biology
ISBN 978-1-4939-8118-2   ISBN 978-1-4939-3718-9   (eBook)
DOI 10.1007/978-1-4939-3718-9

Preface

Gene delivery is the science of transferring genetic material, either DNA or RNA, into cells to alter specific cellular function or structure at a molecular level [1]. Cloned genes can be delivered to cells for biochemical characterization, mutational analyses, investigation of the effects of gene expression on cell growth, understanding of gene regulatory elements, and producing specific proteins. Inversely, the delivery of RNA can be used either to induce protein expression or to repress it using antisense or RNA interference (RNAi) [2].

As the delivery of "naked" nucleic acids is the safest but the least efficient way to transfect mammalian cells and tissues [3], a variety of different vectors, which can be roughly categorized into viral and nonviral systems, have been extensively investigated over the last three decades. Unfortunately, none of them can be applied to any different kind of cells type with no limitation and side effects [4]. That is mainly because gene delivery pathways are complex combinations of multiple, potentially rate-limiting, biological processes and approaches to the design of delivery vehicles focusing on any single barrier individually will likely be suboptimal [5]. Furthermore, many current approaches are frustrated both by mislocalization and by sequestration in nontarget sites [6]. No matter what their origin, strain, and family, viruses have naturally evolved exquisite strategies to reach and penetrate specific target cells where they hijack the cellular machinery to express genes [7]. Even though engineered replication-defective viral vectors outperform nonviral systems and their inherent cell-specific tropism reduces off-target transduction, this, together with other shortcomings, has hitherto precluded the delivery of nucleic acids to alternative cell types and tissues [8]. Recent years have thus witnessed a surge of interest in nonviral delivery systems [9]. Cationic lipids and polymers are nowadays relatively safe, with tunable chemistries and cell targeting moieties, and potential for large-scale production with high reproducibility and at acceptable costs [10]. Nevertheless, despite transfectants are becoming increasingly optimized (at least) for benchtop laboratory research, nonviral gene delivery is still arguably in its infancy. First binary complexes between cationic lipids and polymers with the DNA date back to the mid-70s [11, 12]. Since then several scientists have made substantial contributions to this domain by developing more and more sophisticated, still conventional or classical, chemicals and formulations [13, 14]. Additionally, drawing inspiration from processes naturally occurring in vivo, major strides forward have been made in the development of more effective transfectants. Specifically, smart vectors sensitive to a variety of physiological stimuli such as cell enzymes, redox status, and pH are substantially changing the landscape of gene delivery by helping to overcome some of the systemic and intracellular barriers that viral vectors naturally evade [9]. Stimuli-responsive transfectants are now at the forefront of gene delivery vectors technology [15]. Clearly, existing vectors need to be streamlined further [16]. The promises are still great, and the problems have been identified (and they are surmountable) [17].

Some other fellows and I trust that a key pitfall that plagues science, among other worthy causes, is the difficulty in reproducing results because of the huge amount of variability existing not only between labs but also from time to time in the same lab and never reported in peer-reviewed papers [18, 19]. Furthermore, members of our thriving scientific community come from different backgrounds and are not historically accustomed to talking a common scientific language with each other. It therefore follows that a handbook of best laboratory practices and detailed experimental procedures including organic synthesis going through chemical-physical characterization to biological testing is badly needed.

The volume of the *Methods in Molecular Biology* series provides the readers with a wide collection of the latest and foremost, readily reproducible technical protocols available in the field of nonviral gene delivery vectors, written such that a competent scientist unfamiliar with these methods can carry out the technique(s) successfully at the first attempt by simply following the detailed practical procedure(s) being described.

Such a collection of chapters is organized into three major parts: (1) Part I on conventional bolus gene delivery vectors (*see* Chapters 1–13) introduces typical transfection approaches relying on the addition of transfectants to the cell culture medium where the cells grown in; (2) another one on stimuli-responsive bolus transfectants (*see* Chapters 14–17) covers advanced topics on gene delivery complexes delivered by dripping onto cells, made of smart polymers or stimuli-responsive polymers that undergo changes depending on the environment they are in; (3) an example of substrate-mediated gene delivery (*see* Chapter 18), also termed reverse transfection, or solid-phase delivery concerns the immobilization of a gene delivery vector onto a surface as opposed to more typical bolus delivery from the medium.

Each chapter covers the development and/or characterization and/or testing of a typical transfectant, as apparent by the very specialized title, representative of a wide class of nonviral gene delivery systems. It is worthy of note that it is the running title that will provide readers with general information about the specialty subset of nonviral gene delivery vectors they are going to read and learn about. In this respect, the complete set of information comprises pure cationic lipid-based lipoplexes (*see* Chapter 1), cationic and zwitterionic lipid-based lipoplexes (*see* Chapters 2 and 3), anionic and zwitterionic lipid-based lipoplexes (*see* Chapter 4), non-ionic surfactant-based lipoplexes (*see* Chapter 5), stealth lipoplexes (*see* Chapter 6), targeted lipoplexes (*see* Chapter 7), anionic polymer-strengthened lipoplexes (*see* Chapter 8), pure cationic polymer-based polyplexes (*see* Chapters 9 and 10), stealth polyplexes (*see* Chapter 11), cationic lipid-coated polyplexes (*see* Chapter 12), anionic lipid-coated polyplexes (*see* Chapter 13), redox-responsive lipoplexes (*see* Chapter 14), pH-responsive polyplexes (*see* Chapter 15), photo-responsive polyplexes (*see* Chapter 16), thermo-responsive polyplexes (*see* Chapter 17), and surface-tethered polyplexes (*see* Chapter 18). New and future gene delivery vectors will be dealt with on the basis of this body of knowledge.

The structure of each single chapter, organized in four consecutive and interrelated sections each encompassing different types of information, is the real hallmark typifying the *Methods in Molecular Biology* series. Each chapter opens with a coherent and authoritative account of the very idea underlying the method(s) being described. The Materials section lists all the raw materials, buffers, disposables, and equipment necessary for carrying out every protocol claimed. As the overall aim of this volume is to provide researchers with a full account of the practical steps necessary for carrying out each protocol successfully, the Methods section contains detailed and lucid step-by-step descriptions of every protocol for the successful completion of each method undertaken. The Notes are intended to complement Materials and Methods sections, highlighting critical experimental details and how best to troubleshoot issues that might arise when executing the protocol(s). Finally, a comprehensive list of all the References contains a great deal of useful material in addition to the main text, best provide readers with entry to the literature.

As this volume has been written for experimentalists, it is my most sincere hope that *Nonviral Gene Delivery Vectors: Methods and Protocols* will be an essential part of many laboratory bookshelves and would help novice and professionals alike succeed in their research in this field.

Mere words cannot express my sincere appreciation and gratitude to all and each of the authoritative contributors for providing this volume with such high-quality manuscripts and to Prof. John Walker, the Editor-in-Chief of the *Methods in Molecular Biology* series, for his timely help and guidance.

Milan, Italy   *Gabriele Candiani*

References

1. Pezzoli D, Chiesa R, De Nardo L, Candiani G (2012) We still have a long way to go to effectively deliver genes! J Appl Biomater Funct Mater 10(2):82–91
2. Wickstrom E (2015) DNA and RNA derivatives to optimize distribution and delivery. Adv Drug Deliv Rev 87:25–34
3. Wolff JA, Rozema DB (2008) Breaking the bonds: Non-viral vectors become chemically dynamic. Mol Ther 16(1):8–15
4. Nayerossadat N, Maedeh T, Ali PA (2012) Viral and nonviral delivery systems for gene delivery. Adv Biomed Res 1:27
5. Varga CM, Hong K, Lauffenburger DA (2001) Quantitative analysis of synthetic gene delivery vector design properties. Mol Ther 4(5):438–446
6. Chen HH, Cawood R, Seymour LW (2008) Toward more effective gene delivery. Genome Biol 9(1):301
7. Vannucci L, Lai M, Chiuppesi F, Ceccherini-Nelli L, Pistello M (2013) Viral vectors: a look back and ahead on gene transfer technology. New Microbiol 36(1):1–22
8. Jang JH, Schaffer DV, Shea LD (2011) Engineering biomaterial systems to enhance viral vector gene delivery. Mol Ther 19(8):1407–1415
9. Pezzoli D, Candiani G (2013) Non-viral gene delivery strategies for gene therapy: a "menage a trois" among nucleic acids, materials, and the biological environment Stimuli-responsive gene delivery vectors. J Nanopart Res 15(3):1–27
10. Davis ME (2002) Non-viral gene delivery systems. Curr Opin Biotech 13(2):128–131
11. Wu GY, Wu CH (1987) Receptor-mediated in vitro gene transformation by a soluble DNA carrier system. J Biol Chem 262(10):4429–4432
12. Felgner PL, Gadek TR, Holm M, Roman R, Chan HW, Wenz M, Northrop JP, Ringold GM, Danielsen M (1987) Lipofection: a highly efficient, lipid-mediated DNA-transfection procedure. Proc Natl Acad Sci USA 84(21):7413–7417
13. Mintzer MA, Simanek EE (2009) Nonviral vectors for gene delivery. Chem Rev 109(2):259–302
14. Scomparin A, Polyak D, Krivitsky A, Satchi-Fainaro R (2015) Achieving successful delivery of oligonucleotides - from physico-chemical characterization to in vivo evaluation. Biotechnol Adv 33(6):1294–1309
15. Tanzi MC, Bozzini S, Candiani G, Cigada A, De Nardo L, Fare S, Ganazzoli F, Gastaldi D, Levi M, Metrangolo P, Migliavacca F, Osellame R, Petrini P, Raffaini G, Resnati G, Vena P, Vesentini S, Zunino P (2011) Trends in biomedical engineering: focus on Smart Bio-Materials and Drug Delivery. J Appl Biomater Biomech 9(2):87–97
16. Pezzoli D, Zanda M, Chiesa R, Candiani G (2013) The yin of exofacial protein sulfhydryls and the yang of intracellular glutathione in in vitro transfection with SS14 bioreducible lipoplexes. J Control Release 165(1):44–53
17. Verma IM, Somia N (1997) Gene therapy -- promises, problems and prospects. Nature 389(6648):239–242
18. Malloggi C, Pezzoli D, Magagnin L, De Nardo L, Mantovani D, Tallarita E, Candiani G (2015) Comparative evaluation and optimization of off-the-shelf cationic polymers for gene delivery purposes. Polymer Chem 6(35):6325–6339
19. Bergese P, Hamad-Schifferli K (2013) Nanomaterial interfaces in biology methods and protocols preface. Methods Mol Biol 1025:V–Vi

Contents

Contributors

DANIEL G. ABEBE • *Department of Chemistry, The University of Memphis, Memphis, TN, USA*

MIREIA AGIRRE • *NanoBioCel Group, University of the Basque Country (UPV-EHU), Vitoria-Gasteiz, Spain; Biomedical Research Networking Center in Bioengineering, Biomaterials and Nanomedicine (CIBER-BBN), Vitoria-Gasteiz, Spain*

EMILIO AICART • *Grupo de Química Coloidal y Supramolecular, Departamento de Química Física I, Facultad de Ciencias Químicas, Universidad Complutense de Madrid, Madrid, Spain*

ACHIM AIGNER • *Clinical Pharmacology, Rudolf-Boehm-Institute for Pharmacology and Toxicology, Leipzig, Germany*

MARIO ARIATTI • *Discipline of Biochemistry, University of KwaZulu-Natal, Durban, South Africa*

DANIELLE CAMPIOL ARRUDA • *Dep Faculdade de Farmácia, Universidade Federal de Minas Gerais, Belo Horizonte, Brazil*

ANA L. BARRÁN-BERDÓN • *Grupo de Química Coloidal y Supramolecular, Departamento de Química Física I, Facultad de Ciencias Químicas, Universidad Complutense de Madrid, Madrid, Spain*

SANTANU BHATTACHARYA • *Department of Organic Chemistry, Indian Institute of Science, Bangalore, India; Indian Association for the Cultivation of Science, Kolkata, India*

PASCAL BIGEY • *UTCBS, CNRS UMR8258, INSERM U1022, Université Paris Descartes, Chimie ParisTech, Paris, France*

GABRIELE CANDIANI • *INSTM (Italian National Consortium for Materials Science and Technology), Research Unit Milano Politecnico, Milan, Italy; Department of Chemistry, Materials and Chemical Engineering "Giulio Natta," Politecnico di Milano, Milan, Italy; 'The Protein Factory' Research Centre, Politecnico di Milano and University of Insubria, Milan, Italy*

MARGARIDA I. SIMÃO CARLOS • *UCL School of Pharmacy, London, UK*

HONG CHEN • *Department of Polymer Science and Engineering, College of Chemistry, Chemical Engineering and Materials Science, Soochow University, Suzhou, People's Republic of China*

JIANJUN CHENG • *Department of Materials Science and Engineering, University of Illinois at Urbana–Champaign, Urbana, IL, USA*

MAHA ELSAYED • *Department of Pharmaceutical Sciences, Wayne State University, Detroit, MI, USA*

VIRGINIE ESCRIOU • *UTCBS, CNRS UMR8258, INSERM U1022, Université Paris Descartes, Chimie ParisTech, Paris, France*

ALEXANDER EWE • *Clinical Pharmacology, Rudolf-Boehm-Institute for Pharmacology and Toxicology, Leipzig, Germany*

KAI K EWERT • *Physics Department, University of California at Santa Barbara, Santa Barbara, CA, USA; Materials Department, University of California at Santa Barbara, Santa Barbara, CA, USA; Molecular, Cellular and Developmental Biology Department, University of California at Santa Barbara, Santa Barbara, CA, USA*

SARA FALSINI • *Department of Chemistry "Ugo Shiff"& CSGI, University of Florence, Florence, Italy*

TOMOKO FUJIWARA • *Department of Chemistry, The University of Memphis, Memphis, TN, USA*

ZHISHEN GE • *CAS Key Laboratory of Soft Matter Chemistry, Department of Polymer Science and Engineering, University of Science and Technology of China, Hefei, China*

WILLIAM P.D. GOLDRING • *Department of Science and Environment, Roskilde University, Roskilde, Denmark*

XIAOMENG HUANG • *Pharmaceutics and Pharmaceutical Chemistry, College of Pharmacy, The Ohio State University, Columbus, OH, USA*

EMILE JUBELI • *Faculté de pharmacie, Université Paris-Sud, Châtenay Malabry, France*

ELENA JUNQUERA • *Grupo de Química Coloidal y Supramolecular, Departamento de Química Física I, Facultad de Ciencias Químicas, Universidad Complutense de Madrid, Madrid, Spain*

RIMA KANDIL • *Department of Pharmaceutical Sciences, Wayne State University, Detroit, MI, USA*

TERESA KRAUS • *Department of Pharmaceutical Sciences, Wayne State University, Detroit, MI, USA*

ULRICH LÄCHELT • *Pharmaceutical Biotechnology, Center for System-Based Drug Research, Ludwig-Maximilians-University Munich, Munich, Germany; Nanosystems Initiative, Munich, Germany*

ROBERT J. LEE • *Pharmaceutics and Pharmaceutical Chemistry, College of Pharmacy, The Ohio State University, Columbus, OH, USA*

L. JAMES LEE • *Pharmaceutics and Pharmaceutical Chemistry, College of Pharmacy, The Ohio State University, Columbus, OH, USA*

JUNJIE LI • *CAS Key Laboratory of Soft Matter Chemistry, Department of Polymer Science and Engineering, University of Science and Technology of China, Hefei, China*

YANG LIU • *Department of Materials Science and Engineering, University of Illinois at Urbana–Champaign, Urbana, IL, USA*

RAMSEY N. MAJZOUB • *Physics Department, University of California at Santa Barbara, Santa Barbara, CA, USA; Materials Department, University of California at Santa Barbara, Santa Barbara, CA, USA; Molecular, Cellular and Developmental Biology Department, University of California at Santa Barbara, Santa Barbara, CA, USA*

MOHAMED MASHAL • *NanoBioCel Group, University of the Basque Country (UPV-EHU), Vitoria-Gasteiz, Spain*

OLIVIA M. MERKEL • *Department of Pharmaceutical Sciences, Wayne State University, Detroit, MI, USA*

SANTOSH K. MISRA • *Department of Organic Chemistry, Indian Institute of Science, Bangalore, India; Department of Bioengineering, University of Illinois at Urbana-Champaign, Champaign, IL, USA*

STEPHAN MORYS • *Pharmaceutical Biotechnology, Center for System-Based Drug Research, Ludwig-Maximilians-University Munich, Munich, Germany*

EDILBERTO OJEDA • *NanoBioCel Group, University of the Basque Country (UPV-EHU), Vitoria-Gasteiz, Spain; Biomedical Research Networking Center in Bioengineering, Biomaterials and Nanomedicine (CIBER-BBN), Vitoria-Gasteiz, Spain*

JINGJING PAN • *Department of Polymer Science and Engineering, College of Chemistry, Chemical Engineering and Materials Science, Soochow University, Suzhou, People's Republic of China*

JOSE L. PEDRAZ • *NanoBioCel Group, University of the Basque Country (UPV-EHU), Vitoria-Gasteiz, Spain; Biomedical Research Networking Center in Bioengineering, Biomaterials and Nanomedicine (CIBER-BBN), Vitoria-Gasteiz, Spain*

DANIELE PEZZOLI • *INSTM (Italian National Consortium for Materials Science and Technology), Research Unit Milano Politecnico, Milan, Italy*

CHANTAL PICHON • *Centre de Biophysique Moléculaire, UPR4301 CNRS affiliated to the University of Orléans, Orléans, France*

MICHAEL D. PUNGENTE • *Premedical Unit, Weill Cornell Medical College in Qatar, Education City, Doha, Qatar*

GUSTAVO PURAS • *NanoBioCel Group, University of the Basque Country (UPV-EHU), Vitoria-Gasteiz, Spain; Biomedical Research Networking Center in Bioengineering, Biomaterials and Nanomedicine (CIBER-BBN), Vitoria-Gasteiz, Spain*

SANDRA RISTORI • *Dipartimento di Scienze della Terra, Università di Firenze, Florence, Italy*

ELENA ROSINI • *Department of Biotechnology and Life Sciences, University of Insubria, Varese, Italy; 'The Protein Factory' Research Centre, Politecnico di Milano and University of Insubria, Milan, Italy*

CYRUS R. SAFINYA • *Physics Department, University of California at Santa Barbara, Santa Barbara, CA, USA; Materials Department, University of California at Santa Barbara, Santa Barbara, CA, USA; Molecular, Cellular and Developmental Biology Department, University of California at Santa Barbara, Santa Barbara, CA, USA*

ANDREAS SCHÄTZLEIN • *UCL School of Pharmacy, London, UK; Nanomerics Ltd., London, UK*

ANNE SCHLEGEL • *UTCBS, CNRS UMR8258, INSERM U1022, Université Paris Descartes, Chimie ParisTech, Paris, France*

ELENA TALLARITA • *Department of Chemistry, Materials and Chemical Engineering "Giulio Natta", Politecnico di Milano, Milan, Italy*

IJEOMA UCHEGBU • *UCL School of Pharmacy, London, UK; Nanomerics Ltd., London, UK*

ILIA VILLATE-BEITIA • *NanoBioCel Group, University of the Basque Country (UPV-EHU), Vitoria-Gasteiz, Spain; Biomedical Research Networking Center in Bioengineering, Biomaterials and Nanomedicine (CIBER-BBN), Vitoria-Gasteiz, Spain*

ERNST WAGNER • *Pharmaceutical Biotechnology, Center for System-Based Drug Research, Ludwig-Maximilians-University Munich, Munich, Germany; Nanosystems Initiative, Munich, Germany*

HONGWEI WANG • *Department of Polymer Science and Engineering, College of Chemistry, Chemical Engineering and Materials Science, Soochow University, Suzhou, People's Republic of China*

XINMEI WANG • *Pharmaceutics and Pharmaceutical Chemistry, College of Pharmacy, The Ohio State University, Columbus, OH, USA*

MAGDALENA WYTRWAL • *Academic Centre for Materials and Nanotechnology, AGH University of Science and Technology, Krakow, Poland; Department of Physical Chemistry and Electrochemistry, Faculty of Chemistry, Jagiellonian University, Kraków, Poland*

LIN YUAN • *Department of Polymer Science and Engineering, College of Chemistry, Chemical Engineering and Materials Science, Soochow University, Suzhou, People's Republic of China*

JON ZARATE • *NanoBioCel Group, University of the Basque Country (UPV-EHU), Vitoria-Gasteiz, Spain; Biomedical Research Networking Center in Bioengineering, Biomaterials and Nanomedicine (CIBER-BBN), Vitoria-Gasteiz, Spain*

ZENGSHI ZHA • *CAS Key Laboratory of Soft Matter Chemistry, Department of Polymer Science and Engineering, University of Science and Technology of China, Hefei, China*

MENGZI ZHANG • *Pharmaceutics and Pharmaceutical Chemistry, College of Pharmacy, The Ohio State University, Columbus, OH, USA*

NAN ZHENG • *Department of Materials Science and Engineering, University of Illinois at Urbana–Champaign, Urbana, IL, USA*

Part I

Conventional Bolus Gene Delivery Vectors

Physical Chemical and Biomolecular Methods for the Optimization of Cationic Lipid-Based Lipoplexes In Vitro for the Gene Therapy Applications

Santosh K. Misra and Santanu Bhattacharya

Abstract

Preparation and application protocols play a very important role while optimizing the cationic lipid-based lipoplexes in vitro. These protocols serve as the basis for the betterment of the lipoplexes with regard to their successful application in animals and eventually human subjects. Starting from the chemical structures of used cationic lipids (CLs), optimization of the additive inclusions, methods of nanoparticle (lipoplex) formation, presence of blood serum, time intervals of lipoplex incubation, and type of efficiency read-outs in various conditions play important roles in reaching insightful conclusions. Such steps of summarizing protocols and requirements of the pertinent events focus on getting improved lipoplexes for achieving optimal effects in terms of post transfection gene and protein expression. The progression of optimization and efficiency evaluation lead to predictable structure-method-activity relationship with involvement of various feedback principles including physical chemical and biomolecular evaluations before and after the use of lipoplexes in biological systems. This chapter discusses some of the focused strategies for the establishment of lipoplexes for a better post transfection activity with reduced risk of failure.

Key words Cationic lipids, Liposomes, Lipoplexes, Plasmid DNA, Transfection, In vitro culture

1 Introduction

Therapeutic Bioactives (TpBs) are generally small molecules with molecular weights (MW) below several hundred units till the beginning of the fourth generation of medicines, when polynucleotides, high MW biopolymers, were included in category of bioactives (drugs/genes) [1, 2]. It is explored under gene therapy protocols which employs "Gene as medicine" [3]. This line of treatment offers hitherto unknown hope for survival against many diseases which have origin in genetic pool like cancer [4], diabetes [5], cystic fibrosis [6], AIDS [7], cardiovascular diseases [8], etc. Many of the nucleotide-based bioactives (NBs) are generally administered systemically, and the administration generally involves three processes, i.e. transport within a blood vessel (e.g., blood circulation),

Gabriele Candiani (ed.), *Non-Viral Gene Delivery Vectors: Methods and Protocols*, Methods in Molecular Biology, vol. 1445,
DOI 10.1007/978-1-4939-3718-9_1, © Springer Science+Business Media New York 2016

transport across vasculature walls into surrounding tissues, and transport through interstitial spaces within an organ. These barriers pose major impediments in the success of the NBs and necessitate their encasement in different carrier systems, which are of significant importance in the fields of drug delivery and therapeutic imaging [9–11]. These carrier systems vary from the natural viral particles [12–14] to synthetic molecular assemblies (SCAs). Among these available SCAs, cationic lipids (CLs) are among the most studied for the in vitro delivery of NBs. After the synthesis of various molecular architectures of CLs, including pseudoglyceryl lipids [15–19], cholesterol derivatives [20–25], and other molecular templates [26], it has been observed that CLs-based DNA transfer agents turn out to be particularly attractive due to their easy amenability to structural modifications at the molecular level to improve the gene transfer efficiency (Fig. 1). However, optimization of various components plays a significant role in getting improved transfection efficiency out of a certain gene carrier composition. Correlation of the physical chemical data with the in vitro transfection efficiency suggests that lipoplex instability [27–29], DNA release ability [30], and uptake efficiency [31] are "key factors" toward the transfection efficiency.

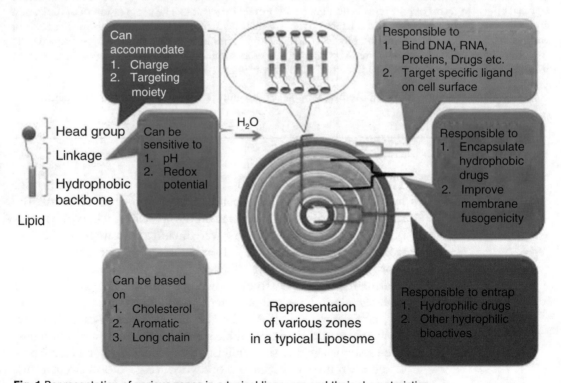

Fig. 1 Representation of various zones in a typical liposome and their characteristics

2 Materials

Prepare all the solutions/suspensions using ultrapure water (using deionized water, dH$_2$O, to attain a sensitivity of 18 MΩ-cm at 25 °C), buffers at a defined pH, and analytical grade reagents. All liposomal preparations should be prepared in a germ-free sterile condition. Preparation and storage of all reagents should be made at temperatures required for each specific experiment. All waste shall be managed in accordance with federal, state, and local regulations. Specific instructions must be followed while working with in vitro cell culture.

2.1 Reagents and Solvents

1. Chloroform (CHCl$_3$).
2. 1:1 (v/v) CHCl$_3$: methanol (MeOH) solution.
3. Cholesterol.
4. 1,2-dioleoyl-sn-glycero-3-phosphoethanolamine   (DOPE) (Avanti Polar Lipids, Alabaster, AL). Store at −20 °C until use.
5. Bovine serum albumin (BSA).
6. Fetal bovine serum (FBS).
7. Sodium dodecyl sulfate (SDS).
8. Sodium hydroxide (NaOH).
9. Sodium chloride (NaCl).
10. Tris(hydroxymethyl)aminomethane (Tris).
11. 4-(2-hydroxyethyl)-1-piperazineethanesulfonic acid (HEPES).
12. Ethylenediaminetetraacetic acid (EDTA).
13. Heparin sulfate.
14. DNase I.
15. Ethidium Bromide (EtBr).
16. pEGFP-c3, pEGFP-N1, PGL-3, and pCEP4-p53 plasmid DNA (pDNA) (ClonTech, DSS Takara Bio India Pvt. Ltd., New Delhi, India).
17. SMAD-2 siRNA (Sigma-Aldrich, St. Louis, MO).
18. 3-(4,5-dimethylthiazol-2-yl)-2,5-diphenyltetrazolium bromide (MTT).
19. Uranyl acetate.

2.2 Buffers

1. 6× DNA loading dye: 30 % (v/v) glycerol, 0.25 % (w/v) bromophenol blue, 0.25 % (w/v) xylene cyanol FF. Store at 4 °C until use.
2. TE buffer: mix 1 mL of 1 M Tris–HCl, pH 8.0, and 200 μL of 0.5 M EDTA, and made up to 100 mL with dH$_2$O. Adjust the pH to 7.5 for RNA and 8.0 for DNA.

3. HEPES buffer: add 2.38 g of HEPES to 80 mL of dH_2O. If necessary, add ~1.5 NaOH to the pellet to adjust the pH to 7.4. Make up to 100 mL with dH_2O. Store at 4 °C until use.

4. DNA binding and release assay buffer: mix 3.5 μL of 7 mM EtBr (final concentration: 25 μM EtBr) to 120 μL of 40 mM HEPES buffer (final concentration: 5 mM HEPES), 200 μL of 0.5 M NaCl (final concentration: 0.1 M NaCl), pH 7.4, in total volume of 1 mL.

5. 50× TAE buffer: add 242 g of Tris to 57.1 mL of glacial acetic acid (CH_3COOH) and 100 mL of 0.5 M EDTA. Make up to 1 L with dH_2O. Store at room temperature (RT).

6. EtBr washing buffer: dilute 50× TAE buffer in dH_2O (1× TAE buffer).

7. EtBr staining buffer: add 300 μg of EtBr to 1 L of 1× TAE.

8. 1× lysis buffer (Promega, Fitchburg, WI).

9. 1% (w/v) agarose gel: dissolve 100 mg of agarose in 100 mL of 1× TAE buffer, then heat the solution by means of a microwave for 1–2 min.

10. LAR II reagent (Promega).

2.3 Instruments and Disposables

1. Dynamic light scattering (DLS) DynaPro apparatus (Artisan Technology Group, Champaign, IL).

2. Transmission electron microscope (TEM) (TECNAI T20, FEI, Hillsboro, OR) operating at an acceleration voltage (DC voltage) of 100 keV.

3. TEM-grid: Formvar-coated, 400 mesh copper grid.

4. UV–Vis spectrophotometer.

5. Spectrofluorimeter.

6. Nuclear magnetic resonance (NMR) spectrometer.

7. High resolution mass spectrometer (HS-MS).

8. High vacuum pump.

9. Vortex.

10. Bath sonicator.

11. Gel imaging system.

12. Cell incubator.

13. Curved-bottom glass vials.

14. 24-well polystyrene cell culture plates.

15. Micropipettes.

16. Elemental (CHN) analyzer (LECO Corp., St. Joseph, MI).

17. BD FACSCalibur™ for flow assisted cell sorting (BD biosciences, Franklin Lakes, NJ).

18. Luminometer.

2.4 Cell Culture	1. HeLa cells (ATCC® CCL-2™) (American Type Culture Collection, ATCC, Manassas, VA).
	2. Cell culture medium: high-glucose Dulbecco's Modified Eagle Medium (DMEM) stored at 4 °C and used after thawing at 37 °C.
	3. Complete cell culture medium: cell culture medium containing 10% (v/v) FBS.
	4. Dulbecco's phosphate buffered saline (PBS).
	5. 1× trypsin solution.

3 Methods

3.1 Preparation of Lipid Assemblies

3.1.1 Solvent Evaporation Method

1. Solubilize CLs (*see* **Notes 1** and **2**) in the organic solvent of choice (*see* **Note 3**) based on solubility and immiscibility; i.e. solubilize 1 mg of 1,2-bis(hexadecyl dimethyl ammonium) ethane in 250 μL of THF.

2. Using a magnetic stirring, stir the 1 mL aliquot of dH$_2$O at 60 °C.

3. Add the organic solution of CL dropwise (1 drop/s, variable) while stirring at 60 °C till all the organic solvent evaporates.

3.1.2 Membrane-Freeze-Thaw Method

1. Solubilize the CLs in curved-bottom glass vials using CHCl$_3$ or 1:1 (v/v) CHCl$_3$:MeOH at a concentration of 2 mg/mL.

2. Prepare thin lipid film by evaporating the organic solvent/ mixtures under a steady stream of dry nitrogen (N$_2$) with rotary motion of glass vials (Fig. 2).

3. Evaporate traces of organic solvents under high vacuum for 4–6 h.

4. Add sterile dH$_2$O (or PBS) (*see* **Notes 4** and **5**) to lipid films to achieve a concentration of ~0.5 mg/mL (*see* **Note 6**).

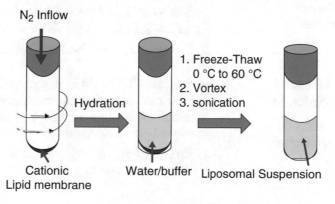

Fig. 2 A representation of freeze-thaw method of liposome preparation

5. Incubate hydrated lipid aggregates for ~12 h at 4 °C to achieve optimal hydration.

6. Subject hydrated lipid membranes to at least three freeze-thaw cycles by incubating the aqueous suspension on ice bath and slightly above the phase transition (melting) temperature of CL or its mixture with helper lipid or any other required additive for 5 min each with intermittent vortexing for ~2 min in between.

7. After ~3 cycles of freeze-thaw, disperse the membranes by bath sonication at RT and slightly above the phase transition temperature of the CL for up to 30 min to obtain lipid vesicles, then store at 4 °C until use (*see* **Notes 7** and **8**).

8. Mildly bath-sonicate lipid vesicles for ~1 min before using them for any experiments (*see* **Notes 8** and **9**).

3.2 Lipoplex (Complex Between CLs and Oligo/Polynucleotides) Formation

3.2.1 Electrostatic Complexation

1. Dilute polynucleotides (e.g., pEGFP-C3) or oligonucleotides (e.g., SMAD-2 siRNA) in sterile dH_2O or TE buffer to achieve a final concentration of 100 ng/μL (*see* **Note 10**).

2. Mix the diluted solution of oligo/polynucleotides with lipid vesicles to get a CL/nucleotide molar ratio (L/D) or charge ratio (N/P) on amine groups of the CL (N) and phosphate units of the DNA (P) varying as 0.125, 0.25, 0.5, 0.75, 1, 1.5, 2, 2.5, 3, and 4 as L/D or N/P (*see* **Note 11**).

3. Mix the CLs and nucleotides carefully by tapping and brief spinning.

4. Incubate the mixtures for 30 min at RT to allow the cationic charges of the CLs and the negative charges of the phosphate backbone of nucleotides to complex by electrostatic interaction (*see* **Note 12**).

3.2.2 Pre-preparative Incorporation to Improve Incorporation of Nucleotides in Liposomes

1. Follow the procedure described in Subheading 3.1.2, **steps 1–3**.

2. Add appropriate amount of polynucleotide in aqueous solution to achieve final L/D or N/P as 0.125, 0.25, 0.5, 0.75, 1, 1.5, 2, 2.5, 3, and 4 (*see* **Note 11**).

3. Continue as described in Subheading 3.1.2, **step 4** onwards.

3.3 Lipoplex Characterization

3.3.1 Evaluation of the Hydrodynamic Diameter

1. Prepare ~0.33 mM lipid and ~0.2 mM lipoplex (respect to the lipid concentration) suspensions in dH_2O (or TE buffer) as described in Subheading 3.1.2, **steps 1–8** and Subheading 3.2.1, **steps 1–4**, respectively.

2. Run samples on DLS machine following the manufacturer's instructions (*see* **Note 13**).

3.3.2 Evaluation of the Anhydrous Diameter

1. Drop-coat 10 μL of 1 mM CLs or 0.2 mM of lipoplex suspensions on carbon-coated copper grids.

2. Add 5 μL of 0.1% (w/v) uranyl acetate in dH_2O on drop-coated cationic liposome suspension, and incubate for 5 min at RT.

3. After 5 min-incubation at RT, wick-off the excess liquid from the grid.

4. Air dry the samples under covered lid for ~2 h.

5. Carefully vacuum dry the samples for ~6 h.

6. Perform recording images under a TEM following the manufacturer's instructions.

3.3.3 DNA Binding Assay with and Without Serum

The steps of the DNA binding assay are reported in Fig. 3.

1. Add the DNA binding assay buffer to makeup a total volume of 1 mL of water [33]. In order to evaluate the DNA binding in the presence of serum, add 10% (v/v) FBS to the DNA binding assay buffer.

2. Record the fluorescence emission of plain EtBr at $\lambda_{em} = 592$ nm using a spectrofluorimeter upon excitation at $\lambda_{ex} = 526$ nm (F_o).

3. Add 16.6 μL of 1 μg/μL of pEGFP-C3 (50 μM) and incubate for 10 min at RT.

4. Record the fluorescence emission of EtBr upon complexation with duplex DNA (F_{max}).

5. Add a 7.8 μL aliquot of 0.8 mM CL suspension to preformed EtBr/pDNA complexes in 5 mM HEPES buffer (*see* **Note 14**).

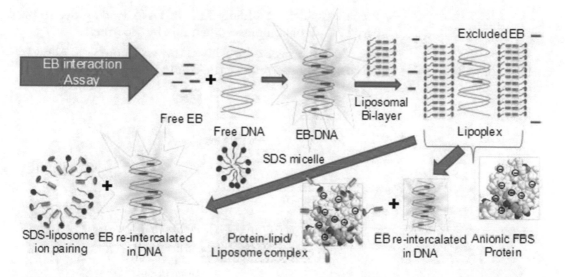

Fig. 3 A typical EtBr interaction assay for evaluating DNA binding with cationic lipid and micellar SDS induced release from a cationic lipid/DNA lipoplex

6. Add other 7.8 μL aliquots of 0.8 mM CL suspension till reaching the saturation of fluorescence quenching (F_x for different lipid/DNA ratios).

7. Calculate the DNA binding (percentage) by using the following formula:

$$\text{DNA binding}(\%) = \left(F_x - F_o\right) / \left(F_{\max} - F_o\right) \times 100$$

3.3.4 DNA Release Assay with and Without Serum

1. Follow the procedure reported in Subheading 3.3.3, **steps 1–5**.

2. Add a 7.8 μL aliquot of SDS (8.0 mM) to CL/DNA complexes formed by addition of CL aliquots in EtBr/pDNA complexes.

3. Add 7.8 μL of SDS aliquots till reaching the saturation of fluorescence increase (F_x for different lipid/DNA ratios).

4. Calculate the DNA release (percentage) by using the following formula:

$$\text{DNA release}(\%) = \left(F_x - F_o\right) / \left(F_{\max} - F_o\right) \times 100$$

3.3.5 Gel Electrophoresis for DNA Binding Assay

The steps of the gel electrophoresis for DNA binding assay are reported in Fig. 4.

1. Add 2 μL of 0.1 μg/μL pDNA to an aliquot of cationic liposome giving different N/Ps as obtained in EtBr intercalation assay reported in Subheading 3.3.3, **steps 1–5**.

2. Incubate the mixture for ~30 min at RT to allow complexation.

3. Prepare cocktail by adding 3 μL of DNA loading dye to prepared 20 μL of complexes, then mix by pipetting.

4. Pour 1 % (w/v) agarose gel in gel tray with comb on. Allow the gel to solidify and remove the comb.

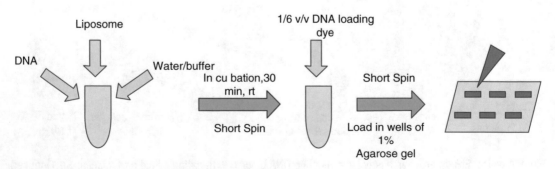

Fig. 4 A typical gel electrophoresis experiment

5. Load the prepared cocktail (*see* **Note 15**) into the well of 1 % agarose gel along with uncomplexed DNA.

6. Dip the gel in 1× TAE buffer and run the electrophoresis at 100 V for 20–30 min (*see* **Note 16**).

7. Follow the tracking dye for DNA mobility.

8. After DNA migration, dip the gel in chamber filled with gel running buffer (1× TAE solution of 300 µg/L EtBr) for ~5 min.

9. Wash the excess EtBr in washing buffer (1× TAE buffer) for 5 min.

10. Image the gel by means of the imaging system under exposure at $\lambda = 362$ nm for 0.5–2 s to visualize and photograph white bands of EtBr intercalated DNA or lipoplexes.

11. Determine the DNA band density by means of the analysis software.

12. Calculate the DNA binding (percentage) using the following formula (*see* **Note 17**):

$$\text{DNA binding}(\%) = (\text{Band intensity from lipoplex} - \text{background intensity}) /$$
$$(\text{band intensity from un} - \text{complexed DNA} - \text{background intensity}) \times 100$$

3.3.6 Gel Electrophoresis for DNA Release Assay

1. Add 2 µL of 0.1 µg/µL pDNA to an aliquot of CLs giving N/P with maximum DNA binding, as evaluated in Subheading 3.3.5, **step 10** (*see* **Note 18**).

2. Incubate the mixture for 30 min at RT to allow complexation.

3. Add SDS to achieve mole ratios of lipid/SDS, 0.5, 1, 1.5, 2, and 2.5.

4. Incubate the mixture for 30 min at RT (*see* **Note 18**).

5. Prepare the samples (*see* **Note 19**) and perform the gel electrophoresis as described in Subheading 3.3.5, **steps 3–9**.

6. Calculate the DNA release (percentage) by using the formula:

$$\text{DNA release}(\%) = (\text{Band intensity from SDS} / \text{lipoplex mixture} - \text{background intensity}) /$$
$$(\text{band intensity from free DNA} - \text{background intensity}) \times 100$$

3.3.7 Gel Electrophoresis and Effect of DNase I

1. Prepare lipoplexes as described in Subheading 3.3.6, **step 1**.

2. Incubate the mixture for 30 min at RT to allow complexation.

3. Add 1 µL (0.1 U) of DNase I, and incubate for 10 min at 37 °C.

4. Add 1 µL of 1 mM EDTA solution to quench the reaction.

5. Prepare the samples and perform the gel electrophoresis as described in Subheading 3.3.6, **step 4**.

6. Image the gel for any cleaved DNA under exposure at $\lambda = 362$ nm for 0.5–2 s (*see* **Note 20**).

3.3.8 Stability
of Lipoplexes with FBS,
BSA, and Heparin Sulfate

1. Prepare lipoplexes as described in Subheading 3.3.6, **step 1**.

2. Incubate the mixture for 30 min at RT to allow complexation.

3. Add variable amounts (0.2–2 μL, 1–10 %) of FBS or an equivalent amount of BSA (*see* **Note 21**) or 10–100 μM of heparin sulfate, then incubate for 30 min at 37 °C.

4. Prepare the samples and perform the gel electrophoresis as described in Subheading 3.3.5, **steps 3–9**.

5. Calculate the DNA release (percentage) by using the following formula (*see* **Note 22**):

$$\text{DNA release}(\%) = (\text{Band intensity from lipoplex mixture} - \text{background intensity}) / (\text{band intensity from free DNA} - \text{background intensity}) \times 100$$

3.4 Liposomal
Stabilization Steps

3.4.1 Inclusion of Helper
Lipid DOPE or Cholesterol

1. Add DOPE or cholesterol to solid lipid samples in molar ratios increasing from 1:0 to 1:6 including 1:1, 1:2, 1:3, 1:4, 1:5, as appropriate (*see* **Note 23**).

2. Follow Subheading 3.1.2, **steps 1–8**, to prepare co-liposomes with DOPE or cholesterol.

3. Check the stability of the resulting suspensions by DLS measurements as described in Subheading 3.3.1, **steps 2** and **3** as a function of time.

3.5 In Vitro
Transfection

The steps of the in vitro cell transfection are described in Fig. 5. Cells are grown in standard culture flasks before being plated typically in 24-well plates [34].

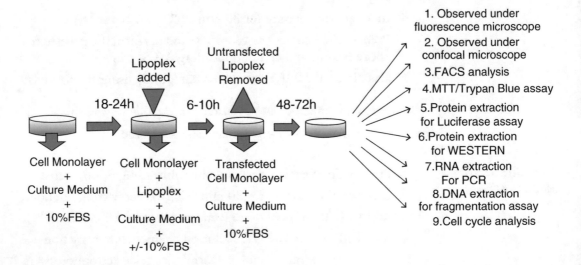

Fig. 5 A typical cell transfection protocol

1. Seed HeLa cells in a 24-well cell culture plate at a density of 3.2×10^4 cells/cm^2, and add 400 μL/well of antibiotic-free complete cell culture medium.

2. Grow cells at 37 °C, 99 % humidity with regular supply of 5 % CO_2 till ~80 % confluence (*see* **Note 24**).

3. Add 0.4, 0.8, 1.2, 1.6, or 2.0 μg of pEGFP-C3 or pGL-3 or pCEP4-p53/well to prepare lipoplexes at different DNA ratios (*see* **Note 25**).

4. Mix 100 μL of the DNA aliquots and 100 μL of liposomal aliquots to achieve N/Ps optimized by EtBr interaction assay (*see* Subheading 3.3.3) and gel electrophoresis assay (*see* Subheading 3.3.5).

5. Incubate the mixture for about 30 min at RT to allow lipoplex formation.

6. Add 200 mL/well of cell culture medium or complete cell culture medium to the lipoplexes.

7. Short spin and collect the lipoplex suspension.

8. Discard the old medium from the 24-well cell culture plate and wash cells once with cell culture medium.

9. Add 200 μL/well of lipoplex suspension to cells and incubate for 6–10 h at 37 °C, 99 % humidity with regular supply of 5 % CO_2.

10. After incubation, replace the entire lipoplex suspension with 400 μL/well of complete cell culture medium.

11. Incubate at 37 °C, 99 % humidity with regular supply of 5 % CO_2 for 48–72 h.

12. After incubation, harvest the cells according to the required end point experiment as reported here below in Subheadings 3.6, 3.7 and 3.8.

3.6 Flow Assisted Cell Sorting (FACS) for Estimating Transfected Cells with pEGFP-C3

1. Transfect cells with lipoplexes containing pEGFP-C3 as described in Subheading 3.5, **steps 1–10**, then wash them with 100 μL/well of PBS.

2. Add 100 μL/well of 1× trypsin solution and incubate for 3 min at 37 °C.

3. After incubation, add 400 μL/well of PBS containing 0.2 % (v/v) FBS to stop the trypsin activity.

4. Collect the cell suspension in 400 μL/well of PBS containing 0.2 % (v/v) FBS

5. Transfer the cell sample on FACS apparatus.

6. Quantify the transfected cells (percentage) according to the following formula:

$$\text{Transfected cells}\,(\%) = (\text{Total cells} - \text{Cells with only residual fluorescence})\,/$$
$$\text{Total cells} \times 100$$

7. Measure the extent of fluorescence analyzing also the mean fluorescence intensity (MFI).

3.7 Luciferase Assay for Estimating Transfection Efficiency with PGL-3

1. Transfect cells with lipoplexes containing pGL-3 as described in Subheading 3.5, **steps 1–10**, then wash them with 100 µL/well of PBS.

2. Lyse the cells with 40 µL/well of 1× lysis buffer.

3. Assay gene expression using LAR II reagent in equal volume with cell lysate solutions and by means of a luminometer.

4. Quantify the protein amount in each well by means of Bradford assay and following the manufacturer's instructions.

5. Evaluate the transfection efficiency in terms of luciferase activity/µg protein per sample.

3.8 MTT Assay for Estimating Cell Viability with pCEP4-p53

1. Transfect cells with lipoplexes carrying pCEP4-p53 as described in Subheading 3.5, **steps 1–10**.

2. Incubate cells with 10 % (v/v) of MTT (5 mg/mL) in complete cell culture medium for 4 h at 37 °C.

3. After incubation, dissolve formazan crystals by adding 400 µL/well of DMSO.

4. By means of a microplate reader acquire absorption at $\lambda = 592$ nm after 5 min of incubation of dissolved formazan crystals on a rocker.

5. Evaluate the cell viability (percentage) according to the following formula:

$$\text{Cell viability}\,(\%) = (\text{A592Lipoplex treated}_{\text{cells}} - \text{A592}_{\text{background}})\,/$$
$$(\text{A592}_{\text{untreated cells}} - \text{A592}_{\text{background}}) \times 100$$

---

4   Notes

1. Some CLs used for gene delivery purposes are: 1,2-bis(hexadecyl dimethyl ammonium) ethane, 1,2-bis(hexadecyl dimethyl ammonium) propane, 1,2-bis(hexadecyl dimethyl ammonium) pentane, and 1,2-bis(hexadecyl dimethyl ammonium) dodecane.

2. Characterize individual lipid molecules by HS-MS, NMR spectroscopy and elemental analysis to identify the purity of such materials as even a low percentage of impurity might lead to unwanted aggregation, instability, and loss of gene delivery efficiencies.

3. Organic solvents most commonly used to solubilize cationic lipids are tetrahydrofuran (THF), chloroform ($CHCl_3$), CH_2Cl_2, etc.

4. Hydration has to be performed in dH_2O or PBS buffer based on stability of liposomes.

5. Perform vesicle preparation in sterile conditions including autoclaved sample vials, germ-free surface, in a laminar flow hood.

6. Optimize the CLs concentration, ratio of organic and aqueous solvents and time of stirring to produce lipid vesicles of desired physical properties as followed by various physical methods of characterizations.

7. Brief bath sonication typically gives multi-lamellar vesicles (MLVs) which on continuous or probe sonication, change into single-lamellar vesicles (SLVs). Optimize the time period for bath sonication to get appropriate size of lipid vesicles that have to be characterized by DLS.

8. We suggest sonication at 40 W into a water bath.

9. Store each formulation at 4 °C and never freeze them. Pre-warm all liposome suspensions at RT before using them in any experimental procedure.

10. Adjust the concentration of polynucleotides or oligonucleotide to 0.33 nmol/µL as per base molarity considering an average base MW of 330 g/mol.

11. Optimize the dilution of nucleotides, L/D or N/P and the duration of complexation to achieve the desired physiochemical and morphological properties.

12. Use lipoplexes for desired physiochemical and morphological experiments immediately after preparation.

13. The mean diameter of liposomes and lipoplexes is expressed in terms of hydrodynamic diameter. Fluctuation of the hydrodynamic diameter over time indicates instability.

14. The electrostatic interaction of liposomes with pDNA results in fluorescence quenching due to EtBr (F_x) removal from the DNA duplex.

15. Avoid any bubble in the cocktail which might induce a brighter background. Remove any eventual bubble by spinning the cocktail for 5 s.

16. The gel must be completely submerged before running gel electrophoresis.

17. Lower band intensity of free DNA in gel from electrophoresed lipoplex compared to uncomplexed DNA indicates DNA binding.

18. The total volume should be decided based on the volume capacity of each well of the agarose gel.

19. It should not be spun for longer time to avoid any possible aggregation of the lipoplexes.

20. Decrease in DNA cleavage for lipoplexes indicates the protection ability of liposomes against DNase I.

21. FBS contains 30% of BSA.

22. Any released DNA from lipoplex indicates the destabilization of liposomes against FBS, BSA, or heparin sulfate.

23. The incorporation of a helper lipid like DOPE or cholesterol [32] may improve the stability of cationic liposomal suspensions.

24. Lower or higher levels of cell confluence may induce variations in transfection effectiveness of a given liposome formulation.

25. Prepare working stocks of DNA and liposome in plain cell culture media without adding any FBS.

References

1. "Disease" at Dorland's Medical Dictionary

2. "Mental Illness—Glossary". US National Institute of Mental Health. Retrieved 18 Apr 2010

3. Anderson WF (1998) Human gene therapy. Nature 392:25–30

4. Hattori Y, Maitani Y (2005) Folate-linked nanoparticle-mediated suicide gene therapy in human prostate cancer and nasopharyngeal cancer with herpes simplex virus thymidine kinase. Cancer Gene Ther 12:796–809

5. Chae HY, Lee BW, Oh SH, Ahn YR, Chung JH, Min YK, Lee MS, Lee MK, Kim KW (2005) Effective glycemic control achieved by transplanting non-viral cationic liposome-mediated VEGF-transfected islets in streptozotocin-induced diabetic mice. Exp Mol Med 37:513–523

6. Yang Y, Nunes FA, Berencsi K, Goenczoel E, Engelhardt JF, Wilson JM (1994) Inactivation of E2a in recombinant adenoviruses improves the prospect for gene therapy in cystic fibrosis. Nat Genet 7:362–369

7. Curiel TJ, Piche A, Kasono K, Curiel DT (1997) Gene therapy strategies for AIDS-related malignancies. Gene Ther 4:1284–1288

8. Yla-Herttuala S, Martin JF (2000) Cardiovascular gene therapy. Lancet 355:213–222

9. Vasir JK, Labhestwar V (2007) Biodegradable nanoparticles for cytosolic delivery of therapeutics. Adv Drug Deliv Rev 59:718–728

10. Ow H, Larson DR, Srivastava M, Baird BA, Webb WW, Wiesner U (2005) Bright and stable core–shell fluorescent silica nanoparticles. Nano Lett 5:113–117

11. Jin S, Ye K (2007) Nanoparticle-mediated drug delivery and gene therapy. Biotechnol Prog 23:32–41

12. Breyer B, Jiang W, Cheng H, Zhou L, Paul R, Feng T, He TC (2001) Adenoviral vector-mediated gene transfer for human gene therapy. Curr Gene Ther 1:149–162

13. Anderson WF (1984) Prospects for human gene therapy. Science 226:401–409

14. Robbins PD, Tahara H, Ghivizzani SC (1998) Viral vectors for gene therapy. Trends Biotechnol 16:35–40

15. Felgner PL, Gadek TR, Holm M, Roman R, Chan HW, Wenz M, Northrop JP, Ringold GM, Danielsen M (1987) Lipofection: a highly efficient, lipid-mediated DNA-transfection procedure. Proc Natl Acad Sci U S A 84:7413–7417

16. Bhattacharya S, Bajaj A (2009) Advances in gene delivery through molecular design of cationic lipids. Chem Commun 31:4632–4656

17. Bhattacharya S, De S (1999) Synthesis and vesicle formation from dimeric pseudoglyceryl lipids with $(CH_2)_m$ spacers: pronounced m-value dependence of thermal properties, vesicle fusion, and cholesterol complexation. Chem Eur J 5:2335–2347

18. Dileep PV, Antony A, Bhattacharya S (2001) Incorporation of oxyethylene units between hydrocarbon chain and pseudoglyceryl backbone in cationic lipid potentiates gene trans-

fection efficiency in the presence of serum. FEBS Lett 509:327–331

19. Bhattacharya S, Dileep PV (2004) Cationic oxyethylene lipids. Synthesis, aggregation, and transfection properties. Bioconjugate Chem 15:508–519

20. Gao X, Huang L (1991) A novel cationic liposome reagent for efficient transfection of mammalian cells. Biochim Biophys Res Commun 179:280–285

21. Ghosh YK, Visweswariah SS, Bhattacharya S (2000) Nature of linkage between the cationic headgroup and cholesteryl skeleton controls gene transfection efficiency. FEBS Lett 473:341–344

22. Hasegawa S, Hirashima N, Nakanishi M (2002) Comparative study of transfection efficiency of cationic cholesterols mediated by liposomes-based gene delivery. Bioorg Med Chem Lett 12:1299–1302

23. Nakanishi M (2003) Strategy in gene transfection by cationic transfection lipids with a cationic cholesterol. Curr Med Chem 10:1289–1296

24. Bajaj A, Mishra SK, Kondaiah P, Bhattacharya S (2008) Effect of the headgroup variation on the gene transfer properties of cholesterol based cationic lipids possessing ether linkage. Biochim Biophys Acta 1778:1222–1236

25. Bajaj A, Kondaiah P, Bhattacharya S (2008) Effect of the nature of the spacer on gene transfer efficacies of novel thiocholesterol derived gemini lipids in different cell lines: a structure–activity investigation. J Med Chem 51:2533–2540

26. Kumar K, Maiti B, Kondaiah P, Bhattacharya S (2015) Efficacious gene silencing in serum and significant apoptotic activity induction by survivin downregulation mediated by new cationic gemini tocopheryl lipids. Mol Pharm 12:351–361

27. Hirsch-Lerner D, Min Z, Eliyahu H, Ferrari ME, Wheeler CJ, Barenholz Y (2005) Effect of "helper lipid" on lipoplex electrostatics. Biochim Biophys Acta 1714:71–84

28. Kerner M, Meyuhas O, Hirsch-Lerner D, Rosen L, Min Z, Barenholz Y (2001) Interplay in lipoplexes between type of pDNA promoter and lipid composition determines transfection efficiency of human growth hormone in NIH3T3 cells in culture. Biochim Biophys Acta 1532:128–136

29. Simberg D, Danino D, Talmon Y, Minsky A, Ferrari M, Wheeler CJ, Barenholz Y (2001) Phase behavior, DNA ordering, and size instability of cationic lipoplexes. Relevance to optimal transfection activity. J Biol Chem 276:47453–47459

30. Candiani G, Pezzoli D, Ciani L, Chiesa L, Ristori S (2010) Bioreducible liposomes for gene delivery: from the formulation to the mechanism of action. PLoS One 5:e13430

31. Sarah R, Paul P, Alain TR (2009) Physicochemical characteristics of lipoplexes influence cell uptake mechanisms and transfection efficacy. PLoS One 4:e6058

32. Hong K, Zheng W, Baker A, Papahadjopoulos D (1997) Stabilization of cationic liposome-plasmid DNA complexes by polyamines and poly(ethylene glycol)-phospholipid conjugates for efficient in vivo gene delivery. FEBS Lett 400:233–237

33. Bhattacharya S, Mandal SS (1998) Evidence of interlipidic ion-pairing in anion induced DNA release from cationic amphiphile-DNA complexes. Mechanistic implications in transfection. Biochemistry 37:7764–7777

34. Misra SK, Biswas J, Kondaiah P, Bhattacharya S (2013) Gene transfection in high serum levels: case studies with new cholesterol based cationic gemini lipids. PLoS One 8:e68305

Chapter 2

Cationic Lipid-Based Nucleic Acid Vectors

Emile Jubeli, William P.D. Goldring, and Michael D. Pungente

Abstract

The delivery of nucleic acids into cells remains an important laboratory cell culture technique and potential clinical therapy, based upon the initial cellular uptake, then translation into protein (in the case of DNA), or gene deletion by RNA interference (RNAi). Although viral delivery vectors are more efficient, the high production costs, limited cargo capacity, and the potential for clinical adverse events make nonviral strategies attractive. Cationic lipids are the most widely applied and studied nonviral vectors; however, much remains to be solved to overcome limitations of these systems. Advances in the field of cationic lipid-based nucleic acid (lipoplex) delivery rely upon the development of robust and reproducible lipoplex formulations, together with the use of cell culture assays. This chapter provides detailed protocols towards the formulation, delivery, and assessment of in vitro cationic lipid-based delivery of DNA.

Key words Nucleic acid delivery, Lipoplexes, Cationic lipids, Co-lipids, Particle size, Charge ratio, Transfection efficiency, Cytotoxicity

1 Introduction

The seminal work of Felgner, beginning in the late 1980s, heralded a new era in our understanding of nonviral gene delivery by employing cationic lipid-DNA complex (lipoplex) assemblies. This began with the synthesis and application of the cationic lipid N-[1-(2,3-dioleyloxy)propyl]-N,N,N-trimethylammonium chloride (DOTMA) [1], and has continued to this day with a variety of cationic structures based on lipids [2, 3], polymers [4, 5], and dendrimers [6, 7], to name a few.

Although the use of viral vectors to deliver therapeutic genes remains the most effective approach for gene therapy, the high cost, complexity, limitations in cargo capacity, and potential for immunological complications make nonviral carriers an attractive alternative. In order to improve upon nonviral gene delivery through nanotechnology, an increasing effort has been witnessed in recent decades [8]. Comprehensive reviews detailing the breadth and scope of existing nonviral gene delivery systems are

Gabriele Candiani (ed.), *Non-Viral Gene Delivery Vectors: Methods and Protocols*, Methods in Molecular Biology, vol. 1445, DOI 10.1007/978-1-4939-3718-9_2, © Springer Science+Business Media New York 2016

reported elsewhere [9, 10]. Herein, we confine our discussion to the use of cationic lipids as carriers of plasmid DNA (pDNA), considered the most promising and extensively studied vehicles for nucleic acids [11].

Despite the commercial availability of numerous cationic lipid vectors, investigations continue to explore new and novel lipid architectures [12]. The general cationic lipid design includes four common domains, a positively charged head group, a hydrophobic domain, a backbone region, and a chemical linker moiety to connect the various domains. The head group typically bears one or more cationic units, commonly amino-based moieties that facilitate binding to the genetic material. The backbone structure, often based on glycerol, influences the overall shape of the cationic lipid and thus the structure of the lipoplex. The hydrophobic domain plays a critical role in the assembly and organization of the lipoplex, and finally the chemical linker used to join these groups together is commonly an ether, ester, or amide bond.

Structural modifications within these four domains are employed to increase the cell tolerance of the cationic lipid, while at the same time enhancing the transfection efficiency. The cell tolerance, or biocompatibility of the lipids is typically addressed through the judicious choice of the chemical linker moiety such that the lipid is rendered biocompatible after successful delivery of the DNA cargo. Enhancing the transfection efficiency of a lipid-DNA formulation depends very much on the chosen route of administration—each of which presents unique barriers to be overcome [13]. As an example, for in vivo delivery using intravenous methods, the barriers to be considered when choosing an appropriate lipid design include poor circulation time due to opsonization followed by rapid clearance, a lack of cell selectivity, poor cellular uptake, endosomal escape, and nuclear entry. Generally, cationic lipid-based gene delivery is a highly inefficient and wasteful approach, and requires an improved understanding of structure efficiency relationships to achieve lower cytotoxicity together with higher transfection efficiency.

Attempts to overcome many of the barriers that have thus far impeded progress towards safe and efficient in vivo delivery of therapeutic nucleic acids, and moving beyond the discrete cationic lipid structure, include the emergence of purpose-designed lipoplex formulations of a modular nature [14–16]. Within these nanoparticle formulations, the modular components are chosen such that the nucleic acid cargo is condensed within functional concentric layers of chemical components designed for delivery into cells and intracellular trafficking, biological stability, and biological cell targeting.

Developments in lipoplex formulations and components that have moved the field towards more effective delivery include the use of neutral co-lipids such as cholesterol or 1,2-dioleoyl-*sn*-glycero-3-phosphoethanolamine (DOPE) to facilitate membrane fusion and endosomal escape [17]. The application of polyethylene glycol (PEG) to modify the liposomal surface results in longer circulation times [18]. Additives, such as protamine or chloroquine, enhance transfection [19]. Finally, targeting ligands, such as carbohydrates [20] or folic acid [21], promote cell selectivity. Nanoparticles that include such modular components have enabled the functional in vivo delivery of nucleic acids to lung, liver, and tumors [22, 23].

Cell-based assays are employed to evaluate the relative in vitro transfection efficiency and cytotoxicity of lipoplexes based on cationic lipids. In support of this key data, additional assays and measurements determine particle size, DNA binding, and protection from degradative enzymes. Therefore, the methods employed in the lipoplex formulation, preparation, and characterization play a key role in the development of safe, efficient, and reproducible cationic lipid-based gene delivery systems.

Herein, we present materials and methods for the preparation of lipoplex formulations from pDNA and liposomes generated from thin films, together with key assay protocols employed in the evaluation of in vitro cytotoxicity and transfection efficiency. Specifically, the chapter describes lipid stock solution preparation, liposome formulation and lipoplex preparation, and the characterization of these nanoparticles based on particle size and zeta potential (ζ-potential). Furthermore, gel assay protocols are described which evaluate lipid-DNA binding and the capacity to protect the genetic material from enzymatic degradation over a range of cationic lipid:DNA molar charge ratios (CRs). Finally, protocols used to perform in vitro assays that evaluate cytotoxicity and transfection efficiency, over a range of CRs, are described. In all, this chapter presents a detailed set of protocols for the successful, reproducible preparation, characterization, and evaluation of lipoplexes, based on cationic lipids, for in vitro gene delivery.

2 Materials

The preparation of all solutions employed deionized water (dH$_2$O) and analytical grade reagents. Unless indicated otherwise, all solvents were obtained from Sigma–Aldrich (St. Louis, MO, USA) and all reagents were prepared and stored at room temperature (RT). Commercial assay solutions and kits are described below. When disposing waste materials, diligently follow all waste disposal regulations.

2.1 Cationic Liposome and Lipoplex Preparation and Characterization

1. Novel or commercial cationic lipid. Store as appropriate.

2. DOPE (Avanti Polar Lipids, Alabaster, USA). Store at –20 °C.

3. Cholesterol (Avanti Polar Lipids, Alabaster, USA). Store at –20 °C.

4. Dichloromethane (CH_2Cl_2).

5. Rotary evaporator.

6. Round-bottom flasks.

7. Polypropylene microcentrifuge tubes.

8. pDNA containing β-galactosidase (β-gal) gene, pCMVBeta Mammalian lacZnls12co (Marker Gene Technologies, Inc, Oregon, USA).

9. Zetasizer Nano ZS (Malvern Instruments, Worcestershire, UK) for particle size determination by dynamic light scattering (DLS) and ζ-potential measurement, or Zetasizer APS (Malvern Instruments, Worcestershire, UK) for particle size determination by DLS at 25 °C.

10. Capillary cells for ζ-potential measurement.

11. Agarose.

12. Tris-borate-ethylenediaminetetraacetic acid (EDTA) buffer (TBE).

13. Ethidium bromide (EtBr).

14. 6× gel loading solution (0.25 % (w/v) bromophenol blue, 0.25 % (w/v) xylene cyanol FF, 40 % (w/v) sucrose in dH_2O).

15. 5 % (w/v) sodium dodecyl sulfate (SDS) in dH_2O.

16. Geliance 200 Gel Imaging System (PerkinElmer Life and Analytical Sciences, Shelton, CT, USA).

2.2 Cell Culture

1. Chinese hamster ovarian (CHO-K1) cell line (Health Protection Agency Culture Collections, Salisbury, UK).

2. Roswell Park Memorial Institute (RPMI) 1640 media (Gibco™ supplied by Life Technologies).

3. Phenol red-free Dulbecco's Modified Eagle Medium (DMEM) (Gibco™ supplied by Life Technologies) (*see* **Note 1**).

4. Phenol red-free Opti-MEM® reduced Serum Media (Gibco™ supplied by Life Technologies) (*see* **Note 1**).

5. Fetal calf serum (FCS).

6. 100× penicillin-streptomycin solution (10,000 U penicillin and 10 mg/mL streptomycin) (Gibco™ supplied by Life Technologies).

7. Amphotericin B.

8. Dulbecco's Phosphate Buffered Saline (PBS) (Gibco™ supplied by Life Technologies).

2.3 Transfection Experiments and Post-transfection Assays

1. BCA Protein Assay (Pierce Biotechnology, Rockford, IL, USA).
2. Beta-Glo® Assay System (Promega, Madison, WI, USA).
3. CellTiter96® Aqueous One Solution Cell Proliferation Assay (Promega, Madison, WI, USA).
4. Absorbance and luminescence microplate reader.

3 Methods

The delivery of pDNA, whether it occurs via in vivo gene transfer for potential therapeutic treatments, or in vitro for cell culture applications, aims to achieve the expression of a protein that is lacking in the cells. In cell culture applications, an assessment of gene delivery efficiency depends upon the expression of the reporter gene (see **Note 2**) employed for this purpose and is matched to the specific application (see **Note 3**). This protocol describes the lipid-based delivery of a pDNA that contains a gene encoding the enzyme, β-gal. Upon successful cellular uptake, the relative efficiency of the delivery vehicle (or transfection efficiency) is assayed using 6-O-β-galactopyranosyl-luciferin, which the pDNA-derived β-gal cleaves to yield luciferin. The subsequent conversion of luciferin, mediated by luciferase in the presence of cofactors, results in the emission of light detected for quantitative analysis. The following protocols will be restricted to cationic lipid formulations that contain a single cationic lipid (see **Note 4**) combined in a 3:2 molar ratio with a neutral co-lipid. Finally, it is important to optimize each lipoplex formulation for each specific cell type (see **Note 5**). Here we outline protocols used in our laboratory that employ CHO cells (specifically, CHO-K1 cells) (see **Note 6**), an easy-to-transfect cell line that is the preferred choice for gene and genome-based research [24].

3.1 Lipid Ethanolic Stock Solutions

1. Dissolve a known amount of each lipid (cationic lipids and co-lipids) separately in CH_2Cl_2 in round-bottom flasks (see **Note 7**).
2. Remove the CH_2Cl_2, in each flask, on a rotary evaporator (see **Note 8**) at 35 °C bath temperature until a dry thin lipid film appears.
3. Dissolve the film in sufficient anhydrous ethanol (EtOH) to achieve a final 1 mM lipid EtOH stock solution (see **Note 9**). Subsequently store the solution at −80 °C until use.

3.2 Liposome Formulation from Thin Film

1. Combine 900 µL of 1 mM stock solution of cationic lipid (see Subheading 3.1) with 600 µL stock solution of the co-lipid in EtOH into a round-bottom flask to achieve a 3:2 molar ratio of cationic lipid to co-lipid, respectively (see **Note 10**).

2. Remove the organic solvent on a rotary evaporator (*see* **Note 8**) to obtain a thin film (*see* **Note 11**).

3. Dry the thin film under high vacuum for at least 2 h, or overnight, to remove all traces of organic solvent.

4. Hydrate the thin lipid film with a known amount (e.g. 450 μL) of sterile dH_2O (or Opti-MEM®) to achieve final hydrated multilamellar vesicle (liposome) stock solution with 2 mM cationic lipid concentration.

5. Upon addition of dH_2O or medium, warm the mixture above the lipid transition temperature for 15 min prior to vortexing for 30 s. Store the liposome stock solution overnight at 4 °C (*see* **Note 12**).

3.3 Liposome Particle Size Reduction

Liposome sonication, freeze-thaw, and extrusion are techniques employed, either separately or in combination, to reduce or homogenize liposome particle size. Each technique involves warming the sample above the phase transition temperature of the lipid.

3.3.1 Sonication

1. Sonicate the hydrated liposome stock solution (*see* Subheading 3.2) stored in the round-bottom flask for 30 min in a sonic bath in order to transform the multilamellar vesicles into liposomes of homogenous particle size (*see* **Note 13**).

2. Store the samples at 4 °C before use.

3.3.2 Freeze-Thaw

1. Transfer 450 μL of the multilamellar liposomes (*see* Subheading 3.2) into a 5 mL glass tube and lower it into liquid nitrogen (N_2) for rapid cooling.

2. After 2–3 min, transfer the frozen formulation to a water bath set at 60 °C and allow it to thaw for 3 min.

3. Freeze the preparation again in liquid N_2.

4. Repeat the freeze-thaw operation (above **steps 2** and **3**) ten times in total.

5. Store the samples in a refrigerator at 4 °C before use.

3.3.3 Extrusion

It is possible to extrude the multilamellar liposomes (*see* Subheading 3.2) at RT or above the phase transition temperature of the lipids (*see* **Note 14**). In the latter case, the extrusion of liposome formulations at elevated temperatures relies upon the use of the heating block provided with the extruder or a formulation pre-incubated in a water bath of adequate temperature.

1. Load 450 μL of the multilamellar vesicle solution into one of the two syringes and carefully place it into one end of the extruder (*see* **Notes 15** and **16**).

2. Place the second, empty syringe into the other end of the extruder.

3. Gently push the plunger of the filled syringe until the lipid solution has completely transferred into the second syringe.

4. Gently push the plunger of the second syringe until the lipid solution has completely transferred back into the original (first) syringe.

5. Repeat the above **steps 3** and **4** until the lipid solution has passed through the membrane a total of ten times or more (*see* **Notes 17** and **18**).

6. Inject the extruded lipid solution into a clean sample vial and store in a refrigerator at 4 °C before use.

3.4 Liposome Characterization

3.4.1 Particle Size

1. Transfer 450 μL of the final liposome solution into disposable square polystyrene cuvettes (dilute it to 1 mL with dH$_2$O) or in disposable 96-well plates (50 μL of liposome solution diluted to 100 μL with dH$_2$O).

2. Measure the liposome particle size (hydrodynamic diameter, dH) and polydispersity (*see* **Note 19**) by quasi-elastic DLS apparatus at 25 °C (*see* **Notes 20** and **21**).

3.4.2 ζ-Potential

1. Liposome suspensions should be prepared in 1 mM NaCl (i.e., in a low ionic strength medium).

2. Combine 350 μL of the liposome sample with 350 μL of 2 mM NaCl.

3. Transfer the sample to a 1 mL disposable syringe, dislodge any air bubbles, and insert the syringe to one of the ports on the ζ-cell.

4. Transfer the mixture into capillary ζ-cell and measure the ζ-potential at 25 °C (*see* **Notes 20** and **22**).

3.5 Preparation of Lipid/pDNA Complexes (Lipoplexes)

The formation of lipoplexes involves combining liposomes with pDNA (*see* **Note 23**).

1. Dilute 14.4 μL of pDNA (250 ng/μL in elution buffer) with 57.6 μL of Opti-MEM giving a final pDNA volume of 72 μL.

2. Dilute a set of five liposome suspensions in dH$_2$O such that the final concentration of net positive charge across the set is 0.5, 1.5, 3, 5, and 10 times higher than the phosphate concentration in the pDNA solution (*see* **Note 24**).

3. Combine equal volumes of the DNA solution with each of the liposome suspensions of varying concentration (*see* **Notes 25** and **26**), and then incubate at RT for 30 min to obtain lipoplex suspensions at molar CR (+/−) of 0.5, 1.5, 3, 5, and 10.

4. Take 48 μL of each lipoplex formulation for the gel assays.

5. Add 204 μL of Opti-MEM to each lipoplex formulation to reach a final volume of 300 μL/well (*see* **Note 27**).

3.6 Characterization of Lipoplexes

3.6.1 Particle Size Analysis and ζ-Potential

Measure particle size and ζ-potential of lipoplex suspensions as described above (*see* Subheading 3.4).

3.6.2 Gel Retardation Assay

Gel assays performed using lipoplexes prepared in different CRs (*see* **Notes 28** and **29**).

1. Transfer 20 μL of each lipoplex formulation into a polypropylene microcentrifuge tube.

2. Add 2 μL of 6× gel loading solution and mix.

3. Load 18 μL of each lipoplex sample onto a 1% agarose gel impregnated with EtBr and run at 105 V for 1 h in 1× TBE buffer (*see* **Note 30**).

4. Observe the pDNA bands using a gel imaging system.

3.6.3 DNase I Degradation Assay

A degradation assay characterizes the capacity of the cationic lipids to protect the genetic material from degradation by enzymes that the lipoplex could encounter outside the cells (in vivo) (*see* **Note 31**).

1. Transfer 20 μL of each lipoplex formulation into a polypropylene microcentrifuge tube, add 1 μL of DNase I solution, then incubate at 37 °C for 1 h.

2. After incubation, add 4 μL of 5% SDS solution and incubate for a further 30 min.

3. After incubation, continue as described in Subheading 3.6.2, **steps 2–4**.

3.7 Transfection Experiments and Post-transfection Assays

3.7.1 Cell Culture and Transfection Protocol

1. Grow the CHO cells in RPMI 1640 media supplemented with 10% FCS, 100 U/mL of penicillin/streptomycin, and 0.25 μg/mL amphotericin B.

2. 24 h before transfection, seed the cells onto an opaque and transparent 96-well plate at a density of (3×10^4 cells/cm^2) 1×10^4 cells per well and incubate at 37 °C in the presence of a 5% CO_2 atmosphere.

3. Once 80% confluence is reached (after approximately 24 h), remove old medium and wash cells with 100 μL of PBS.

4. Add 45 μL/well of each lipid-pDNA complex preparation at different CR (in triplicate) and incubate the plate at 37 °C in the presence of a 5% CO_2 atmosphere for 4 h.

5. After 4 h of incubation, remove the lipoplex-containing medium and wash the cells with PBS.

6. Add 100 μL/well of RPMI, then incubate at 37 °C in the presence of a 5% CO_2 atmosphere for an additional 44 h.

3.7.2 BCA Assay

1. 48 h after transfection, remove old medium and wash cells with 100 μL of PBS.

2. Add 10 μL/well of passive lysis buffer and incubate at RT for 30 min.

3. Dilute the contents of a Bovine Albumin Standard (BSA) ampule of Promega BCA kit using dH$_2$O to obtain serial dilutions with a range of 20–2000 μg/mL.

4. Use the calibration curve obtained from these dilutions to determine the cellular protein content per well.

5. Add 200 μL/well of BCA working solution, gently mix by pipetting, and incubate at RT for 1 h.

6. Read the absorbance at $\lambda = 562$ nm using a microplate reader.

7. Determine the cellular protein content per well by extrapolation from the standard curve.

3.7.3 β-Galactosidase Assay

1. 48 h after transfection, remove old medium and wash cells with 100 μL of PBS.

2. Add 50 μL/well of phenol red-free DMEM media, and mix thoroughly.

3. Add 50 μL/well of Beta-Glo™ working solution and mix thoroughly.

4. Incubate at RT for 1 h.

5. Read the luminescence at $\lambda = 562$ nm on a plate reader. Express β-Galactosidase activity as relative light units (RLU).

6. Normalize luminescence values with protein concentration (determined by the BCA assay described in Subheading 3.7.2) to afford RLUs/mg of proteins.

3.7.4 Cytotoxicity Assay

The cytotoxicity associated with the lipoplex formulations at CRs (+/−) ranging from 0.5 to 10 can be evaluated through the use of a standard assay. The assay described here is based on the 3-(4,5-dimethylthiazol-2-yl)-5-(3-carboxymethoxyphenyl)-2-(4-sulfophenyl)-2H-tetrazolium (MTS) assay [25]. Other methods for the evaluation of cell viability include the 3-[4,5-dimethylthiazol-2-yl]-2,5-diphenyl tetrazolium bromide (MTT) assay [26] (*see* **Note 32**) and the Alamar Blue assay [27], which employs a sensitive oxidation–reduction indicator that fluoresces and changes color upon reduction by living cells.

1. 48 h after transfection, remove old medium and wash cells with 100 μL of PBS.

2. Add 50 μL/well of phenol red-free DMEM media, and mix thoroughly.

3. Add 10 μL/well of CellTiter96® Aqueous One Solution Cell Proliferation Assay and mix by gentle rocking.

4. Incubate at 37 °C in the presence of a 5 % CO_2 atmosphere for 1 h.

5. Read the absorbance at $\lambda = 490$ nm using a microplate reader (*see* **Note 33**).

6. The percentage of viable cells is calculated from the absorbance ratio of treated to untreated cells (Cell viability (%) = [Cell viability of treated cells/Cell viability of untreated cells] × 100).

4 Notes

1. The presence of phenol red will affect the luminescent signal. Therefore, it is strongly recommended that phenol-red-free culture media be employed.

2. Commonly employed gene reporter systems include the following pDNA systems: β-gal; luciferase; or green fluorescent protein (GFP) using a pCMVTnT-GFP pDNA [28].

3. Fluorescent microscopy or fluorescence-activated cell-sorting (FACS) analysis of living cells are methods used to monitor GFP expression. The visualization of GFP by fluorescence microscopy facilitates the assessment of relative transfection efficiency, and thus enables a comparison between different formulations. It is possible to visualize a sample using either an inverted light microscope with epifluorescence optics or a confocal microscope. The possibility of making optical slices with a confocal microscope provide evidence that lipoplexes (or DNA released from them) are indeed inside the cells and not simply associated with the cell surface.

4. Mixed or binary cationic lipid formulations can lead to enhanced gene delivery, however, one must take care when working with binary cationic lipid formulations, as noted by MacDonald and coworkers [29].

5. The optimized molar ratio between the cationic lipid and the neutral co-lipid depends upon the cell line of choice.

6. A number of immortalized or primary cell lines are commercially available. The literature is replete with reports that describe nonviral in vitro gene transfer studies with different cell types.

7. For example, in the case of lipid L1 (molecular weight, MW of 437 g/mol) weigh out 4.37 mg and solubilize in 5 mL of CH_2Cl_2.

8. If the lipids are light sensitive, the use of a foil covered round-bottom flask will reduce light exposure during procedures such as rotary evaporation.

9. For the example lipid L1 mentioned above, solubilize the 4.37 mg thin film in 10 mL of EtOH.

10. The addition of components other than cationic and helper lipids occurs at the step of combining appropriate volumes of the separate EtOH lipid stock solutions. Examples of additional components include 3–5 % (molar ratio) of PEGylated lipid for "stealth" liposomal systems; and/or a lipid with an attached targeting ligand, if desired, for systems that are more complex.

11. For EtOH lipid stock solutions, rotary evaporate for approximately 1 h at 35 °C.

12. Before use, warm the hydrated stock solution to 37 °C and sonicate for 30 min.

13. Depending on the liposome concentration, the solution will be a transparent or milky dispersion.

14. For example, an Avanti Mini-Extruder (Avanti Polar Lipids, Alabaster, USA).

15. To reduce the dead volume, prewet the extruder parts by passing a syringe full of dH_2O or buffer through the extruder, and discard the liquid.

16. Extrusion of multilamellar liposomal suspensions will produce unilamellar liposomes with a pore size of 0.2 μm.

17. Polycarbonate membranes are intended for a single liposome preparation and should not be reused.

18. The final extrusion should fill the second syringe. This reduces the possibility of contamination with larger particles or foreign material.

19. Polydispersity index is a measure of the liposome or lipoplex size distribution. Methods that aim to reduce the size distribution (extrusion for example) are associated with a decrease in the polydispersity index value. Small size lipoplexes (<200 nm) are required for intravenous administration, whereas the administration of larger lipoplexes must occur via other routes (intraperitoneal for example).

20. Report the data as a mean ± standard deviation (SD) derived from three independent measurements.

21. Within the range of concentrations used in this protocol, the samples do not require predilution with water.

22. Cationic liposomes should have a positive ζ-potential in order to interact with negatively charged pDNA.

23. Unlike liposomal delivery of small organic molecules encapsulated within the aqueous core of the liposome, the combination of a cationic liposome and a large pDNA molecule results in a lipid-based complex characterized commonly by a lamellar, inverted hexagonal or cubic structure, or some combination of these morphologies. The determination of lipoplex

morphology commonly employs transmission electron micros-copy (TEM) or small-angle X-ray diffraction (SAXD) studies. It is possible to observe the structure and morphology of lipo-plexes using negatively stained TEM. A drop of liposome or lipoplex suspension is deposited over a carbon coated standard TEM copper grid, and then a droplet of the stain solution (generally uranyl acetate or phosphotungstic acid) is applied to the copper grid. The stained liposome or lipoplex suspension is observed on the grid, using a transmission electron micro-scope. SAXD protocols are dependent on beam source [30].

24. Lipoplexes of concentrations 0.081 mM, 0.243 mM, 0.486 mM, 0.81 mM, and 1.62 mM, corresponding to CRs (+/−) of 0.5, 1.5, 3, 5, and 10 respectively, are prepared from the 2 mM liposome stocks.

25. Greater transfection efficiency has been reported when the nonviral DNA complex is formed by addition of the cationic vector to the DNA solution, as opposed to the reverse [31].

26. The average weight of a single DNA base pair (bp) is 650 Da (Daltons or g/mol), and therefore the MW of a double-stranded DNA (dsDNA) molecule equals the number of base pairs multiplied by 650 Da. In terms of the negative charge, for every mole of base pair there are 2 mol of negative phosphorus groups. Therefore, the number of moles of negative phospho-rus groups within a dsDNA molecule equals the number of moles of DNA multiplied by the number of bases within its structure. If the cationic lipid carries one positive charge, the number of moles of positive charge is equal to the number of moles of the lipid itself.

27. Transfection experiments are performed using each of the diluted lipoplex formulations and conducted in triplicates.

28. Based on constant DNA and an increasing amount of cationic lipid, employ a 1% TBE-agarose gel, which separates any remaining nucleic acid not incorporated into the particles. The absence of DNA bands indicates full association of the DNA with the cationic lipid.

29. In addition to the gel retardation assay, it is possible to per-form a competitive binding assay to determine how tightly the DNA and cationic lipid are bound to one another. The nega-tively charged surfactant, SDS, is commonly employed and competes for lipid binding. In practice, the weaker the lipo-plex, the greater the number of cationic lipid molecules that bind to SDS, thus leaving a greater amount of unbound DNA that is visualized on the gel.

30. The electric field impedes the migration of pDNA complexed with the cationic lipid.

31. The exposure of lipoplexes to DNase I leads to cleavage of the unbound and/or unprotected DNA into linear fragments. Separation of the DNA fragments from the cationic lipids, using a detergent, leads to the subsequent detection of the components by agarose gel electrophoresis. The presence of a DNA band is indicative of the proportion of the DNA protected via association with a cationic lipid.

32. In cytotoxicity assays, MTT and MTS function in a similar manner, which involves the reduction of a tetrazolium into a formazan product. The amount of formazan is directly proportional to the number of living cells. In the MTT assay, the formazan product is insoluble, and extra steps are required to dissolve the crystals resulting in the full destruction of cells. The formazan product formed using the MTS assay is soluble in tissue culture medium, hence, the medium can be used for the cell viability evaluation while the cells themselves can be used for other quantitative analyses, such as total protein BCA assay.

33. The absorbance of the converted dye correlates with the number of viable cells.

Acknowledgement

This work was supported in part by the British Council (PMI2 Gulf States Cooperation Grant No. RCGS206), the Biomedical Research Program intramural funding at Weill Cornell Medical College in Qatar, and the Qatar National Research Fund under the National Priorities Research Program, award NPRP08-705-3-144. Its contents are solely the responsibility of the authors and do not necessarily represent the official views of the Qatar National Research Fund.

References

1. Felgner PL, Gadek TR, Holm M, Roman R, Chan HW, Wenz M, Northrop JP, Ringold GM, Danielsen M (1987) Lipofection: a highly efficient, lipid-mediated DNA-transfection procedure. Proc Natl Acad Sci U S A 84: 7413–7417

2. Bhattacharya S, Bajaj A (2009) Advances in gene delivery through molecular design of cationic lipids. Chem Commun:4632–4656

3. Martin B, Sainlos M, Aissaoui A, Oudrhiri N, Hauchecorne M, Vigneron JP, Lehn JM, Lehn P (2005) The design of cationic lipids for gene delivery. Curr Pharm Des 11:375–394

4. Hosseinkhani H, Abedini F, Ou KL, Domb AJ (2015) Polymers in gene therapy technology. Polym Adv Technol 26:198–211

5. Schaffert D, Wagner E (2008) Gene therapy progress and prospects: synthetic polymer-based systems. Gene Ther 15:1131–1138

6. Chaplot SP, Rupenthal ID (2014) Dendrimers for gene delivery - a potential approach for ocular therapy? J Pharm Pharmacol 66: 542–556

7. Dufès C, Uchegbu IF, Schätzlein AG (2005) Dendrimers in gene delivery. Adv Drug Deliv Rev 57:2177–2202

8. Wirth T, Parker N, Ylä-Herttuala S (2013) History of gene therapy. Gene 525:162–169

9. Yin H, Kanasty RL, Eltoukhy AA, Vegas AJ, Dorkin JR, Anderson DG (2014) Non-viral vectors for gene-based therapy. Nat Rev Genet 15:541–555

10. Elsabahy M, Nazarali A, Foldvari M (2011) Non-viral nucleic acid delivery: key challenges and future directions. Curr Drug Deliv 8:235–244

11. Guo X, Huang L (2012) Recent advances in nonviral vectors for gene delivery. Acc Chem Res 45:971–979

12. Junquera E, Aicart E (2014) Cationic lipids as transfecting agents of DNA in gene therapy. Curr Top Med Chem 14:649–663

13. Belmadi N, Midoux P, Loyer P, Passirani C, Pichon C, Le Gall T, Jaffres PA, Lehn P, Montier T (2015) Synthetic vectors for gene delivery: an overview of their evolution depending on routes of administration. Biotechnol J 10:1370–1389

14. Li W, Huang Z, MacKay JA, Grube S, Szoka FC Jr (2005) Low-pH-sensitive poly(ethylene glycol) (PEG)-stabilized plasmid nanolipoparticles: effects of PEG chain length, lipid composition and assembly conditions on gene delivery. J Gene Med 7:67–79

15. Govender D, Ul Islam R, De Koning CB, van Otterlo WAL, Arbuthnot P, Ariatti M, Singh M (2015) Stealth lipoplex decorated with triazole-tethered galactosyl moieties: a strong hepatotropic gene vector. Biotechnol Lett 37:567–575

16. Kostarelos K, Miller AD (2005) Synthetic, self-assembly ABCD nanoparticles; a structural paradigm for viable synthetic non-viral vectors. Chem Soc Rev 34:970–994

17. Pozzi D, Marchini C, Cardarelli F, Amenitsch H, Garulli C, Bifone A, Caracciolo G (2012) Transfection efficiency boost of cholesterol-containing lipoplexes. Biochim Biophys Acta 1818:2335–2343

18. Lee JS, Ankone M, Pieters E, Schiffelers RM, Hennink WE, Feijen J (2011) Circulation kinetics and biodistribution of dual-labeled polymersomes with modulated surface charge in tumor-bearing mice: comparison with stealth liposomes. J Control Release 155:282–288

19. Sanz V, Coley HM, Silva SRP, McFadden J (2012) Protamine and chloroquine enhance gene delivery and expression mediated by RNA-wrapped single walled carbon nanotubes. J Nanosci Nanotechnol 12:1739–1747

20. Kong F, Zhou F, Ge L, Liu X, Wang Y (2012) Mannosylated liposomes for targeted gene delivery. Int J Nanomed 7:1079–1089

21. Huang Y, Yang T, Zhang W, Lu Y, Ye P, Yang G, Li B, Qi S, Liu Y, He X, Lee RJ, Xu C, Xiang G (2014) A novel hydrolysis-resistant lipophilic folate derivative enables stable delivery of targeted liposomes in vivo. Int J Nanomed 9:4581–4595

22. Carmona S, Jorgensen MR, Kolli S, Crowther C, Salazar FH, Marion PL, Fujino M, Natori Y, Thanou M, Arbuthnot P, Miller AD (2009) Controlling HBV replication in vivo by intravenous administration of triggered PEGylated siRNA-nanoparticles. Mol Pharm 6:706–717

23. Kenny GD, Kamaly N, Kalber TL, Brody LP, Sahuri M, Shamsaei E, Miller AD, Bell JD (2011) Novel multifunctional nanoparticle mediates siRNA tumour delivery, visualisation and therapeutic tumour reduction in vivo. J Control Release 149:111–116

24. Wurm FM (2013) CHO Quasispecies—implications for manufacturing processes. Processes 1:296–311

25. Cory AH, Owen TC, Barltrop JA, Cory JG (1991) Use of an aqueous soluble tetrazolium/formazan assay for cell growth assays in culture. Cancer Commun 3:207–212

26. Mosmann T (1983) Rapid colorimetric assay for cellular growth and survival: application to proliferation and cytotoxicity assays. J Immunol Methods 65:55–63

27. Ahmed SA, Gogal RM Jr, Walsh JE (1994) A new rapid and simple non-radioactive assay to monitor and determine the proliferation of lymphocytes: an alternative to [3H]thymidine incorporation assay. J Immunol Methods 170:211–224

28. Parvizi P, Jubeli E, Raju L, Khalique NA, Almeer A, Allam H, Al Manaa M, Larsen H, Nicholson D, Pungente MD, Fyles TM (2014) Aspects of nonviral gene therapy: correlation of molecular parameters with lipoplex structure and transfection efficacy in pyridinium-based cationic lipids. Int J Pharm 461:145–156

29. Wang L, Koynova R, Parikh H, MacDonald RC (2006) Transfection activity of binary mixtures of cationic O-substituted phosphatidylcholine derivatives: the hydrophobic core strongly modulates physical properties and DNA delivery efficacy. Biophys J 91:3692–3706

30. Koynova R (2010) Analysis of lipoplex structure and lipid phase changes. Methods Mol Biol 606:399–423

31. Boussif O, Lezoualc'h F, Zanta MA, Mergny MD, Scherman D, Demeneix B, Behr JP (1995) A versatile vector for gene and oligonucleotide transfer into cells in culture and in vivo: polyethylenimine. Proc Natl Acad Sci U S A 92:7297–7301

Lipoplexes from Non-viral Cationic Vectors: DOTAP-DOPE Liposomes and Gemini Micelles

Sara Falsini and Sandra Ristori

Abstract

This chapter describes the topic of gene therapy based on colloidal drug delivery, as an alternative to the use of viral carriers. Non-viral vectors are promising transfection agents and do not suffer from limitations related to toxicity and immunogenic effects. In particular, lipid-based aggregates are generally considered biocompatible and versatile nanocarriers whose composition can be designed to include a cationic molecule which ensures strong interaction with nucleic acid. Herein the main issues related to complex formation and in vitro administration are illustrated with key examples, such as liposome-DNA plasmid (pDNA) association and micelles-siRNA complexes.

Key words Gene therapy, Cationic micelles, Lipoplex, siRNA, Plasmid transfection

1 Introduction

In the last few decades, gene therapy has gained recognition as an alternative method for the treatment of different and severe pathologies, such as cancer [1], infectious diseases [2], cardiovascular disorders [3], dermatological [4], ocular [5], and respiratory injuries. Gene therapy concerns all the procedures used to treat disease by modifying, silencing, and replacing the abnormal expression of genes in targeting cells [6]. Depending on the genetic material, gene therapy can be classified according to different mechanisms of treatment. For example, the delivery of small interfering RNA (siRNA) and short hairpin RNA (shRNA) promotes sequence specific silencing of gene in human cells, while the transport of pDNA is involved in restoring the normal expression of proteins.

Exogenous siRNA and shRNA pDNAs [7] promote a sequence-specific degradation of messenger RNA (mRNA), operating at different steps in RNA interference (RNAi) pathway. siRNAs are double stranded RNA of ~19–23 bp with impair endings, able to control degradation of mRNA with fully complementary sequence. Once in the cytosol, synthetic siRNAs interact with the

Gabriele Candiani (ed.), *Non-Viral Gene Delivery Vectors: Methods and Protocols*, Methods in Molecular Biology, vol. 1445,
DOI 10.1007/978-1-4939-3718-9_3, © Springer Science+Business Media New York 2016

endogenous RNA Induced Silencing Complex (RISC). One strand of the siRNA duplex (the guide strand) is loaded into a component of RISC, called Argonaute protein (Argo), and then mature RISC locates siRNA on the mRNA with complementary sequence, thus promoting its cleavage [8]. While the effect induced by siRNA is transient, the knocking down promoted by shRNA pDNA is permanent, due to its capability of DNA integration. shRNAs transcribed by RNA polymerase III consist of two complementary 19–22 bp RNA sequences linked by a short loop of 4–11 nt similar to the hairpin. Following transcription, shRNAs are processed by DICER, which removes the terminal loop and leaves a staggered end, allowing its interaction with RISC, where the degradation of mRNA is performed [9].

Gene therapy was originally carried out by delivering pDNAs to restore the normal expression of specific genes, and this line of action is still very active. Recently, the attention of researchers has also been focused on synthetic double-strand small DNAs (~30 bp). Such short fragments are called siDNAs, since they are able to interfere with the signaling of DNA double-strand break (DSB) repair, improving the response to conventional therapies, e.g., radiotherapy [10].

The transport of genetic materials is a widely studied technique in vitro, though major challenge remains for applications in vivo. In all cases the choice of vectors able to carry and release genetic materials into the target cells is a fundamental prerequisite for the success of gene therapy. An ideal vector should provide protection of genetic material, preventing its degradation in the bloodstream. Moreover, the vector should exert its therapeutic role only in target cells, avoiding off-target tissues and facilitating cellular uptake [11].

Two different classes of delivery systems are currently used: viral and non-viral vectors. The former demonstrated high efficiency in transfection, though their use has been hampered by limitations such as cytotoxicity and immunogenicity. Another restriction arises from the large scale production of viruses, which requires high caution for patients and medical staff. Inversely, non-viral vectors are easy to prepare, safe, and can be designed with a rich variety of physico-chemical properties, such as structure, size, and surface charge. In particular, non-viral carriers based on cationic lipids have gained interest in biomedical applications, shaping the scientific landscape in terms of diagnosis, treatment, and prevention [12]. These carriers have been extensively studied, especially in their liposomal formulations or as lipid nanoparticles (NPs), which are scarcely immunogenic, handable and able to carry large amount of DNA. The positive charge of the surface cationic vectors also promotes the interaction with the plasma membrane, thus improving the uptake by cells.

Herein, we focus on selected classes of non-viral carriers based on cationic lipids, starting from micelles and increasing the structural complexity, to liposomes.

1.1 Micellar Vectors

Micelles, composed of amphiphiles, i.e. lipids or surfactants (Fig. 1a), represent the simplest lipid-based nanocarrier. In aqueous media, amphiphilic molecules spontaneously self-assembly into aggregates above a specific amount called Critical Micellar Concentration (CMC). In micelles, the hydrophilic heads are located in contact with the solvent, whereas the hydrophobic tails are mainly confined to the inner region. Similar to classical micelles are polymeric micelles (Fig. 1b). As mentioned above, positively charged head groups represent a critical component of core-shell aggregates for their ability to interact with the negative backbone of nucleic acids. Therefore, for the purpose of gene delivery, an interesting class of polymers is represented by cationic polyelectrolytes. Their use has been reported by several authors [13, 14]. The source of cationic polymers can be synthetic or natural, such as chitosan [15], bovine serum albumin (BSA) [16], and amino modified pectin [17]. Both standard and polymeric micelles are at thermodynamic equilibrium and can be prepared by simply dissolving the starting molecules in the aqueous medium at the desired concentration.

In the following we describe a typical protocol for the preparation of transfection complexes containing cationic micelles and liposomes. These systems are particularly suitable for in vitro cell cultures and with small modifications, can also be adopted for in vivo studies. A possibility for this latter purpose is to add a small amount, i.e. 10–20% (w/w) polyethylene glycol (PEG) in the formulation [18].

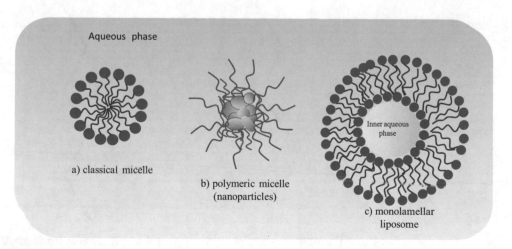

Fig. 1 Scheme of "soft matter" aggregates that can be used for gene delivery

The cationic micelles considered herein are formed by dimeric surfactants called "Gemini" with general formula α, ω-bis (*N*-dodecyl-*N*,*N*-dimethylammonium) m-alkane bromide [19]. They are characterized by two amphiphilic moieties covalently connected by a spacer at the level of the head group. In particular, we used three different Gemini 12-3-12, 12-6-12, and 12-12-12, with spacer of 3-CH_2, 6-CH_2, and 12-CH_2, respectively (Fig. 2) [20].

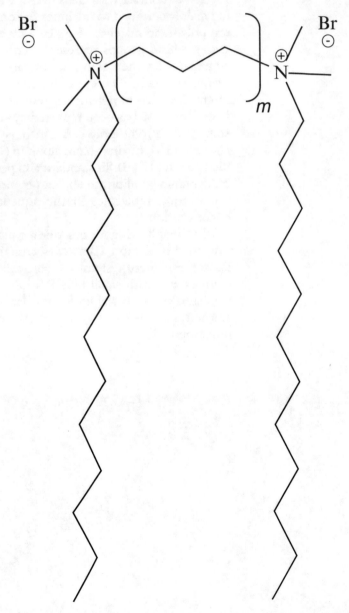

Fig. 2 Chemical structure of 12-m-12 gemini surfactant with tetramethylammonium bromide polar heads

It has been established that Gemini micelles aggregate with siRNA at charge ratio (CR, −/+) of 0.75 and 1.25, where the CR is the ratio between negative charge of the siRNA backbone and positive charge of cationic surfactants [21].

1.2 Liposome Vectors

Liposomes have been used for many years for gene delivery applications (Fig. 1c). As in the case of micelles, the headgroups of lipids used in the formulation play a major role for the docking to cells and tissues. In practice, the positive charge of cationic components facilitates DNA condensation, and governs the first interaction with plasma membranes. The most popular cationic lipids are 1,2-dioleoyl-3-trimethylammoniopropane (DOTAP) (Fig. 3a), used for its well-known ability to give stable and fluid bilayers, and cholesteryl 3β-N-(di-methyl-amino-ethyl)-carbamate hydrochloride (DC-Chol) (Fig. 3b), usually mixed with a neutral co-lipid or helper lipid, which improves structural stability and decreases toxicity. Other suitable components are cholesterol and its derivatives, whose main function is to increase the similarity between liposomes and mammalian cell membranes. It has been found that cholesterol addition also prolongs the circulation of liposomes in vivo, though it is not clear if this property stems from the smaller size generally obtained for cholesterol containing liposomes or

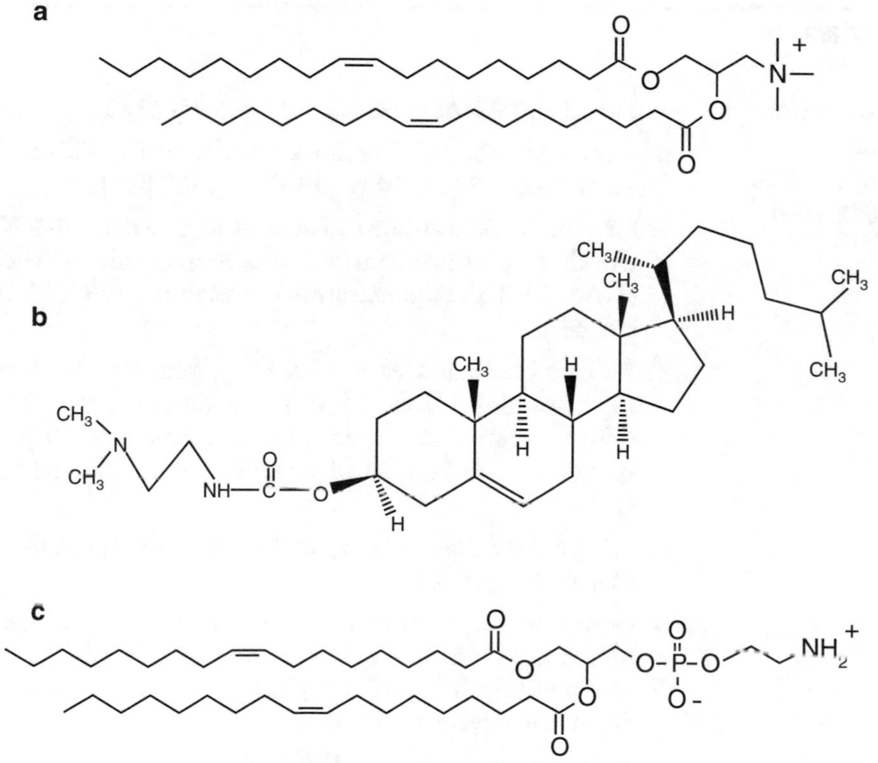

Fig. 3 Chemical structure of DC-Chol, DOPE and DOTAP

from the higher rigidity that cholesterol imparts to the lipid bilayers [22]. Among the preferred lipid chains used for lipid-based drug delivery, unsaturated fatty acids are generally used, due to their fluid state at room temperature (RT) and in operative conditions. This characteristic feature promotes a better incorporation of huge molecules and confers higher flexibility to the vector surface during all the transfection steps. A common helper lipid is 1,2-dioleoyl-sn-glycerol-phosphoethanolamine (DOPE) (Fig. 3c), whose fusogenic properties have been recognized about two decades back [23, 24].

The preparation of liposomes for gene delivery usually consists of: (i) obtaining dried films from all the different lipids and helpers previously dissolved in volatile organic solvents; (ii) rehydrating these films with the desired culture medium, also containing the genetic material to be transfected; (iii) downsizing by means of extrusion or sonication with high power ultrasound apparatus. This procedure usually results in unilamellar or oligolamellar liposomes, whose shelf life may vary from few days to several months, depending on the specific composition and size. However, in the case of cationic formulations, the tendency towards fusion, which is the main destabilizing effect, is attenuated by the positive surface charge and consequent repulsions among liposomes.

2   Materials

2.1   Consumables, Disposables, and Equipment Used for siRNA/Micelles

1. Sterile and RNAse free MilliQ® water (dH$_2$O).

2. Home-synthesized Gemini surfactants [25] (12-3-12, 12-6-12 and 12-12-12). Store powders at RT [21].

3. Gemini stock solution: dissolve the powders in RNAse free dH$_2$O at a concentration of 2.5 mM, above their CMC [**Note 1**]. This concentration corresponds to 5 mM in positive charges.

4. AllStars Hs Cells Death siRNA (Qiagen, Venlo, Netherlands) stock solution [**Note 2**]: dissolve the powder in RNAse free dH$_2$O in order to obtain a stock solution of 20 μM, corresponding to 0.84 mM of negative charge. Stored at –20 °C until use.

5. HEK293 (*Homo sapiens*, embryonic kidney) cells (ATCC©, Manassas, VA) [26].

6. Complete cell culture medium: Dulbecco's Modified Eagle Medium (DMEM) supplemented with 10% (v/v) fetal bovine serum (FBS), 1% (w/v) L-glutamine, and 1% (w/v) penicillin/streptomycin antibiotics.

7. Transfection medium: DMEM/F12 medium containing 25 mM of HEPES and 10% (v/v) fetal calf serum (FCS).

8. 96-well polystyrene cell culture plates.

9. Inverted microscope.

2.2 Consumables, Disposables, and Equipment Used for Lipoplexes Containing pDNA

1. >99 % pure DOTAP (Avanti Polar Lipids, Alabaster, AL). Use without further purification.

2. >99 % pure DOPE (Avanti Polar Lipids). Use without further purification.

3. >99 % pure DC-Chol (Avanti Polar Lipids). Use without further purification.

4. >99 % pure chloroform ($CHCl_3$) (Sigma-Aldrich, Saint Louis, MO). Use without further purification.

5. 10 mM Tris(hydroxymethyl)aminomethane-hydrochloride (Tris–HCl) buffer, pH 7.4.

6. Polycarbonate membranes with pore diameter of 100 nm.

7. LiposoFast apparatus (Avestin, Ottawa, Canada).

8. Sterile dH_2O.

9. pEGFP-pcDNA (Invitrogen, insert length 4.7 kb) extracted from *E. coli DH5α* cells with the Qiagen MIDI kit, according to the manufacturer's instructions, contains the reporter gene encoding the Enhanced Green Fluorescent Protein (EGFP).

10. CHO Chinese hamster ovary cells (ATCC©) [26].

11. 24-well polystyrene cell culture plates.

12. Complete cell culture medium.

13. Transfection medium.

14. 4 % (w/v) paraformaldehyde (PFA) in phosphate buffered-saline (PBS).

15. Inverted microscope.

16. Fluorescence microscope.

3 Methods

3.1 siRNA/Micelle Complexation

An example of protocol to obtain siRNA/Gemini complexes, suited for in vitro transfection experiments is reported here.

1. Dilute AllStars Hs Cells Death siRNA stock solution to obtain a 29.8 µM of siRNA solution, corresponding to 1.25 mM in terms of negative charge.

2. Combine equal volumes of Gemini stock solution and diluted **Note 3** siRNA stock solution in order to obtain aggregates with positive CR []. For example, to obtain complexes with CR 0.25, add 100 µL of 2.5 mM Gemini stock solution to 100 µL of 29.8 µM diluted siRNA solution. The final concentra-

tions of Gemini and siRNA are 1.25 mM and 14.88 μM, respectively.

3. Dilute 20 μL of the solution obtained in **step 2** in 500 μL of complete cell culture medium in order to obtain 50 μM Gemini (595 nM of siRNA).

4. Dilute the complexes in order to obtain the following concentrations: 10 μM of Gemini (119 nM of siRNA), 1 μM of Gemini (23.8 nM of siRNA), and 0.5 μM of Gemini (4.76 nM of siRNA).

3.2 Lipoplex Preparation

An example of the protocol to obtain DOTAP/DOPE-pDNA or DOTAP/DOPE-pDNA lipoplexes [27, 28] suited for in vitro transfection experiments is reported in the following.

Large unilamellar vesicles (LUVs) are formulated with DOTAP (or DC-Chol) and DOPE at 1:1 (mol/mol), as described in ref. 27.

1. Dissolve the mixture of lipid powders in $CHCl_3$ in order to obtain a total lipid concentration of 2.8 mM.

2. Allow the solvent to carefully evaporate. For this purpose the final step should be drying in a vacuum pump with temperature set at 30 °C for at least 20–30 min.

3. Swell the obtained mixed lipid film with 10 mM of Tris–HCl buffer, pH 7.4, at RT.

4. Vortex to obtain multilamellar vesicles.

5. Perform eight freeze/thaw cycles by plunging the sample in liquid nitrogen (N_2), followed by warming in a water-bath at 40 °C and vortexing [**Notes 4** and **5**].

6. Reduce liposomes in size and convert to LUV by extrusion [**Note 6**] through 100 nm polycarbonate membranes.

7. Perform 27 runs with the LiposoFast apparatus.

8. Dilute the obtained LUV solution 1:10 with sterile dH_2O and then filter through 200 μm pore sterile membranes.

9. Dissolve pEGFP in sterile dH_2O at the concentration of 35 mM in negative charges.

10. Add 500 μL of pEGFP solution to an equal volume of liposomes to form lipoplexes [**Note 7**]. The final cationic lipid concentration is 0.7 mM, and the final pEGFP$^-$/lipid$^+$ CR is 0.25 [**Note 8**].

3.3 Transfection Experiments Mediated by siRNA Complexes

1. Grow HEK 293 in complete cell culture medium at 37 °C in a 5 % CO_2 atmosphere.

2. One day before transfection, seed into a 96-well plate HEK 293 at a density of 10^4 cells/cm^2 in 200 μL of complete cell culture medium. Incubate at 37 °C in a 5 % CO_2 atmosphere for 24 h.

3. After 24 h, remove the old medium from cells, wash the cells with PBS, then add 200 μL/well of medium containing Gemini complexes. Incubate at 37 °C in a 5 % CO_2 atmosphere for 72 h. Perform the experiments at least in duplicate.

4. After 72 h, perform standard microscopy evaluation to quantify the vector efficacy.

3.4 Transfection Experiments Mediated by Lipoplexes

1. Grow CHO cells in 100-mm Petri dishes in transfection culture medium at 37 °C in a 5 % CO_2 atmosphere.

2. Seed CHO cells into a 24 multi-well plate at a cell density of 7.5×10^4 cells/cm^2 in 500 μL/well of culture medium. Incubate at 37 °C in a 5 % CO_2 atmosphere for 24 h.

3. After 24 h of cell culture, add the pDNA/liposome mixture to the cells. Incubate at 37 °C in a 5 % CO_2 atmosphere for additional 24 h.

4. After 24 h, remove the old medium, and wash the cells with PBS.

5. Fix the cells with 4 % (w/v) PFA in PBS for 20 min at RT.

6. Following fixation, analyze cells under an inverted microscope. The ratio of fluorescent to total cells visible by means of a fluorescence microscope ($\lambda_{ex} = 488$ nm) is the parameter used to estimate the transfection efficacy of lipoplexes [**Note 9**].

4   Notes

1. The suggested concentration of Gemini stock solution has to be above CMC. In our case, the CMC values are the following: 0.96 mM, 1 mM, and 0.37 mM for 12-3-12, 12-6-12, and 12-12-12, respectively. We choose to prepare stock solution with concentration of 2.5 mM where micelles are already formed.

2. AllStars Hs Cells Death siRNA, distributed by Qiagen, contains a mixture of siRNAs targeting cell survival genes. For this reason AllStars Hs Cells Death siRNA allows a rapid screening of different formulations.

3. The formation of complexes appears after few sec, becoming visible to the naked eye due to the increase of suspension turbidity. Following this preparation procedure, the complexes are stable for more than 45 min. Before the delivery to culture cells, we suggest to wait 20 min to allow full complexation of micelles with siRNA molecules. If the cell density in the wells treated with siRNA/Gemini complexes is significantly reduced in comparison with control wells, the transfection experiment is successful.

4. Freeze/thaw is recommended to improve the homogeneity of size distribution in the final suspension.

5. To perform safe freeze-thawing, the solution must be placed in a glass tube with round bottom and thick walls. Lab goggles and gloves are mandatory throughout these manipulations.

6. Liposomes prepared using the cationic component DC-Chol appear hard to be extruded. In this case it is suggested to reduce slightly the content of DC-Chol in the formulation or to replace extrusion with sonication for the downsizing step. The use of membranes with pore size larger than 100 nm should be avoided, since it favors the formation of oligolamellar liposomes.

7. As the preparation procedure may have an effect on the structure and size of the final aggregates, in all experiments DNA was injected into the cationic liposome solution and not vice versa. This is also compatible with the non-equilibrium nature, generally attributed to transfection complexes.

8. The DNA - /lipid + CR was the range 0-1. In each sample the lipid concentration was taken as constant and the DNA concentration varied to obtain the desired charge ratio.

9. The success of the transfection process is easy to detect since the pDNA allows the cells to acquire a fluorescent signal due to the presence of EGFP.

Acknowledgments

We would like to thank Laura Ciani (Department of Chemistry University of Florence), Anna Salvati (Research Institute of Pharmacy, University of Groningen), and Angelo Fortunato (Center for Evolution and Cancer, University of California San Francisco) for the optimization of experimental protocols.

References

1. Koldehoff M (2015) Targeting bcr-abl transcripts with siRNAs in an imatinib-resistant chronic myeloid leukemia patient: challenges and future directions. Methods Mol Biol 1218:277–292

2. Geisbert TW, Lee AC, Robbins M, Geisbert JB, Honko AN, Sood V, Johnson JC, de Jong S, Tavakoli I, Judge A, Hensley LE, Maclachlan I (2010) Postexposure protection of non-human primates against a lethal Ebola virus challenge with RNAinterference: a proof-of-concept study. Lancet 375(9729):1896–1905

3. Evans CH, Huard J (2015) Gene therapy approaches to regenerating the musculoskeletal system. Nat Rev Rheumatol 11:234–242

4. McLean WH, Hansen CD, Eliason MJ, Smith FJ (2011) The phenotypic and molecular genetic features of pachyonychia congenita. J Invest Dermatol 131(5):1015–1017

5. Pechan P, Wadsworth S, Scaria A (2014) Gene therapies for neovascular age-related macular degeneration. Cold Spring Harb Perspect Med 5(7):a017335

6. Amer MH (2014) Gene therapy for cancer: present status and future prespective. Mol Cell Ther 2:27

7. Moore CB, Guthrie EH, Tze-Han Huang M, Taxman DJ (2010) Short hairpin RNA (shRNA): design, delivery, and assessment of gene knockdown. Methods Mol Biol 629:141–158

8. Elbashir SM, Lendeckel W, Tuschl T (2001) RNA interference is mediated by 21-and 22-nucleotide RNAs. Genes Dev 15:188–200

9. Kutter C, Svoboda P (2008) miRNA, siRNA, piRNA: knows of the unknown. RNA Biol 5:181–188

10. Quanz M, Berthault N, Roulin C, Roy M, Herbette A, Agrario C, Alberti C, Josserand V, Coll JL, Sastre-Garau X, Cosset JM, Larue L, Sun JS, Dutreix M (2009) Small-molecule drugs mimicking DNA damage: a new strategy for sensitizing tumors to radiotherapy. Clin Cancer Res 15(4):1308–1316

11. Davis ME (2002) Non-viral gene delivery systems. Curr Opin Biotechnol 13(2):128–131

12. Chawla JP, Iyer N, Soodan KS, Sharma A, Khurana SK, Priyadarshni P (2015) Role of miRNA in cancer diagnosis, prognosis, therapy and regulation of its expression by Epstein-Barr virus and human papillomaviruses: with special reference to oral cancer. Oral Oncol 51(8):731–737

13. Wang S, Fengting L (2013) Functionalized conjugated polyelectrolytes: design and biomedical applications. Springer, Berlin. ISBN 978-3-642-40540-2

14. Bielke W, Erbacher C (2010) Nucleic acid transfection, vol 296, Topics in current chemistry. Springer, Berlin. ISBN 978-3-642-16430-9

15. Desbrieres J (2013) Amphiphilic systems as biomaterials based on chitin, chitosan, and their derivatives. In: Dumitriu S, Popa VI (eds) Polymeric biomaterials: structure and function, vol 1. CRC Press, Boca Raton, FL, pp 243–270

16. Eisele K, Gropeanu RA, Zehendner CM, Rouhanipour A, Ramanathan A, Mihov G, Koynov K, Kuhlmann CR, Vasudevan SG, Luhmann HJ, Weil T (2010) Fine-tuning DNA/albumin polyelectrolyte interactions to produce the efficient transfection agent cBSA-147. Biomaterials 31(33):8789–8801

17. Katav T, Liu L, Traitel T, Goldbart R, Wolfson M, Kost J (2008) Modified pectin-based carrier for gene delivery: cellular barriers in gene delivery course. J Control Release 130(2):183–191

18. Guo X, Huang L (2012) Recent advances in nonviral vectors for gene delivery. Acc Chem Res 45(7):971–979

19. Zana R (2002) Dimeric (Gemini) surfactants: effect of the spacer group on the association behavior in aqueous solution. J Colloid Interface Sci 248:203–220

20. Falsini S, Ciani L, Arcangeli A, Di Cola E, Spinozzi F, Ristori S (2015) Physico-chemical properties of gemini micelles studied by X-ray scattering and ESR spectroscopy. Colloids Surf A Physicochem Eng Asp 472:101–108

21. Falsini S, Ristori S, Ciani L, Di Cola E, Supuran CT, Arcangeli A, In M (2014) Time resolved SAXS to study the complexation of siRNA with cationic micelles of divalent surfactants. Soft Matter 10(13):2226–2233

22. Farhood H, Serbina N, Huang L (1995) The role of dioleoyl phosphatidylethanolamine in cationic liposome mediated gene transfer. Biochim Biophys Acta 1235:289–295

23. Koltover JO, Salditt I, Radler T, Safinya CR (1998) An inverted hexagonal phase of cationic liposome-DNA complexes related to DNA release and delivery. Science 281:78–81

24. In M, Bec V, Anguerre-Chariol O, Zana R (2000) Quaternary ammonium bromidesurfactant oligomers in aqueous solution: self-association and microstructure. Langmuir 16:141–148

25. http://www.lgcstandards-atcc.org/

26. Ciani L, Ristori S, Salvati A, Calamai L, Martini G (2004) DOTAP/DOPE and DC-Chol/DOPE lipoplexes for gene delivery: zeta potential measurements and electron spin resonance spectra. Biochim Biophys Acta 1664:70–79

27. Salvati A, Ciani L, Ristori S, Martini G, Masi A, Arcangeli A (2006) Physico-chemical characterization and transfection efficacy of cationic liposomes containing the pEGFP plasmid. Biophys Chem 121:21–29

28. Ciani L, Ristori S, Bonechi C, Rossi C, Martini G (2007) Effect of the preparation procedure on the structural properties of oligonucleotide/cationic liposome complexes (lipoplexes) studied by electron spin resonance and zeta potential. Biophys Chem 131:80–87

Chapter 4

Anionic/Zwitterionic Lipid-Based Gene Vectors of pDNA

Ana L. Barrán-Berdón, Emilio Aicart, and Elena Junquera

Abstract

The use of anionic lipids (ALs) as non-viral gene vectors depicts a promising alternative to cationic lipids (CLs) since they are more biocompatible and present lower levels of phagocytosis by macrophages. Several experimental methods, such as electrophoretic mobility (ζ-potential), gel electrophoresis, small-angle X-ray scattering (SAXS), fluorescence and confocal fluorescence microscopies (FM and CFM), flow assisted cell sorting-flow cytometry (FACS-FCM), and cell viability/cytotoxicity assays can be used for a complete physicochemical and biochemical characterization of lipoplexes formed by an AL, a zwitterionic lipid (ZL), and a plasmid DNA (pDNA), their electrostatic interaction being necessarily mediated by divalent cations, such as Ca^{2+}. In the present chapter, we summarize the protocols optimized for the mentioned characterization techniques.

Key words Anionic lipids, pDNA, ζ-potential, SAXS, Gel electrophoresis, Fluorescence microscopy, Flow cytometry, Liposomes, Lipoplexes, Non-viral gene vectors

1 Introduction

In order to evaluate the potential of anionic lipids-based non-viral vectors in the presence of divalent cations, it is necessary to perform an extensive characterization using different experimental methods which are described in this section. Due to its intrinsic complexity, the transfection process needs to be addressed from two perspectives: a physicochemical and a biochemical characterization. Thus, the integrated knowledge of both disciplines will permit us to understand each of the steps involved in the transfection, and in turn, to control and improve the efficiency of the process [1–6]. Prior to any biochemical study, such as gene expression and cell viability of the gene vector, a deep physicochemical characterization of the lipoplexes is required in the absence of cells. This may help to better understand its behavior when interacting with the cells. Therefore, the physicochemical characterization of lipoplexes (mixed lipids in presence of divalent cations and DNA) is a key factor in the gene therapy process. It involves a deep study

Gabriele Candiani (ed.), *Non-Viral Gene Delivery Vectors: Methods and Protocols*, Methods in Molecular Biology, vol. 1445, DOI 10.1007/978-1-4939-3718-9_4, © Springer Science+Business Media New York 2016

of several properties of DNA-lipid complexes, such as, their electrochemical properties, aggregation behavior, and structure of the formed complexes. Each of them is analyzed using different methods, which will be described below. The electrochemical behavior of lipoplexes is one of the most important properties to be evaluated, because they must display a neutral-to-positive net charge [4–9] in order to be suitable for interacting with the negatively charged cell membrane, a crucial step in the transfection process. Specific experiments, such as electrophoretic mobility and/or agarose gel electrophoresis, need to be performed in order to analyze the electrochemical properties of lipoplexes and, in particular, the electroneutrality value and the level of plasmid (pDNA) compaction. The structure and aggregation pattern of the complex is also important, since it is well known that structure is normally correlated with the final biological activity of the system (structure-activity relationship, SAR). In this regard, small-angle X-ray scattering (SAXS) is a powerful experimental tool. And finally, it is also mandatory to check how efficient is the non-viral vector to transfect living cells in vitro and its level of cytotoxicity. Techniques such as flow assisted cell sorting-flow cytometry (FACS-FCM), fluorescence microscopies (FMs), and 3(4,5-dimethyl-2-tiazoil)-2,5-dipheniltetrazolic (MTT) assays (cell viability/cytotoxicity) are usually used to get this information.

1.1 Electrophoretic Mobility

The electrophoretic mobility and ζ-potential measurements of lipoplex solutions permit knowing the surface charge of liposomes and lipoplexes, and determining with high accuracy the lipoplex composition for which the net charge between the (anionic lipid/ zwitterionic lipid/Ca^{2+}, AL/ZL/Ca^{2+}) gene vector and the nucleic acid (NA) counterbalances. The knowledge of the surface charge of lipoplexes is important since it allows preparing neutral or positive complexes that will be potentially effective as transfecting agent of the nucleic acids to the cells. Therefore, this technique provides essential information about both the range of composition of the mixed liposome and the lipoplex concentration that may be of interest for transfection purposes [10, 11]. ζ-potential of liposomes and lipoplexes is measured using an interferometric technique that uses light scattering to determine the electrophoretic mobility of the charged colloidal suspensions subjected to an electrical field. Both properties are related through the Henry equation, and the Smoluchovski limit is usually applied [12, 13].

1.2 Agarose Gel Electrophoresis

Similarly to ζ-potential, agarose gel electrophoresis allows to determine the electroneutrality values of lipoplexes in solution. In addition, this technique is specifically useful to analyze the efficacy of the AL/ZL formulations in compacting pDNA mediated by Ca^{2}, since ζ-potential technique is not able to find any lipoplex formulation with a moderate-to-high positive ζ-potential value in this kind of lipoplexes. In fact, the use of agarose gel electrophoresis is required as a complementary method to ζ-potential in order to assure that the DNA is completely compacted by the anionic liposomes. Agarose gel electrophoresis is based on the migration of charged molecules present in a sample through a gel made with agarose, when a charge field is applied to the sample. The migration speed is determined by three factors: agarose concentration in the gel, the voltage applied to the sample, and the molecular properties (such as charge and size) of the formulation. In the case of DNA, the migration speed is determined by the size (number of base pairs, bp) and conformation (linear DNA, coiled DNA, or supercoiled DNA). Ethidium bromide (EtBr) or GelRed are fluorescent probes whose fluorescence emission, almost negligible in polar media, is enhanced around 20 times when they are intercalated within the hydrophobic environment of the DNA helix interior. Besides, it is known that when pDNA is compacted by the lipidic vector, the probe is displaced from the interior to the bulk, where its quantum fluorescent yield experiments a sharp decrease. Thus, the fluorescent emission decay measured as long as the complex is formed, is indicative of the level of pDNA compaction. Accordingly, the disappearance of fluorescent bands along the gel gives information about the composition of the lipoplex for which the pDNA is fully compacted, as required for a later potential success on transfection. This can be distinguished because when DNA is totally complexed, a static fluorescent band appears in the starting position (well) of the agarose gel. On the contrary, the uncomplexed or partially complexed DNA appears as an observable band that moves when subjected to the electric field (Fig. 1). In this way, it is possible to distinguish the different DNA fragments, or the different conformations of the same DNA (in the case of a circular pDNA) present in the sample. The visualization of DNA band with the intercalating dye requires the use of a short wavelength ultraviolet light source (transilluminator).

1.3 Small-Angle X-ray Scattering (SAXS)

When the lipoplexes are formed, they can organize in different lyotropic liquid-crystal phases. Lipoplex structure is strongly dependent on the molecular characteristics of lipids (size, shape of hydrophobic region, and/or type of the headgroups), lipidic composition (AL mole fraction in AL/ZL mixture), complex composition (AL/pDNA ratio), and the solution conditions [7, 14]. It is known that the structure, shape, and morphology of lipoplexes may affect their behavior as transfecting agent. A powerful tool to get insight about the supramolecular structure of the lipoplex is synchrotron SAXS. Two typical phases are commonly found in lipoplexes formed with pDNA: the lamellar $L\alpha$ phase and the inverted hexagonal $H_{II}{}^{C}$ phase (Fig. 2) [15–17]. The lamellar phase is characterized by a multilamellar pattern with alternating layers of mixed lipids and supercoiled pDNA molecules, which results in a

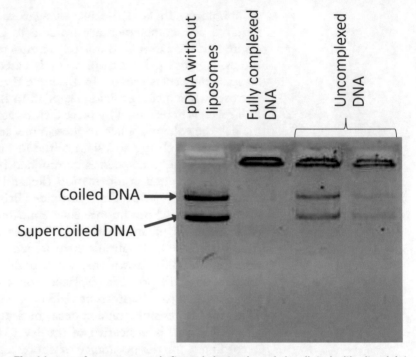

Fig. 1 Image of an agarose gel after gel electrophoresis irradiated with ultraviolet light. In the gel, it can be observed, the DNA in absence of liposomes and Ca^{2+} (*lane 1*), DNA fully complexed (*lane 2*, DOPG/DOPE-Ca^{2+}-pDNA lipoplexes at $\alpha = 0.20$ and AL/pDNA mole ratio of 20 in the presence of 25 mM Ca^{2+}) and DNA uncomplexed in presence of Ca^{2+} (*lanes 3* and *4*, DOPG/DOPE-Ca^{2+}-pDNA lipoplexes at $\alpha = 0.20$ and AL/pDNA mole ratio of 20 in the presence of 5 and 10 mM Ca^{2+}, respectively)

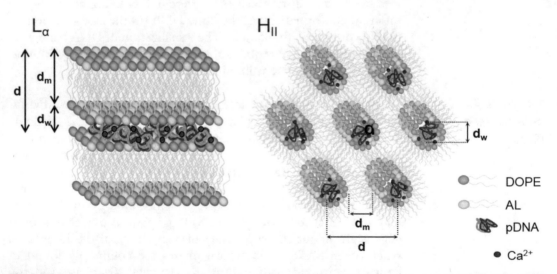

Fig. 2 3D Schematic drawings of the lamellar, L_α, and inverted hexagonal, H_{II}, phases of AL/DOPE-Ca^{2+}-pDNA lipoplexes

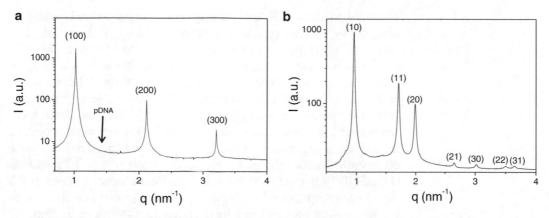

Fig. 3 SAXS diffractograms with Miller indexes (hkl) for: (**a**) lamellar phase, L_α, (DOPG/DOPE-multivalent cation-pDNA lipoplexes, at $\alpha = 0.5$, and AL/pDNA mole ratio of 1 in the presence of 60 μM multivalent cation), and (**b**) inverted hexagonal phase, H_{II}, (DOPG/DOPE-Ca^{2+}-pDNA lipoplexes, at $\alpha = 0.20$, and AL/pDNA mole ratio of 20 in the presence of 25 mM Ca^{2+}). Reprinted (adapted) with permission from Barrán-Berdón AL, Yélamos B, Malfois M, Aicart E, Junquera E (2014) Ca^{2+}-mediated anionic lipid-plasmid DNA lipoplexes. Electrochemical, structural, and biochemical studies. Langmuir 30 (39):11704–11713. Copyright (2014) American Chemical Society

typical scattering pattern where the Miller indexes (hkl) are (100), (200), (300), and so on (Fig. 3a). The "q" factor (x-axis) is directly related to the interlamellar distance "d" ($=2\pi/q_{100}$), that is the sum of the thickness of the lipidic bilayer, "d_m", and that of the aqueous region, "d_w", where the supercoiled pDNA and/or divalent cations are allocated. In this lamellar phase, a smoothed peak corresponding to DNA-DNA correlation can be roughly found. The "q_{pDNA}" factor of this peak allows for the determination of the separation between pDNA molecules within the aqueous monolayer, "d_{pDNA}" ($=2\pi/q_{pDNA}$) [17]. The columnar inverted hexagonal liquid-crystal phase is commonly found when a ZL, as 1,2-dioleoyl-sn-glycero-3-phosphoethanolamine (DOPE) with high packing parameter (i.e., $P > 1$), is used in the liposome formulation. DOPE induces the lamellar to hexagonal structural transition by controlling the spontaneous curvature of the monolayer. The hexagonal structure presents "hkl" of (10), (11), (20), (21), (30), (22), (31), and so on (Fig. 3b); the spacing "a" of the cell unit is also related to the "q" factor ($a = 4\pi/3^{1/2}q_{10}$). In this hexagonal lattice, a monolayer of mixed lipids surrounds the DNA helix resembling an inverted cylindrical micelle. In the hexagonal structure, the DNA-DNA separation is the same than the interlayer distance (Fig. 2) [16].

1.4 Transfection Studies

Once the physicochemical study has been carried out, a test to confirm the transfection efficacy (TE), and, accordingly, the potential of ALs as gene vectors, is required. Transfection studies consist of trials to introduce the nucleic acids into different living mammalian cells. TE levels are dependent on several biological parameters, such as: type of the cell or cell line, confluence degree, and cells population. Therefore, in order to get representative results, it is recommendable to use different kinds of cells and, for each one, to test different transfection conditions. There are two principal techniques used to evaluate the transfection efficacy of a lipid formulation: FM and/or CFM and FACS-FCM. Both techniques are used to evaluate the intracellular fluorescence produced by the actual expression of the pDNA used for transfection, which commonly codifies the green fluorescence protein (GFP), such as the pEGFP-C3 used in this work. The fluorescence microscopy is based on an optical microscope that uses fluorescence to observe the expression and physical localization of GFP protein (Fig. 4). However, this technique is not adequate to quantify in a reliable and reproducible way the transfection levels achieved by a specific lipid formulation. On the other hand, FACS-FCM, a technique based on a laser source for cell counting and cell sorting, is a powerful tool to quantify the transfection levels in terms of percentage of GFP, which gives information about the percentage of transfected cells, and mean fluorescence intensity (MFI), indicative of the averaged fluorescence intensity per cell. In any case, TE levels of gene vectors must always be compared with the results obtained in the same experimental conditions for a positive universal control, which in the case of lipidic formulations is Lipofectamine 2000, a commercial mixture of cationic lipids (CLs).

1.5 Cell Viability

Concerning the biological characterization, the evaluation of cytotoxicity of the lipoplex formulation is as important as TE. In other words, gene vectors must be highly efficient on transfecting cells, but they also must allow cells to be viable after transfection (cell viability). The most common approach to study cell viability is based on the reduction of MMT, a tetrazol (yellow) which is enzymatically reduced to formazan (purple crystals, insoluble in aqueous media) in the mitochondria of living cells. These crystals may be solubilized by the addition of a proper solvent, like dimethyl sulfoxide (DMSO), and their concentration may be quantified by means of a spectrophotometric analysis. The capacity of cells to reduce MTT is indicative of the integrity of the mitochondria and their functional activity, and it can be used as a measure of the cellular viability. Since for most cell populations, the total mitochondrial activity is related to the number of viable cells, this assay is broadly used to measure the in vitro cytotoxic effect of lipoplexes on different cell lines [18]. The viability is determined with a spectrophotometer at a $\lambda = 500–600$ nm.

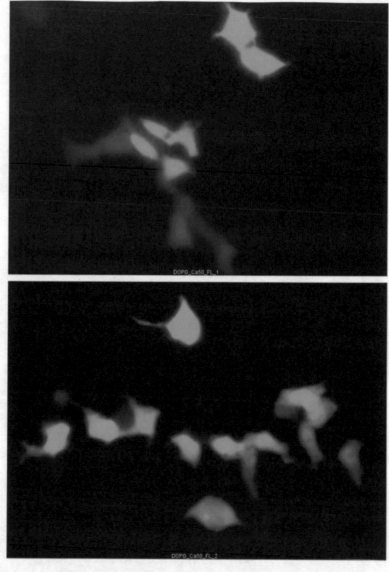

Fig. 4 Fluorescence micrographs showing GFP expression in HEK293T cells after transfection with DOPG/DOPE-Ca^{2+}-pDNA lipoplexes at 50 mM Ca^{2+}. *Green color is indicative of GFP expression*

2   Materials

2.1   Equipments and Materials

1. ζ Potential apparatus.
2. Small-Angle X-ray scattering apparatus (SAXS).
3. UV light illuminator.
4. Flow cytometer (FACS-FCM).

5. Microtiter plate reader.

6. Lab balance.

7. Magnetic stirrer.

8. Vortex.

9. Bath sonicator.

10. Thermobarrel extruder.

11. Vacuum centrifuge.

12. Submerged horizontal electrophoresis cell.

13. UV-transparent gel tray.

14. Microwave oven.

15. Hemocytometer.

16. Incubator.

17. 50 mL Erlenmeyer flask.

18. 1 L volumetric flask.

19. 10 mL glass tubes

20. 1.5 or 2.0 mL polypropylene microcentifuge tubes.

21. 10 and 50 mL polypropylene centrifuge tubes.

22. 5000, 1000, 100, 20, and 10 μL micropipettes.

23. Polycarbonate membranes (400, 200, and 100 nm).

24. 15 mL glass bottles.

25. 1.5 mm diameter glass capillaries.

26. 2 mL ζ-potential cuvettes.

27. 25 cm² cell culture flasks.

28. 10 and 25 mL graduate pipettes.

29. 24-well and 96-well plates.

30. Rotary evaporator.

31. Fluorescence microscopy (FM).

32. Flat rocker

2.2 Reactives and Solutions

All solutions must be prepared using dH_2O, prepared by purifying deionized water to attain a sensitivity of 18 MΩ-cm at 25 °C, and analytical grade reagents. Prepare and store all reagents at room temperature (RT) unless otherwise indicated.

1. Anionic Lipid, L^-.

2. Zwiterionic Lipid, L^0.

3. Chloroform ($CHCl_3$).

4. Agarose powder.

5. Glacial acetic acid (CH_3COOH).

6. Glycerol.

7. GelRed (fluorescent dye).

8. 3-(4,5-dimethylthiazol-2-yl)-2,5-diphenyltetrazolium bromide (MTT).

9. Dimethyl sulfoxide (DMSO).

10. Trypsin.

11. Dulbecco's Phosphate-Buffered Saline (PBS).

12. Penicillin.

13. Streptomycin.

14. 1 L of 10 mM HEPES, pH 7.4. Weigh 1.26 g of 4-(2-hydroxyethyl)-1-piperazineethanesulfonic acid (HEPES-H MW 238.31). Weigh 1.20 g of 4-(2-hydroxyethyl)piperazine-1-ethanesulfonic acid sodium salt (HEPES-Na MW 260.30). Make up to 1 L with dH_2O. Measure the pH and, if necessary, adjust it with hydrochloric acid (HCl) or sodium hydroxide (NaOH).

15. 5 mL of 10 mg/mL DNA stock solution. Weigh 50 mg of DNA (pEGFP-C3 or commercial ct-DNA) in a glass bottle and add 5 mL of 10 mM HEPES, pH 7.4. Mix slowly and leave it for 2 h resting. Keep the solution at 4 °C (*see* **Note 1**).

16. 10 mL of 0.1 mg/mL DNA stock solution. Weigh 1 mg of DNA (pEGFP-C3 or commercial ct-DNA) in a glass bottle. Add 10 mL of 10 mM HEPES, pH 7.4. Mix slowly and leave it for 2 h resting. Keep the solution at 4 °C.

17. 5 mL of 250 mM Ca^{2+} stock solution. Weigh 0.184 g of calcium chloride dihydrated ($CaCl_2 \times 2H_2O$). Dissolve the $CaCl_2$ in 5 mL of 10 mM HEPES, pH 7.4. Keep the solution at RT.

18. 1 L of 50× Tris-Acetate-EDTA (TAE). Weigh 242 g of TRIS base (121 MW). Add 57.1 mL of CH_3COOH. Add 100 mL of 0.5 M ethylenediaminetetraacetic acid (EDTA), pH 8.0. Dissolve in 600 mL of dH_2O and fill to a final volume of 1 L with dH_2O. Keep the solution at 4 °C. Prepare the 1× TAE by diluting to 50× TAE and keep it at RT.

19. 1 mL of 10× DNA sample loading dye. Add 0.5 mL of glycerol to a microcentrifuge tube of 1.5 mL. Weigh 2.5 mg of bromophenol blue and add it in the polypropylene microcentrifuge tube. Weigh and add 2.5 mg of xylene cyanol. Mix and dilute to 1 mL in 1× TAE buffer. Keep the dye solution at 4 °C.

20. 20 mL of complete cell culture medium (Dulbelcco's Modified Eagle Medium (DMEM) containing 10% (v/v) FBS). Add 2 mL of fetal bovine serum (FBS) and 18 mL of DMEM in a 50 mL centrifuge tube. Mix slowly (*see* **Note 2**). Store at 4 °C until use.

21. 20 mL of DMEM containing 20% (v/v) FBS. Add 4 mL of FBS and 16 mL of DMEM in a 50 mL centrifuge tube. Mix slowly. Store at 4 °C until use.

3   Methods

3.1   Preparation of Lipid Films

1. Weigh appropriate amounts of AL, L^-, and zwitterionic lipid, L^0, in order to obtain the desired molar fraction and the AL/pDNA ratio (*see* **Note 3**). Depending on which lipid is used, it will be required to prepare stock solutions from lipids in powder form prior to the preparation of the sample.

2. Dissolve the ALs and ZLs in 1–3 mL of $CHCl_3$ in a glass tube or in a flask.

3. After a brief vortexing, remove $CHCl_3$ by evaporation under high vacuum by using either a centrifuge or a rotary evaporator for at least 3 h, until yielding a dry lipid film.

4. Hydrate the resulting dry lipid film with 2–5 mL of 10 mM HEPES, pH 7.4, and homogenize it by alternating at least 10 repetitive cycles of vigorous vortexing for 3 min each and 2 min of sonication.

5. Place the sample in a bath at 60 °C for 1 h.

6. Vortex again for 1 h to get a homogeneous suspension.

7. Apply a sequential extrusion procedure through a 10 mL-capacity thermobarrel extruder as follows (*see* **Note 4**): pass the suspension 5 times through the 400 nm-pore size, 5 times through the 200 nm-pore size and at least 10 times through the 100 nm-pore size polycarbonate membranes (*see* **Note 5**).

3.2   Preparation of Lipid-Ca^{2+}-pDNA Lipoplexes (See Note 6)

1. Mix adequate volumes of DNA stock solution and $CaCl_2$ stock solution.

2. Add an adequate volume of mixed lipid solution to the DNA/$CaCl_2$ solution (*see* Subheading 3.2, **step 1**) in a small glass bottle.

3. Stir this solution for 10 min at RT.

4. Let the final solution stand at RT for additional 10 min.

3.3   ζ-Potential

1. Prepare a total volume of 800 μL with a constant DNA amount of 12.8 μg, by mixing adequate volumes of $CaCl_2$ stock solution, 128 μL of 0.1 mg/mL DNA stock solution, and appropriate volumes of 10 mM HEPES in a 1.5 mL polypropylene microcentrifuge tube (*see* **Note 7**).

2. In a small glass bottle, add 800 μL of mixed lipid solution to 800 μL of the mixture prepared in Subheading 3.3, **step 1**. Stir vigorously with a magnetic stirrer for 10 min (*see* **Note 8**).

3. Place the lipoplex suspension in the ζ-potential cuvette and proceed carrying out the electrophoretic mobility measurement.

4. Get the experimental data accordingly to the software of the ζ-potential apparatus (*see* **Note 9**).

3.4 Gel Electrophoresis

3.4.1 Preparation of 1% (w/v) Agarose Gel

1. Weigh 0.5 g of agarose powder and add it to an Erlenmeyer flask.

2. Add 50 mL of 1× TAE buffer and swirl it to suspend the agarose powder in the buffer.

3. Melt the agarose in 1× TAE in a microwave oven. Heat at medium power for 2 min. Stop the microwave oven every 30 s and swirl the flask gently to suspend the undissolved agarose (*see* **Note 10**).

4. Let the gel cool down to 60 °C for a couple of min, before adding the fluorescent dye.

5. Add 0.7 μL of GelRed fluorescent dye solution and swirl the flask gently.

6. Pour the gel on the casting tray (7 cm × 10 cm) and place the comb.

7. Allow the gel to solidify for ~20 min at RT.

8. Remove the comb very carefully from the solidified gel.

9. Submerge the gel beneath 2–6 mm of 1× TAE.

3.4.2 Sample Preparation and Running

1. In order to get a final volume of 12.5 μL with a constant DNA amount of 200 ng, mix appropriated amounts of $CaCl_2$ stock solution, 2 μL of 0.1 mg/mL DNA stock solution, and HEPES in a polypropylene microcentrifuge tube (*see* **Note 11**).

2. In order to obtain an adequate AL/pDNA ratio, add 12.5 μL of mixed lipid solution to the solution prepared in Subheading 3.4.2, **step 1**. To favor an optimum lipoplex formation, let the final solution stand for 20 min at RT.

3. Add 1 μL of standard NA sample loading dye, to make dense samples for underlying into sample wells.

4. Using a micropipette, load 20 μL of the samples into the wells.

5. Run the gel for 30 min at 80 mV in 1× TAE.

6. Remove the gel from the gel tray and expose it under UV light illumination at $\lambda = 365$ nm for 1.6 s.

3.5 Small-Angle X-ray Scattering (SAXS)

3.5.1 Capillaries Preparation

1. Add the 45 μL of mixed lipid solution in the 1.5 mm glass capillaries (*see* **Note 12**).

2. Put the capillaries inside of centrifuge plastic tube and centrifuge at 4800 rpm (RCF or *g*-force value of 1900) for 2 min.

3. Add to the capillaries, 45 μL of mixed Ca^{2+}/DNA solution required to obtain the desired AL/pDNA and Ca^{2+} concentration (*see* **Note 13**).

4. Centrifuge at a RCF (*g*-force) of 1900 for 15 min the samples in order to get pellet solid lipoplexes in the bottom of the capillaries.

5. Seal the capillaries (*see* **Note 14**).

3.5.2 SAXS **Measurement**	1. Prior to starting the experiments, fit the beamline configuration. Set the incident beam to have the following characteristics: energy = 12.6 keV, $\lambda = 0.995$ Å; beam size = 100 μm; and distance from the sample to detector = 1.4 m.

2. Place several capillaries in a predesigned holder (*see* **Note 15**).

3. Take a measurement by collecting data on each sample over 10–30 s each (*see* **Notes 16** and **17**).

3.6 Cell Transfection Protocol

3.6.1 Cell Culture

1. Take the preserved cell lines at –80 °C and gradually thaw into a cold water bath until defrosted (*see* **Note 18**).

2. Incubate the cells for 24 h at 37 °C, 99 % humidity with regular supply of 5 % CO_2.

3. Replace the medium with 1 mL of PBS and 1× trypsin (*see* **Note 19**), and incubate for 2 min (*see* **Note 20**).

4. Add 3 mL of complete cell culture medium and 1× penicillin and streptomycin.

5. Take 1 mL of cell culture and transfer to a 25 cm² cell culture flask.

6. Add 3 mL of complete cell culture medium with 1× trypsin and incubate for 48 h at 37 °C, 99 % humidity with regular supply of 5 % CO_2 (*see* **Note 21**).

7. Remove the medium from cell culture flask (*see* **Note 22**).

8. Wash the cells with PBS and discard it.

9. Briefly coat the cells with trypsin and incubate for 2 min.

10. Transfer the cells to 50 mL centrifuge tubes and add 5 mL of complete cell culture medium.

11. Determine the cell density using a hemocytometer.

12. Add 400 μL of complete cell culture medium to each well of a 24-well plate.

13. Calculate the required volume of cell suspension and seed cells into a 24-well plate at 6×10^4 cells/well.

14. Culture the cells at 37 °C and 99 % humidity with regular supply of 5 % CO_2 for 24 h.

15. After 24 h, check if a 70 % of confluence has been reached before running the transfection experiment.

3.6.2 Transfection

1. In an 1.5 mL polypropylene microcentrifuge tube, mix appropriate amounts of $CaCl_2$ stock solution with 0.8 μg of DNA (8 μL of 0.1 μg/μL stock solution) and HEPES buffer to give a final volume of 12.5 μL, with a protocol similar to the one used to prepare the sample for ζ-potential measurements (*see* Subheading 3.3).

2. Add 87.5 μL of DMEM and incubate the lipoplex suspension for 30 min.

3. Dilute with 100 µL of DMEM containing 20 % FBS.

4. Transfer 200 µL of the lipoplex suspension to 1 well of a 24-well plate previously washed with plain DMEM (*see* **Note 23**).

5. After a 6 h-incubation at 37 °C, 99 % humidity with regular supply of 5 % CO_2, remove the old medium from each well.

6. Wash the cells with plain DMEM and add 500 µL/well of complete cell culture medium.

7. Incubate the cells at 37 °C, 99 % humidity with regular supply of 5 % CO_2 for ~48 h.

8. At the end of incubation, observe the 24-well plate under a FM in order to visualize the GFP-positive cells.

9. Wash the cells with 200 µL of PBS and discard it

10. Add 1× trypsin to cells and subsequently 5 % (v/v) FBS solution and collect them in a tube.

11. In order to analyze the transfection results by means of a FACS-FCM, set the instrument laser at $\lambda_{ex} = 488$ nm which allows the quantification of GFP-positive cells (*see* **Note 24**), as well as average intensity of fluorescence per cell (MFI).

12. Analyze the data with appropriate software (*see* **Note 25**) in order to obtain the percentage of GFP-positive cells and MFI.

3.7 Cell Viability Assay

1. Seed the cells at a density of ~1.5×10^4 cells/well into a 96-well plate and let them grow up to ~70 % confluence.

2. Prepare the lipoplexes for each composition using 0.2 µg of DNA/well, following the protocol described elsewhere (*see* Subheading 3.6.2, **steps 1–3**).

3. Incubate lipoplexes with cells at 37 °C, 99 % humidity with regular supply of 5 % CO_2 for 6 h.

4. Wash cells with complete cell culture medium.

5. After 42 h, add 20 µL of MTT to each well and incubate at 37 °C, 99 % humidity with regular supply of 5 % CO_2 for further 4–5 h (*see* **Note 26**).

6. After incubation, discard the medium and add 200 µL/well of DMSO and keep it on flat rocker for 10 min to dissolve the formazan crystals.

7. Measure the absorbance using a microtiter plate reader.

8. Calculate the cell viability with the data taken with a microplate reader using Eq. 1.

$$\% \text{ cell viability} = \frac{A_{590,\text{treated cells}} - A_{590\text{background(DMSO)}}}{A_{590,\text{untreated cells}} - A_{590\text{background(DMSO)}}} \times 100 \quad (1)$$

4   Notes

1. The DNA is easily degraded by nucleases present in the media; thus, the solution should be prepared using gloves under clean conditions. The prepared solution should be stored for 2–3 days at 4 °C. For longer times, keep it at –20 °C.

2. Cell culture medium should be prepared immediately before the transfection studies. Do not store for more than 3 days at 4 °C.

3. The films can be prepared at different molar fractions "α" of the AL/ZL mixture, using the following Equation:

$$\alpha = \frac{\left(L^- / M_{L^-}\right)}{\left[\left(L^- / M_{L^-}\right) + \left(L^0 / M_{L^0}\right)\right]} \tag{2}$$

where L^- and L^0 are the masses of ALs and ZLs, and M_{L^-} and M_{L^0} are the molar masses of ALs and ZLs, respectively. The amount of L^- must be determined given a fixed DNA concentration in order to obtain the desired AL/pDNA molar ratio, following the next Equation:

$$\frac{AL}{pDNA} = \frac{\left(L^-\right)\left(M_{pDNA}\right)}{\left(m_{pDNA}\right)\left(M_{L^-}\right)} \tag{3}$$

where AL and pDNA are the number of moles of L^- and pDNA, respectively; m_{pDNA} is the mass of pDNA and M_{pDNA} are the molar mass of pDNA per bp.

4. The sequential extrusion is required in order to obtain the desired unilamellar liposomes (LUVs).

5. The extrusion process should be performed under pressurized nitrogen (N_2) flow in order to force the solution to pass through a membrane of a selected pore size previously placed within the extruder.

6. For a detailed description of the lipid-Ca^{2+}-pDNA lipoplexes preparation protocols, see each experimental technique.

7. The volume of $CaCl_2$ and HEPES solutions depends on the final Ca^{2+} concentration required (Table 1 shows the µL required to give different final Ca^{2+} concentrations).

8. An agitation speed of 0.2 mL/min is suggested to favor the formation of lipoplexes.

9. Each data point of electrophoretic mobility should be taken as an average of at least 50 independent measurements.

10. Boil and swirl the solution until all the small translucent agarose particles are dissolved.

Table 1
Volumes of Ca^{2+} and HEPES in μL (for stock solution concentrations as appear in the Subheading 2) that must be added to the samples for the ζ-potential experiments

Ca^{2+}(mM)	Ca^{2+} (μL)	HEPES (μL)
5	32	640
10	64	608
25	160	512
50	320	352
100	640	32

Table 2
Volumes of Ca^{2+} and HEPES in μL (for stock solution concentrations as appear in Subheading 2) that must be added to the samples for gel electrophoresis experiments

Ca^{2+} (mM)	Ca^{2+} (μL)	HEPES (μL)
5.0	0.5	10.0
10.0	1.0	9.5
25.0	2.5	8.0
50.0	5.0	5.5
100.0	10.0	0.5

11. Use a similar protocol to the one used to prepare the sample for ζ-potential measurement (*see* Subheading 3.3). Table 2 shows the μL of solution required for different final Ca^{2+} concentrations.

12. The total volume of SAXS capillary (1.5 mm) is around 100 μL; thus, the volumes added in a 1:1 dilution process should be below 50 μL.

13. The optimal DNA concentration for SAXS experiment is 10 μg/capillary.

14. Seal the capillary with the flame. If capillaries are not Pyrex but regular glass, a candle is enough to seal them.

15. The holder is necessary in order to being able to measure several samples without entering to the beam area, and without having to change the capillary each time.

16. Ensure that the samples are placed in the intended space between the beam and the detector.

17. The scattered X-ray is detected and converted to one-dimensional scattering by radial averaging, and represented as a function of the momentum transfer vector "q" ($=4\pi \sin \theta/\lambda$), in which θ is half the scattering angle, and λ the wavelength of the incident X-ray beam. Represent the collected data as vs. "q" factor in a linear or logarithmic plot in order to determine "hkl" and assign them to the correct structure.

18. The cell thawing should be performed gradually to prevent cell damage.

19. All media and solutions that are applied to the cells should be prewarmed to 37 °C in a water bath.

20. Verify that all the cells are detached from the tube walls.

21. After 24 h, check for any contamination.

22. Use a large washing flask connected to water aspirator or pipette.

23. Each experimental condition must be performed in duplicate, i.e., 2 wells for each experimental condition, and the experiment should be performed twice independently for all the compositions.

24. The quantification of GFP-positive cells as compared to residual fluorescence of the cells (due to fluorescent amino acids residues and other bio-macromolecules).

25. *WinMDI2.8* Software is one of the commercially available.

26. The blue formazan crystals can be visualized under microscope.

References

1. Kumar K, Barran-Berdon AL, Datta S, Muñoz-Ubeda M, Aicart-Ramos C, Kondaiah P, Junquera E, Bhattacharya S, Aicart E (2015) A delocalizable cationic headgroup together with an oligo-oxyethylene spacer in gemini cationic lipids improves their biological activity as vectors of plasmid DNA. J Mater Chem B 3:1495–1506

2. Barran-Berdon AL, Yelamos B, Malfois M, Aicart E, Junquera E (2014) Ca(2+)-mediated anionic lipid-plasmid DNA lipoplexes. Electrochemical, structural, and biochemical studies. Langmuir 30(39):11704–11713

3. Barran-Berdon AL, Misra SK, Datta S, Muñoz-Ubeda M, Kondaiah P, Junquera E, Bhattacharya S, Aicart E (2014) Cationic gemini lipids containing polyoxyethylene spacers as improved transfecting agents of plasmid DNA in cancer cells. J Mater Chem B 2(29): 4640–4652

4. Misra SK, Muñoz-Ubeda M, Datta S, Barran-Berdon AL, Aicart-Ramos C, Castro-Hartmann P, Kondaiah P, Junquera E, Bhattacharya S, Aicart E (2013) Effects of a delocalizable cation on the headgroup of gemini lipids on the lipoplex-type nanoaggregates directly formed from plasmid DNA. Biomacromolecules 14(11):3951–3963

5. Muñoz-Ubeda M, Misra SK, Barran-Berdon AL, Data S, Aicart-Ramos C, Castro-Hartmann P, Kondaiah P, Junquera E, Bhattacharya S, Aicart E (2012) How does the

spacer length of cationic gemini lipids influence the lipoplex formation with plasmid DNA? Physicochemical and biochemical characterizations and their relevance in gene therapy. Biomacromolecules 13:3926–3937

6. Muñoz-Ubeda M, Misra SK, Barran-Berdon AL, Aicart-Ramos C, Sierra MB, Biswas J, Kondaiah P, Junquera E, Bhattacharya S, Aicart E (2011) Why is less cationic lipid required to prepare lipoplexes from plasmid DNA than linear DNA in gene therapy? J Am Chem Soc 133:18014–18017

7. Junquera E, Aicart E (2014) Cationic lipids as transfecting agents of DNA in gene therapy. Curr Topics Med Chem 14(5):649–663

8. Barran-Berdon AL, Muñoz-Ubeda M, Aicart-Ramos C, Perez L, Infante MR, Castro-Hartmann P, Martin-Molina A, Aicart E, Junquera E (2012) Ribbon-type and cluster-type lipoplexes constituted by a chiral lysine based cationic gemini lipid and plasmid DNA. Soft Matter 8(28):7368–7380

9. Muñoz-Ubeda M, Rodriguez-Pulido A, Nogales A, Llorca O, Quesada-Perez M, Martin-Molina A, Aicart E, Junquera E (2011) Gene vectors based on DOEPC/DOPE mixed cationic liposomes: a physicochemical study. Soft Matter 7:5991–6004

10. Rodriguez-Pulido A, Martin-Molina A, Rodriguez-Beas C, Llorca O, Aicart E, Junquera E (2009) A theoretical and experimental approach to the compaction process of DNA by dioctadecyldimethylammonium bromide/zwitterionic mixed liposomes. J Phys Chem B 113(47):15648–15661

11. Muñoz-Ubeda M, Rodriguez-Pulido A, Nogales A, Martin-Molina A, Aicart E, Junquera E (2010) Effect of lipid composition on the structure and theoretical phase diagrams of DC-Chol/DOPE-DNA lipoplexes. Biomacromolecules 11(12):3332–3340

12. Delgado AV (2002) Interfacial electrokinetics and electrophoresis, vol 106, Surfactant science series. Marcel Dekker, New York

13. Ohshima H, Furusawa K (1998) Electrical phenomena at interfaces: fundamentals, measurements, and applications. Marcel Dekker, New York

14. Dias RS, Lindman B (2008) DNA interaction with polymers and surfactants. Wiley, Hoboken

15. Safinya CR (2001) Structures of lipid-DNA complexes: supramolecular assembly and gene delivery. Curr Opin Struct Biol 11(4):440–448

16. Koltover I, Salditt T, Rädler JO, Safinya CR (1998) An inverted hexagonal phase of cationic liposome-DNA complexes related to DNA release and delivery. Science 281:78–81

17. Rädler JO, Koltover I, Salditt T, Safinya CR (1997) Structure of DNA-cationic liposome complexes: DNA intercalation in multilamellar membranes in distinct interhelical packing regimes. Science 275:810–814

18. van Meerloo J, Kaspers GL, Cloos J (2011) Cell sensitivity assays: the MTT assay. In: Cree IA (ed) Cancer cell culture, vol 731, Methods in molecular biology. Humana Press, New York, pp 237–245. doi:10.1007/978-1-61779-080-5_20

Chapter 5

Elaboration and Physicochemical Characterization of Niosome-Based Nioplexes for Gene Delivery Purposes

Edilberto Ojeda, Mireia Agirre, Ilia Villate-Beitia, Mohamed Mashal, Gustavo Puras, Jon Zarate, and Jose L. Pedraz

Abstract

Niosome formulations for gene delivery purposes are based on nonionic surfactants, helper lipids, and cationic lipids that interact electrostatically with negatively charged DNA molecules to form the so-called nioplexes. Niosomes are elaborated by different techniques, such as solvent emulsion-evaporation, thin film hydration, hand-shaking, dissolvent injection, and microfluidization method, among many others. In this chapter, we have described some protocols for the elaboration of niosomes and nioplexes and their physicochemical characterization that guarantees the quality criteria of the formulation in terms of size, morphology, ζ-potential, and stability.

Key words Niosomes, Gene delivery, Nonviral vector, Cationic lipid, Nonionic surfactant, Transfection

1 Introduction

Niosomes are drug delivery systems that form vesicles with a bilayer structure and represent an alternative to liposomes where the phospholipids of the liposomes have been substituted by nonionic surfactants [1]. Compared to liposomes, niosomes are recognized for their low cost and superior chemical and storage stabilities. Niosomes have been widely used as carrier vectors to deliver chemotherapy drugs, peptides, antigens, and hormones. Additionally, niosomes are also recognized as gene delivery vectors to promote the desirable gene expression [2]. Consequently, many research groups have focused their attention on the use of niosomes as nonviral carriers for gene delivery [3].

Niosome formulations for gene delivery purposes are based on (1) nonionic surfactants, such as Tween 80, brij, and span, that play an important role in terms of toxicity and stability; moreover, these nonionic surfactants do not have any charge in their headgroups, which makes no interference with the charge of the

Gabriele Candiani (ed.), *Non-Viral Gene Delivery Vectors: Methods and Protocols*, Methods in Molecular Biology, vol. 1445, DOI 10.1007/978-1-4939-3718-9_5, © Springer Science+Business Media New York 2016

niosomes [2]; (2) helper lipids, such as cholesterol or squalene, which enhance the physicochemical properties of the lipid emulsion as they can modify the morphology, permeability, storage time, nucleic acid release, and stability of the formulation [4, 5]; (3) cationic lipids that interact electrostatically with negatively charged nucleic acid to form nioplexes, whose structural and physical properties clearly influence the transfection efficiency and toxicity of the final nioplexes [6]. These cationic lipids contain four functional domains: (1) hydrophobic group: this group is usually derived from aliphatic hydrocarbon chains and often contains two linear aliphatic chains because it has been reported that cationic lipids containing one or three carbon chains tend to be more toxic and show poor transfection efficiencies [7]; (2) linker group: this part affects the flexibility, stability, and biodegradability of the cationic lipid and, its length determines the level of hydration; thus, it has been hypothesized that the replacement of the ether bonds by ester bonds in the cationic lipids could lead to a better tolerated niosome formulation since ether bonds are too stable to be biodegraded [8]; (3) backbone: it separates the polar head-group from the hydrophobic group; serinol and glycerol groups are the most popular units [9]; (4) hydrophilic head-group: this domain is responsible for the interaction and condensation of the nucleic acid to form nioplexes due to electrostatic interactions. Additionally, this domain especially affects transfection efficiencies and it clearly affects the stability and physicochemical parameters of the niosomes [6, 10].

Once the niosomes and nioplexes are prepared, it is important to characterize them to ensure that the formulations meet our needs. Such characterization can be defined in terms of size, size distribution, morphology, ζ-potential, and stability, among many others [6].

In this chapter, we will describe step by step our laboratory protocols to prepare niosomes for gene delivery purposes, formation of nioplexes and their subsequent characterization.

2 Materials

Prepare and use all reagents at room temperature (RT). Carefully follow all the waste disposal regulations when disposing waste materials. Prepare all solutions using ultrapure water (dH$_2$O).

1. 5 mg of the desired cationic lipid (Fig. 1a).

2. Polysorbate 80 (0.5 % (w/w) Tween 80 in dH$_2$O) (*see* **Note 1**).

3. Squalene.

4. Dichloromethane (CH$_2$Cl$_2$).

5. Branson Sonifier 250 sonicator (Branson Ultrasonics Corp., Danbury, CT) (Fig. 2a2).

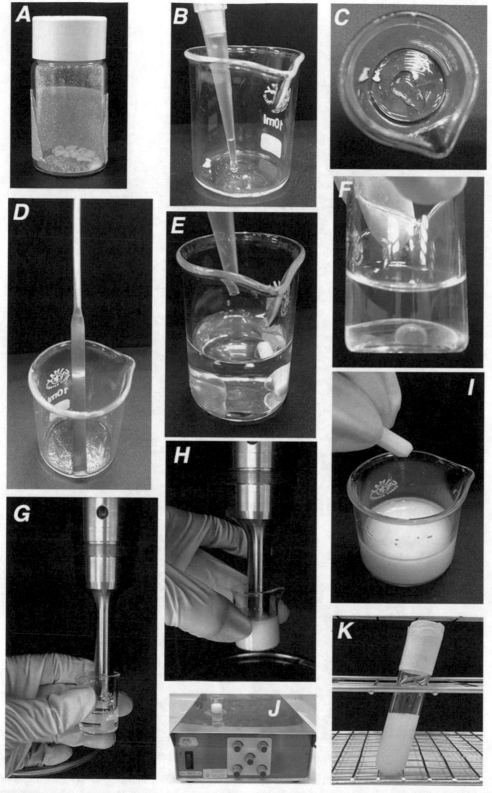

Fig. 1 Materials and preparation procedure for niosome elaboration. (**a**) Cationic lipid, (**b**) addition of squalene to cationic lipid, (**c**) cationic lipid, squalene added, (**d**) mix of squalene and cationic lipid, (**e**) addition of Polysorbate 80 to the mix of squalene, cationic lipid, and CH Cl, (**f**) organic (at the bottom) and aqueous (at the top) phases, (**g**) formulation prior to sonication, (**h**) formulation post sonication, (**i**) placing magnetic stirring bar into the formulation, (**j**) placing the glass beaker with the emulsion on the magnetic stirrer, and (**k**) niosome formulation

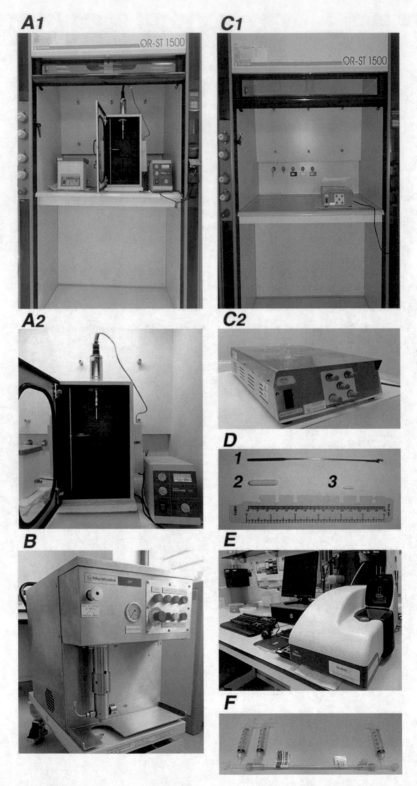

Fig. 2 Required materials and equipment for niosome preparation. (**a1**) Extraction hood and sonicator, (**a2**) sonicator, (**b**) microfluidics, (**c1**) extraction hood and magnetic stirrer, (**c2**) magnetic stirrer, (**d**) (1) spatula, (2) magnetic stirring bar 4 cm L × 0.8 cm ⌀, (3) magnetic stirring bar 1.2 cm L × 0.4 cm ⌀, (**e**) Zetasizer-nano, and (**f**) filters

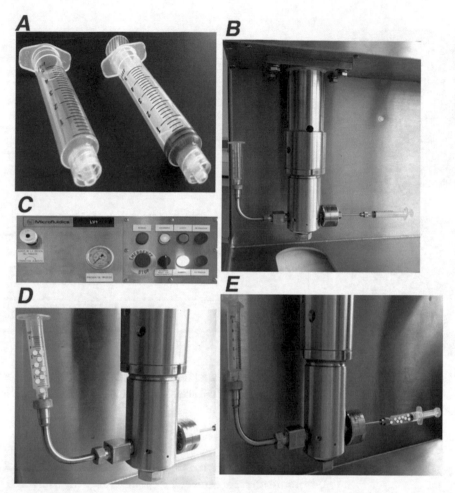

Fig. 3 Materials and procedure for microfluidization. (**a**) Two 5 mL syringes, (**b**) syringes attached to the entry and exit conduits, (**c**) control center, (**d**) loaded sample into the syringe in the entry conduit, and (**e**) collected niosomes in the syringe in the exit conduit

6. LV1 microfluidizer (Microfluidics International Corp., Westwood, MA) (Fig. 2b).

7. Magnetic stirrer (Fig. 2c2).

8. Magnetic stirring bar 1.2 cm L × 0.4 cm Ø (Fig. 2d, 3).

9. Magnetic stirring bar 4 cm L × 0.8 cm Ø (Fig. 2d, 2).

10. 10 mL glass beaker.

11. Spatula (Fig. 2d, 1).

12. Parafilm.

13. Two 5 mL syringes (Fig. 3a).

14. 10 mL glass beaker.

15. 0.05 μm Ø polycarbonate filters (Spectrum Laboratories, CA, USA) (Fig. 2f).

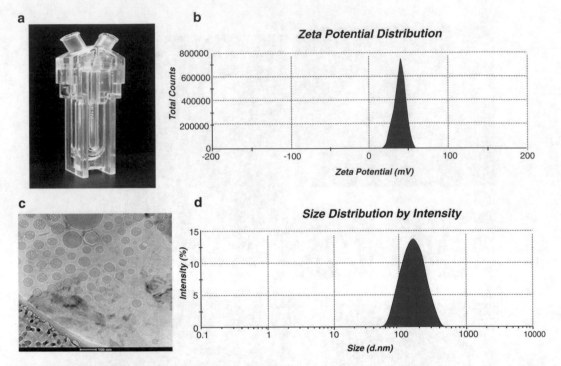

Fig. 4 Materials and data for characterization of niosomes. (**a**) Clear disposable size and ζ-cell, (**b**) graph indicating ζ-potential distribution of the niosomes, (**c**) Cryo-TEM image of niosomes, and (**d**) characterizing graph of size distribution of niosomes in nanometers

16. Zetasizer-nano dynamic light scattering (DLS) and ζ-potentiometer (Malvern Instruments Ltd, Malvern, UK).

17. Clear disposable size and ζ-cell (Fig. 4a).

18. 0.5 mg/mL of pCMS-EGFP (PlasmidFactory GmbH & Co., Bielefeld, Germany) plasmid DNA (pDNA).

19. Opti-MEM transfection medium.

20. 0.1 mM sodium chloride (NaCl).

3   Methods

It is important to mention that all the techniques described below may be combined to obtain the desirable niosomes, such as the preparation of niosomes based on cationic lipids by thin film-hydration and microfluidization methods.

According to our criteria and experience in preparing niosome formulations, the following techniques have been adapted from the original methods to specifically prepare cationic niosome formulations for gene delivery purposes. However, these techniques can be modified according to the employed components.

3.1 Niosome Elaboration Techniques

3.1.1 Solvent Emulsion-Evaporation Technique

1. Weigh 5 mg of the cationic lipid in a 10 mL glass beaker.

2. Add 23 μL of squalene (Fig. 1b, c).

3. Gently mix the squalene with the cationic lipid (Fig. 1d).

4. Quickly add 1 mL of CH_2Cl_2 and mix it by magnetic stirring in the glass (Fig. 2d, 3). The glass beaker must be inside the extraction hood (Fig. 2c1).

5. Once the lipid and squalene are dissolved, remove the magnetic stirring bar with the help of another magnetic stirring bar (Fig. 2d, 2).

6. Add 5 mL of aqueous phase containing the nonionic surfactant Polysorbate 80 (Fig. 1e).

7. Once the two phases are observed in the beaker (Fig. 1f, g), sonicate them for 30 s at 50 W to obtain the final emulsion (Fig. 1h). The sonicator must be inside the extraction hood (Fig. 2a1).

8. Remove the organic solvent from the emulsion by evaporation under magnetic agitation for 3 h (Fig. 1i, j). The magnetic stirrer must be inside the extraction hood (Fig. 2c1). Upon CH_2Cl_2 evaporation, a dispersion containing the nanoparticles (NPs) is formed by precipitation of the cationic NPs in the aqueous medium (Fig. 1k).

9. Harvest the niosomes and store them at 4 °C until use to keep their properties (stability depends on the storage time and temperature). The final concentration is 1 mg of cationic lipid/ mL (*see* **Notes 2** and **3**).

10. Characterize the niosomes by size, polydispersity index (PDI), ζ-potential (Fig. 2e), and stability over the time.

3.1.2 Thin Film-Hydration Technique

1. Weigh 5 mg of the cationic lipid in a 10 mL glass beaker.

2. Add 23 μL of squalene (Fig. 1b, c).

3. Gently mix the squalene with the cationic lipid (Fig. 1d).

4. Quickly add 1 mL of CH_2Cl_2 and thoroughly mix it by magnetic stirring (Fig. 2d, 3) to obtain the organic phase.

5. Evaporate the solvent under magnetic agitation for 3 h. The glass beaker and magnetic stirrer must be inside the extraction hood (Fig. 2c1).

6. Once CH_2Cl_2 evaporates, remove the magnetic stirring bar with the help of another magnetic stirring bar (Fig. 2d, 2).

7. Hydrate the obtained lipid film with 5 mL of aqueous phase containing the nonionic surfactant, Polysorbate 80.

8. Sonicate the mix for 30 s at 50 W to obtain the emulsion (Fig. 1h).

9. Harvest the niosomes and store them at 4 °C until use to keep their properties (stability depends on the storage time and temperature). The final concentration of cationic lipid in the formulations is 1 mg cationic lipid/mL (*see* **Notes 2** and **3**).

10. Characterize the niosomes by size, PDI, ζ-potential (Fig. 2e), and stability over the time.

3.1.3   Hand Shaking Method

1. Weigh 5 mg of the cationic lipid in a 10 mL glass beaker.

2. Add 23 µL of squalene (Fig. 1b, c).

3. Gently mix the squalene with the lipid (Fig. 1d).

4. Quickly add 1 mL of CH_2Cl_2 and thoroughly mix it by magnetic stirring (Fig. 2d, 3) to obtain the organic phase.

5. Allow the solvent to evaporate under magnetic agitation for 3 h. The glass beaker and magnetic stirrer must be inside the extraction hood (Fig. 2c1).

6. Once CH_2Cl_2 evaporates, remove the magnetic stirring bar with the help of another magnetic stirring bar (Fig. 2d, 2).

7. Hydrate the obtained lipid film with 5 mL of aqueous phase containing the nonionic surfactant Polysorbate 80.

8. Cover the top of the beaker with parafilm and gently agitate it to form the niosomes.

9. Harvest the niosomes and store them at 4 °C until use to keep their properties (stability dependents on storage time and temperature). The final concentration is 1 mg of cationic lipid/mL (*see* **Notes 2** and **3**).

10. Characterize the niosomes by size, PDI, ζ-potential (Fig. 2e), and stability over the time.

3.1.4   Dissolvent Injection Method

1. Weigh 5 mg of the cationic lipid in a 10 mL glass beaker.

2. Add 23 µL of squalene (Fig. 1b, c).

3. Gently mix the squalene with the lipid (Fig. 1d).

4. Quickly add 1 mL of CH_2Cl_2 and mix it by magnetic stirring (Fig. 2d, 3). The glass beaker must be inside the extraction hood (Fig. 2c1).

5. Once the lipid and squalene are dissolved, remove the magnetic stirring bar with the help of another magnetic stirring bar (Fig. 2d, 2).

6. In another glass beaker with one magnetic stirring bar, add 5 mL of aqueous phase containing the nonionic surfactant Polysorbate 80.

7. Under magnetic agitation, slowly add the solution obtained in **step 5** to the nonionic surfactant solution glass.

8. Allow the solvent to evaporate under magnetic agitation for 3 h. The glass beaker and magnetic stirrer must be inside the extraction hood (Fig. 2c1). Upon CH_2Cl_2 evaporation, a dispersion containing the NPs is formed by precipitation of the cationic NPs in the aqueous medium (Fig. 1k).

9. Harvest the niosomes and store them at 4 °C until use to keep their properties (stability depends on the storage time and temperature). The final concentration is 1 mg of cationic lipid/mL (*see* **Notes 2** and **3**).

10. Characterize the niosomes by size, PDI, ζ-potential (Fig. 2e), and stability over the time.

3.1.5 Microfluidization Technique

This technique is used to decrease the PDI values of the niosome preparation with the aim of obtaining more homogeneous niosomes.

1. Place the emulsion into the microfluidic system (Fig. 2b).

2. Connect the 2 mL syringes to the microfluidics conducts as follow: connect one syringe without the syringe plunger to the inlet port (Fig. 3b); connect the second syringe with the syringe plunger to the outlet to collect the sample (Fig. 3b).

3. Set the desired pressure on the central control (Fig. 3c).

4. Pour the sample into the microfluidic system (Fig. 3d) and allow the sample to pass through it.

5. Once the sample is processed, collect the niosomes in the syringe connected to the outlet port (Fig. 3e).

6. Store the niosomes at 4 °C until use to keep their properties (stability dependents on the storage time and temperature).

7. Characterize the niosomes by size, PDI, ζ-potential (Fig. 2e), and stability over time.

3.2 Preparation of Nioplexes

Once the niosomes are prepared, they can be complexed with DNA to form nioplexes. The niosome/DNA proportions are expressed as the (w/w) ratio of cationic lipid/DNA. In order to exemplify the preparation of nioplexes, we will use 30:1 cationic lipid:DNA ratio. Stock niosome formulation contains 1 mg cationic lipid/mL and 0.5 mg/mL stock pDNA solution.

1. In a small tube, add 30 μL (30 μg) of niosome formulation and 20 μL of dH_2O or transfection medium to obtain a final volume of 50 μL (*see* **Note 4**).

2. In a separate tube, add 2.5 μL (1.25 μg) of pDNA stock solution and add 47.5 μL of dH_2O or transfection medium to obtain a final volume of 50 μL (*see* **Note 4**).

3. Add 50 μL of the pDNA solution to the niosome solution. The final volume obtained is 100 μL (*see* **Note 5**).

4. Mix by pipetting up and down 3–4 times.

5. Leave the niosome/DNA suspension for 30 min at RT to enhance electrostatic interactions between the cationic lipids and the negatively charged pDNA (*see* **Note 6**).

6. Characterize the nioplexes by size, PDI, and ζ-potential (Fig. 2e).

3.3 Characterization of Niosomes and Nioplexes

3.3.1 Size and PDI

Niosomes are usually spherically-shaped (Fig. 4c) and they show different sizes according to the technique and materials used for their preparation. Additionally, differences in terms of size are also found in the same niosome suspension due to high polydispersity of the preparation method. In order to analyze the size and polydispersity, we can use different instruments, such as the Zetasizer-nano that measures the size of the particles by DLS.

1. Turn the Zetasizer-nano on and start the software.

2. In a small tube, add 50 μL of niosome formulation or nioplexes (*see* **Note 7**).

3. Add 950 μL of 0.1 mM NaCl.

4. Pipette up and down 3–4 times and add 1 mL of the mix in a size/ζ-cell (*see* **Note 8**) (Fig. 4a).

5. Place the cell into the instrument.

6. Measure the size according to the equipment protocol for size and PDI characterization (*see* **Note 9**).

3.3.2 ζ-Potential

ζ-potential is the measurement obtained by the combination of electrophoresis and laser Doppler velocimetry techniques, where the data obtained indicates the charge of our niosome formulation or nioplexes (Fig. 4b). We can also use other instruments, such as those previously mentioned to obtain this information.

1. Turn on the Zetasizer-nano and open the software.

2. In a small tube, add 50 μL of niosome or nioplexes (*see* **Note 10**) and 950 μL of 0.1 mM NaCl (*see* **Note 11**).

3. Mix pipetting up and down 3–4 times, then add the 1 mL of the mixture in a size/ζ-cell (*see* **Note 12**) (Fig. 4a).

4. Place the cell into the instrument.

5. Measure the ζ-potential according to the equipment protocol (*see* **Notes 9** and **13**).

3.3.3 Stability

Periodic measurements of size, PDI, and ζ-potential of niosomes at different storage temperatures are necessary to avoid unwanted process, such as aggregation that could hamper the performance of the formulation.

1. Aspirate 800 μL of niosomes from the main batch, and transfer into two small tubes (400 μL/tube). Store one tube at RT and the other one at 4 °C.

2. Perform the first size and ζ-potential measurement right on fresh niosomes.

3. Perform periodic measurements of size, PDI, and ζ-potential of the niosomes (e.g., every 30 days up to 100 days) as indicated elsewhere (*see* Subheadings 3.3.1 and 3.3.2) (*see* **Notes 14** and **15**).

4 Notes

1. We find that it is best to prepare fresh nonionic surfactant solution each time.

2. The evaporation technique can be used to obtain a higher concentrated formulation. Once the niosomes are formed, keep the sample under magnetic agitation until desired concentration is reached (e.g., three more hours). The rpm of the magnetic stirrer will affect the evaporation time; we suggest employing around 1400 rpm. Attach the glass to the stirrer plate with adhesive tape to avoid spilling the sample.

3. The filtration technique is employed to obtain higher concentrated formulations. When the niosomes are formed, place the sample inside the filters (Fig. 2f) (filters can be found at different diameters) and drain the sample through the filters until the desired concentration is reached (check on the manufacturer website, spectrumlabs.com, for protocol details).

4. Use dH_2O or transfection medium to prepare the nioplexes. We use dH_2O when nioplexes are prepared for characterization purposes (e.g., size, ζ-potential, agarose gel assays) while we use transfection medium, such as Opti-MEM [6], when nioplexes are prepared for transfection purposes (e.g., cell transfection, cell uptake, cell viability).

5. Use the same volumes of DNA solution and noisome suspensions to enhance the cationic lipid to pDNA interaction.

6. Use nioplexes as soon as possible to avoid DNA degradation.

7. Smaller amounts of niosomes or nioplexes can be used to measure the size and PDI, especially when working with more concentrated niosome formulations. The Zetasizer-nano is able to measure the size and PDI in small amounts of sample. Thus, if you exceed the required amount of sample, the size and PDI might not be accurate. PDI indicates the size distribution of the particles, where the maximum value is 1.0. A sample displaying a PDI value close to 1.0 suggests a broad size distribution and the presence of large particles or aggregates. In such a case, the sample is not suitable for DLS measurements.

8. If you do not want to waste valuable sample, we suggest using the ζ-potential cell. Additionally, the ζ-potential cell only requires 1 mL of final volume compared to other cells that require greater amounts of sample.

9. It is recommendable to repeat the measurements on the same sample at least thrice.

10. Smaller amounts of niosomes or nioplexes can be used to measure the ζ-potential, especially for those niosome formulations that have been concentrated. The Zatasizer-nano is able to perform measurements employing small amounts of sample. Thus, if you exceed the required amount of sample, the ζ-potential might not be accurate.

11. Conductivity can be a problem when the saline solution used to measure the ζ-potential is highly concentrated. In order to avoid wrong ζ-potential data, we suggest using 0.1 mM NaCl.

12. Before pouring the sample into the cell, make sure that the electrodes are not black. Due to the constant use of the cells, the electrodes turn black (burned aspect) impeding accurate measurements.

13. The ζ-potential is an important factor to be considered for niosome aggregation. The ζ-potential is also important when the niosomes are bound with DNA through electrostatic interactions to form nioplexes. Moreover, positively charged nioplexes are desired in order to facilitate their interaction with the negatively charged cell surfaces and encourage the endocytic process.

14. The stability of niosomes is a relevant aspect since, with time, niosomes can show modifications due to poor stability that directly affects their size, ζ-potential, and polydispersity.

15. Acquisition time of size and ζ-potential data will depend on the desired storage time. We recommend measuring size and ζ-potential up to 100 days.

Acknowledgments

This project was partially supported by the University of the Basque Country UPV/EHU (UFI 11/32), the National Council of Science and Technology (CONACYT), Mexico, Reg. # 217101, the Spanish Ministry of Education (Grant CTQ2010-20541, CTQ2010-14897), the Basque Government (Department of Education, University and Research, pre-doctoral PRE-2014-1-433 and BFI-2011-2226 grants) and by Spanish grants MAT2012-39290-C02-01 and IPT-2012-0574-300000. Technical and human support provided by SGIker (UPV/EHU) is gratefully acknowledged. Authors also wish to thank the intellectual and technical assistance from the ICTS "NANBIOSIS", more specifically by the Drug Formulation Unit (U10) of the CIBER in Bioengineering, Biomaterials & Nanomedicine (CIBER-BBN) at the University of Basque Country (UPV/EHU).

References

1. Rajera R, Nagpal K, Singh SK et al (2011) Niosomes: a controlled and novel drug delivery system. Biol Pharm Bull 34(7):945–953

2. Moghassemi S, Hadjizadeh A (2014) Nanoniosomes as nanoscale drug delivery systems: an illustrated review. J Control Release 185:22–36

3. Puras G, Mashal M, Zarate J et al (2014) A novel cationic niosome formulation for gene delivery to the retina. J Control Release 174:27–36

4. Junyaprasert VB, Teeranachaideekul V, Supaperm T (2008) Effect of charged and non-ionic membrane additives on physicochemical properties and stability of niosomes. AAPS PharmSciTech 9(3):851–859

5. Spanova M, Zweytick D, Lohner K et al (2012) Influence of squalene on lipid particle/droplet and membrane organization in the yeast Saccharomyces cerevisiae. Biochim Biophys Acta 1821(4):647–653

6. Ojeda E, Puras G, Agirre M et al (2015) Niosomes based on synthetic cationic lipids for gene delivery: the influence of polar headgroups on the transfection efficiency in HEK-293, ARPE-19 and MSC-D1 cells. Org Biomol Chem 13(4):1068–1081

7. Byk G, Dubertret C, Escriou V et al (1998) Synthesis, activity, and structure--activity relationship studies of novel cationic lipids for DNA transfer. J Med Chem 41(2):229–235

8. Mahidhar YV, Rajesh M, Chaudhuri A (2004) Spacer-arm modulated gene delivery efficacy of novel cationic glycolipids: design, synthesis, and in vitro transfection biology. J Med Chem 47(16):3938–3948

9. Zhi D, Zhang S, Wang B et al (2010) Transfection efficiency of cationic lipids with different hydrophobic domains in gene delivery. Bioconjug Chem 21(4):563–577

10. Karmali PP, Chaudhuri A (2007) Cationic liposomes as non-viral carriers of gene medicines: resolved issues, open questions, and future promises. Med Res Rev 27(5): 696–722

Chapter 6

Quantitative Intracellular Localization of Cationic Lipid–Nucleic Acid Nanoparticles with Fluorescence Microscopy

Ramsey N. Majzoub, Kai K. Ewert, and Cyrus R. Safinya

Abstract

Current activity in developing synthetic carriers of nucleic acids (NA) and small molecule drugs for therapeutic applications is unprecedented. One promising class of synthetic vectors for the delivery of therapeutic NA is PEGylated cationic liposome (CL)–NA nanoparticles (NPs). Chemically modified PEG-lipids can be used to surface-functionalize lipid–NA nanoparticles, allowing researchers to design active nanoparticles that can overcome the various intracellular and extracellular barriers to efficient delivery. Optimization of these functionalized vectors requires a comprehensive understanding of their intracellular pathways. In this chapter we present two distinct methods for investigating the intracellular activity of PEGylated CL–NA NPs using quantitative analysis with fluorescence microscopy.

The first method, spatial localization, describes how to prepare fluorescently labeled CL–NA NPs, perform fluorescence microscopy and properly analyze the data to measure the intracellular distribution of nanoparticles and fluorescent signal. We provide software which allows data from multiple cells to be averaged together and yield statistically significant results. The second method, fluorescence colocalization, describes how to label endocytic organelles via Rab-GFPs and generate micrographs for software-assisted NP–endocytic marker colocalization measurements. These tools will allow researchers to study the endosomal trafficking of CL–NA NPs which can guide their design and improve their efficiency.

Key words Nucleic acid carriers, PEGylated nanoparticles, Rab GTPase, Particle tracking, Image analysis, Endosomal escape, Transfection, Liposomes, Liquid crystals

1 Introduction

1.1 Background

Lipids are a class of amphiphilic molecules that self-assemble into liquid crystalline phases in aqueous environments at high concentrations [1]. The structures of lipid phases are determined by the physical and chemical properties of the individual lipid molecules [2]. Energetically favorable assemblies of lipids with distinct shapes are those that minimize exposure of the hydrophobic tails to water due to the hydrophobic effect. Numerous intracellular organelles, along with the cell itself, are enclosed within lipid membranes. These biological membranes are two-dimensional (2D) bilayer structures that are impermeable to water and house membrane-bound proteins

Gabriele Candiani (ed.), *Non-Viral Gene Delivery Vectors: Methods and Protocols*, Methods in Molecular Biology, vol. 1445,
DOI 10.1007/978-1-4939-3718-9_6, © Springer Science+Business Media New York 2016

which play a variety of essential roles in cellular function [3]. Their inherent impermeability allows cellular membranes to act as a barrier so that organelles maintain chemically distinct environments. Shortly after their initial discovery as the major component in plasma membranes [4], biomedical researchers used lipid vesicles, or liposomes, as drug carriers by loading the hydrophobic regions and aqueous interiors with hydrophobic and hydrophilic drugs, respectively [5–7]. This marked the beginning of lipids as carriers of therapeutic drugs in delivery applications. Although in vitro results were promising [8, 9], in vivo studies showed that the phagocytic system and filtering activity of the liver and kidneys made circulation times brief and impractical [10, 11]. One approach to prolonging the circulation time of lipid-based drug or nucleic acid (NA) carriers is through surface modification with hydrophilic polymers [12, 13]. Polyethylene glycol (PEG) satisfies a number of requirements for use as a surface modification agent in nano-therapeutics; it is charge-neutral, hydrophilic, and biologically inert [14]. When PEG is grafted to surfaces it inhibits adhesion of macromolecules by inducing a repulsive interaction between the surface and macromolecules [15–17]. By the same mechanism, PEG-modification of particles in solution prevents aggregation induced by van der Waals forces, imparting colloidal stability to the modified particles [18]. These attributes make PEG-modification (a process often called PEGylation) a promising strategy for developing lipid-based vectors for delivery applications in vivo.

Figure 1 shows the evolution of lipid-based carriers that has occurred in recent decades [19]. Initially, liposomes lacking surface modification were used as vectors for hydrophobic and hydrophilic drugs (Fig. 1a). These carriers were replaced by surface-modified liposomes containing polymer lipids (Fig. 1b). The polymer chains, which extend beyond the surface in a brush conformation, provide a platform for covalent attachment of targeting ligands, allowing liposomes to target specific cell types and facilitate receptor-mediated endocytosis [20, 21]. Finally, as shown in Fig. 1c, condensed lipid–DNA particles containing both targeting moieties and chemically responsive polymers capable of undergoing cleavage in the low pH environments of late endosomes are being developed as future therapeutics. Lipid vectors using such chemically modified PEG-lipids are promising candidates for targeted and effective delivery of NA to specific cell types.

1.2 Effects of PEGylation on the Structure and Assembly of Cationic Liposome (CL)–DNA Complexes

Cationic liposomes and NA spontaneously self-assemble into ordered structures which have been extensively characterized via small angle X-ray scattering [21–28]. The CL–DNA complexes' structures are predicted by the curvature elastic theory of membranes [29]. The shape of the lipid, which determines the preferred phase of the lipid self-assembly (i.e., L_α, H_I, H_{II}) [30–32], can also determine the phase of the CL–DNA complex. In many lipid systems the

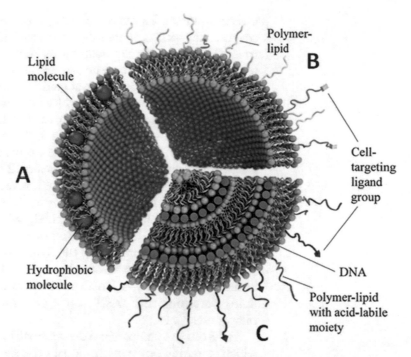

Fig. 1 Evolution of lipid-based drug carriers. (**a**) Initially liposomes, formed with lipid molecules (shown with *blue headgroups* and *gold tails*), were used to trap hydrophobic drugs (*red spheres*) within the bilayer and hydrophilic drugs in the aqueous interior. (**b**) Surface-functionalized liposomes typically contain polymer lipids to inhibit protein binding to the surface. The distal end of the polymer can be chemically modified with a targeting ligand for organ- and cell-specific targeting. (**c**) CLs mixed with DNA form condensed CL–DNA complexes with well ordered structure. Polymer lipids can be synthesized with an acid-labile moiety to promote shedding of the polymer at low pH. Reproduced from ref. 19 by permission of The Royal Society of Chemistry (RSC) on behalf of the Centre National de la Recherche Scientifique (CNRS) and the RSC

"shape" of the molecule determines the spontaneous curvature of the membrane ($C_o = 1/R_o$) and also determines the actual curvature $C = 1/R$. The actual curvature describes the structure of the lipid self-assembly where $C = 0$ corresponds to lamellar (L_α), $C < 0$ corresponds to inverted hexagonal (H_{II}) and $C > 0$ corresponds to hexagonal (H_I). This model successfully predicts the phase behavior of systems where the rigidity of the membrane is large ($\kappa/k_B T \gg 1$) such that significant deviations of C from C_o would cost elastic energy ($\kappa/2)\cdot(1/R - 1/R_o)^2$ [29]. If the bending cost is low ($\kappa \approx k_B T$), then C can deviate from C_o without a large elastic energy cost. This behavior is further driven by the lowering of other energies in the process (e.g., the electrostatic energy between DNA and CL). In the case of DOTAP–DOPC–DNA complexes, the membrane rigidity $\kappa/k_B T$ is of order 10 resulting in the complex assembling into the lamellar L_α^C phase (DOTAP/DOPC membranes have a zero spontaneous curvature [22]). However, the addition of a cosurfactant such as pentanol (molar ratio of about 4:1 cosurfactant to lipid [33]) lowers the bending rigidity ($\kappa \approx k_B T$) so that the system will prefer the inverse hexagonal H^C_{II} phase [23]. This occurs because the electrostatic energy gain in transitioning from the L_α^C to H^C_{II} is greater than the energy loss due to C deviating from C_o.

Figure 2 shows three structures that have been reported for different combinations of cationic and neutral lipids with DNA. The lamellar phase shown in Fig. 2a (as well as in Fig. 1c) contains DNA sandwiched between lipid bilayers [22]. Figure 2b shows the H^C_{II} phase where hexagonally packed, inverted cylindrical micelles contain DNA in their aqueous interior [23]. Figure 2c shows the H^C_I phase where hexagonally packed, cylindrical micelles form a dual lattice with DNA packed in a honeycomb pattern [26]. In the case of lamellar complexes, the compositional parameters ρ_{chg} (charge ratio of CL to anionic base pairs (bp)) and σ_m (the membrane charge density, a function of the ratio of cationic to neutral lipid) determine the DNA spacing by modulating the available bilayer area [24].

CLs can also complex and deliver small interfering RNA (siRNA), which is used in posttranscriptional gene silencing [34]. Along with the lamellar and hexagonal phases shown in Fig. 2a, b, synchrotron X-ray scattering has shown that CLs containing glycerol mono-oleate (GMO) can form cubic phases when mixed with siRNA [35, 36]. Figure 3a shows the unit cell of the double gyroid cubic phase where siRNA is contained in distinct water channels (green and orange) that are separated by a lipid surface (grey). The silencing efficiency of vectors in the cubic phase is shown in Fig. 3b where optimal silencing corresponds to K_T (total gene knockdown including sequence

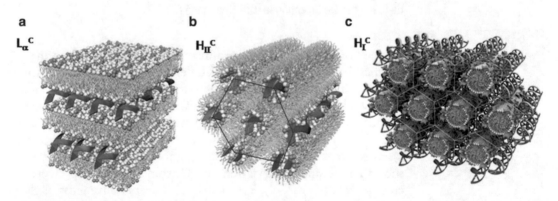

Fig. 2 Internal nanoscale structures of lipid–DNA complexes. (**a**) The lamellar (L^C_α) phase forms when the neutral lipid has a cylindrical shape and prefers surfaces with spontaneous curvatures of zero (e.g., DOPC). (**b**) The inverted hexagonal (H^C_{II}) forms when neutral lipids that prefer negative spontaneous curvature such as DOPE are used. (**c**) The hexagonal (H^C_I) phase was discovered upon mixing DOPC and DNA with a custom-synthesized dendritic cationic lipid, MVLBG2 (+16). (**a**) and (**b**) reprinted with permission from ref. 23. (**c**) reprinted with permission from ref. 26. Copyright 2006 American Chemical Society

specific and nonspecific) equals 1 and K_{NS} (nonspecific knockdown) equals 0. From Fig. 3b we observe that the cubic phase with $0.6 < K_T < 0.7$ and $K_{NS} < 0.1$ (black squares where the GMO mol fraction Φ_{GMO} is greater than 0.75) significantly outperforms lamellar complexes which are formed with DOPC (black circles). The observed high silencing efficiency of cubic phase complexes at low membrane charge density stands out because lamellar phase CL–DNA complexes only show high efficiency at a high membrane charge density. The nonspecific silencing (K_{NS}), a measure of toxicity, is low for both phases (red curves). The proposed mechanism for the high silencing efficiency of cubic phases is that the negative Gaussian curvature of the cubic phase can promote fusion of the complex with the endosomal membrane and subsequent pore formation, resulting in delivery of siRNA molecules to the cytoplasm.

When liposomes are pre-grafted with PEG-lipids and subsequently combined with DNA, the resulting CL–DNA complexes contain PEG-lipid on their interior and exterior. The interior PEG moieties can reduce the DNA–DNA spacing by inducing a depletion attraction force [25]. This effect was found to be most pronounced at low membrane charge densities where the DNA–DNA spacing in the absence of PEG-lipid is large and can be reduced by a factor of 2 when 10 mol% of PEG-lipid is incorporated. PEG-lipids not only alter the DNA spacing but can also influence the size of the complexes as well as the total number of

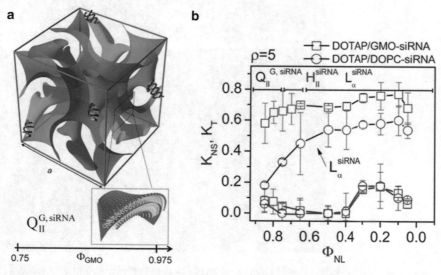

Fig. 3 Double gyroid cubic phase for the delivery of siRNA (**a**) The unit cell of the cubic phase contains a negative Gaussian surface of lipids (*grey*) separating two water channels that contain siRNA (*orange* and *green*). (**b**) Both lamellar complexes (L$_\alpha$^siRNA, *circles*) and cubic complexes (Q$_{II}$^{G, siRNA}, *squares*) show low nonspecific silencing (*red curves*) at low membrane charge density but the cubic phase significantly outperforms the lamellar phase at total gene knockdown (*black curves*). Reprinted with permission from ref. 35. Copyright 2010 American Chemical Society

layers [25, 28, 37]. In 150 mM NaCl solution, the electrostatic repulsion of like-charged CL–DNA complexes is screened, resulting in fusion of smaller complexes into large aggregates (*see* Fig. 4a). Incorporating PEG-lipids into these complexes provides a repulsive steric force that prevents fusion and promotes the assembly of stable, sub-100 nm CL–DNA nanoparticles (NPs, *see* Fig. 4b) that can maintain their size for at least 24 h post-complexation [37]. Steric stabilization of CL–DNA particles is essential for developing lipid-based NPs for in vivo applications, where NPs are exposed to high-ionic-strength plasma and subject to filtration by organs upon reaching a critical size.

The polymer-induced steric repulsion also modulates the average number of layers or lamellae in each NP [28]. Using small angle

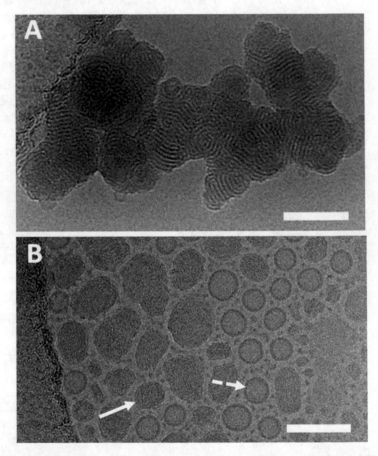

Fig. 4 Cryo-EM micrographs of CL–DNA complexes with and without PEGylation. (**a**) Complexes formed with DOTAP–DOPC at a molar ratio of 80:20 with a charge ratio of 10 in 50 mM NaCl fuse together, forming a large aggregate. (**b**) Stable sub-100 nm NPs form when DNA is mixed with liposomes containing PEG-lipid. Complexes formed with 80:15:5 (molar ratio) DOTAP–DOPC–PEG2K-lipid and a charge ratio of 10 in 50 mM NaCl. Electron-dense CL–DNA NPs (*solid arrow*) coexist with cationic liposomes (*dotted arrow*). Scale bars correspond to 100 nm. Adapted and reprinted with permission from ref. 37; copyright Elsevier

X-ray scattering, Silva et al. showed that NP formation is pathway-dependent: the ionic strength of the formation buffer can alter the average number of layers per NP [28]. PEGylated liposomes and DNA complexed in the presence of physiological salt concentrations result in NPs containing five or fewer layers while complexation in pure water, in the absence of added salt (dH₂O), followed by transfer of NPs into solutions near physiological salt concentrations results in a bimodal distribution of NPs containing either 20–30 or 2–3 layers. The phase diagram provided in [28] shows that by tuning the membrane charge density, PEG grafting density, charge ratio, and buffer ionic strength, it is possible to form NPs with a desired number of layers between 2 and 30. While all in vitro and in vivo applications of PEGylated CL–DNA NPs require they be transferred to physiological buffer, the study by Silva et al. demonstrated that forming NPs in water and transferring them to salt solution enables the preparation of kinetically trapped particles which are unable to reach their equilibrium configuration of only a sparse number of layers at the higher salt concentrations.

A recent cryo-EM study has found that the DNA length and topology can also influence the average number of layers found in each particle [38]. NPs formed with long, linear DNA (48 kbps, lambda DNA) or circular plasmid (2 kbps, pDNA) results in more layers than NPs formed with polydisperse, linear DNA (2 kbps, salmon DNA). Furthermore, NPs formed with lambda DNA at low charge ratios (i.e., with excess DNA) in the presence of dH₂O results in DNA-induced tethering of NPs into polymer-mediated flocs.

1.3 Effects of Structure and PEGylation of CL–DNA Complexes on Transfection Efficiency (TE)

The significance of the discovery of the structure of CL–DNA complexes was highlighted by the finding that the structure of CL–DNA complexes affects their function [39]. Confocal imaging and TE assays showed that while H^C_{II} (inverse hexagonal) complexes are capable of undergoing direct fusion with the plasma membrane, lamellar complexes are taken up by cells through endocytosis [39]. Upon endocytosis, complexes are trafficked via endosomes and their efficacy is limited due to their degradation in lysosomes barring their escape from endosomes into the cytoplasm [37, 40]. Endosomal escape, the bottleneck to efficient therapeutic delivery, occurs through fusion of the endosomal membrane and outer cationic bilayer of the complex. Complexes with high membrane charge density (σ_m = total charge per membrane area, a parameter that depends on the ratio of cationic to neutral lipids as well as lipid valency and headgroup area) escape endosomes more efficiently and exhibit higher TE [40]. Figure 5a shows the TE of various CL–DNA complexes plotted against their membrane charge density. The data is divided into three regimes: at low membrane charge density (Regime 1), complexes mostly remain trapped in endosomes; at moderate membrane charge density (Regime 2), complexes escape endosomes and undergo disassociation (release of DNA from the complex); finally, at high membrane charge densities (Regime 3), complexes escape endosomes but fail to undergo complete disassociation due to a strong electrostatic interaction between CLs and DNA. As mentioned above, the TE of H^C_{II} complexes (hollow symbols in Fig. 5a) does not depend on their membrane charge density, implying that endosomal escape is not a bottleneck to efficient transfection for these complexes. The dependence of TE on structure and membrane charge density (in the case of lamellar complexes) provides guidelines for the optimal formulation of effective CL–DNA complexes.

For in vivo applications of CL–DNA complexes, PEGylation is required to extend circulation times. However, the addition of PEG-lipids significantly alters the interactions of CL–DNA complexes with cellular membranes such as the plasma membrane and the compositionally related endosomal membrane [37]. Figure 5b shows the TE of CL–DNA NPs with moderate membrane charge density as a function of mol% PEG2K-lipid. As PEG-lipid increases beyond 5 mol% (coinciding with the grafting density that marks the transition of the PEG chains from the mushroom to the brush conformation), a significant drop in TE occurs. Two plausible explanations for this drop in TE are (1) the PEG corona around individual NPs obstructs adhesion of NPs to the plasma membrane, reducing cell uptake and (2) PEG-induced steric repulsion between the NP and endosomal membrane inhibits fusion between the two.

Custom-synthesized PEG-lipids allow the formulation of NPs designed to overcome these barriers to efficient transfection. Cellular attachment may be recovered by grafting a ligand or peptide sequence to the distal of the PEG moiety, allowing NPs to bind to receptors on the plasma membrane [37]. One class of targeting peptides that has shown significant success both in vitro and in vivo is based on the arginine-glycine-aspartic acid (RGD) motif [41]. RGD peptides specifically interact with integrin receptors (which are frequently over-expressed in cancer cells), making them an ideal candidate for peptide-mediated targeting of tumors [42, 43]. As shown in Fig. 5c, RGD-tagging of CL–DNA NPs partially recovers the TE that is lost when CL–DNA complexes are PEGylated. PEG-lipids with a pH-sensitive linker that is capable of undergoing hydrolysis (named HPEG: hydrolyzable PEG-lipid) in the late endosomal environment allow NPs to shed their PEG corona, fuse with the endosomal membrane and access the cytoplasm for efficient release of cargo [44]. Figure 5d shows the TE of HPEGylated CL–DNA NPs as a function of ρ_{chg}. As observed for RGD-tagged NPs, TE partially recovers.

The similarity of the TE results for RGD-tagged NPs and HPEGylated NPs despite their differing chemistry and design concepts highlights the need for a more informative experimental technique for studying NP uptake and intracellular processing. While the TE assay is a high-throughput and sensitive technique for measuring the efficacy of gene transfer and subsequent expression,

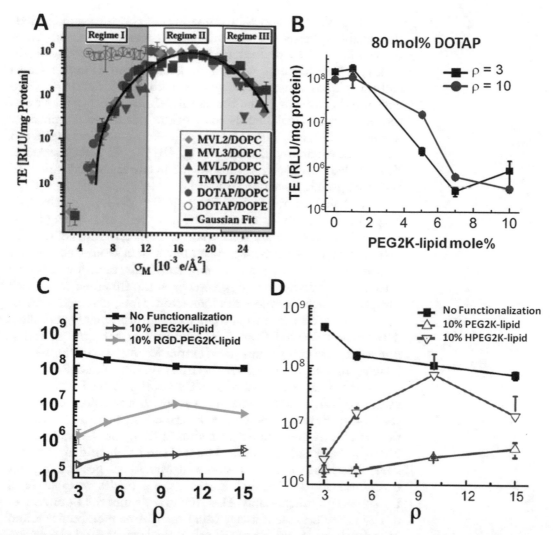

Fig. 5 Transfection Efficiency (TE) of CL–DNA complexes with and without surface functionalization (**a**) The TE of lamellar CL–DNA complexes without functionalization follows a universal curve when plotted against membrane charge density. *Filled symbols* are different cationic lipids (*see* legend) and *hollow symbols* are hexagonal complexes which do not show membrane charge density-dependent TE. (**b**) TE of 80/20-x/x DOTAP–DOPC–PEG2K-lipid complexes where x is noted on the x-axis. (**c** and **d**) The effect of PEGylation, RGD-tagging, and HPEG-modification on TE compared to complexes lacking surface modification. (**a**) is reprinted with permission from ref. 40; copyright 2005 John Wiley & Sons. (**b**) and (**c**) are adapted and reprinted with permission from ref. 37; copyright Elsevier. (**d**) is adapted with permission from ref. 44, copyright Elsevier

robust optimization of vectors requires the ability to discriminate between the major bottlenecks to transfection.

1.4 Quantitative Intracellular Imaging of Fluorescently Labeled CL–DNA NPs

Fluorescence microscopy has been instrumental in understanding biological processes. Specific labeling of biological components through fluorescent tagging allows direct observation of biological interactions in situ. Fluorescence microscopy of cells incubated with CL–DNA NPs allows investigations of pathways and barriers, thus enabling better chemical design and formulation. One common strategy when performing fluorescence microscopy with NA vectors is dual labeling, where a fluorescent lipid is used to label and track lipids while a separate dye (with distinct excitation and emission) is covalently attached to the NA for tracking the fate of the NA cargo. Dual fluorescent labeling permits discrimination between CL–DNA NPs and cationic liposomes lacking DNA (which coexist at equilibrium, *see* Fig. 4b) [24, 38]. Furthermore, dual-labeled CL–DNA complexes allow direct visualization of vector-cargo disassociation [39, 45].

The value of qualitative imaging for yielding mechanistic insights is limited in systems as complex as cells undergoing transfection. Rather, a comprehensive understanding of intracellular NP behavior requires extracting quantitative data from fluorescence micrographs. One issue in obtaining statistically meaningful results through quantitative imaging of cells is the inherent cell-to-cell variability which produces random error. Thus, it is necessary to use computer software to automate the measurements and allow data to be extracted from large numbers of cells. As of today, numerous research groups use quantitative analysis of fluorescent imaging to study gene delivery vectors [37, 38, 44, 46–51].

Intracellular localization is an interesting feature that can be measured using fluorescence microscopy. Localization allows the spatial distribution of NPs to be measured, so that the accumulation of NPs in the perinuclear region (a frequent characteristic of NPs with poor early endosomal escape) can be quantified. We have developed image analysis routines in Matlab for performing this quantification [37, 38, 44]. Figure 6a, b provides an example of the software's functionality. First, the user defines the boundary of a cell in the fluorescent image using the plasma membrane-bound NPs that form an outline of the cell in the current focal plane (Fig. 6a). Alternatively, the cell boundary can be determined via a bright-field image. Second, the nuclear membrane is identified by the user in the bright field image so that it may be used as a reference point, allowing data from multiple cells to be averaged (Fig. 6b). Next, the routine automatically detects and localizes fluorescent NPs using algorithms from [52]. Finally, the software defines regions of the cell which are equidistant to the nuclear membrane and counts the number of NPs in each region [37]. The routine is also capable of measuring the total number of NPs per cell by integrating over the localization curves at each time point [37]. This feature is use-

---

Fig. 6 (continued) distance to the nuclear membrane for CL–DNA NPs containing PEG2K-lipid, RGD-PEG2K-lipid, and HPEG2K-lipid. The *inset* shows total NPs/cell for PEGylated, RGD-tagged and HPEG-modified NPs. (**d–i**) DIC and fluorescent micrographs of representative live cells used to generate the data in (**c**). The surface functionalization is indicated above the micrographs. All scale bars are 10 μm. (**a**, **b**, *right panel* of **c**) and (*left* and *middle panel* of **c**, **d**, **e**, **g**, **h**) are adapted and reprinted with permission from refs. 44 and 37, respectively; copyright Elsevier

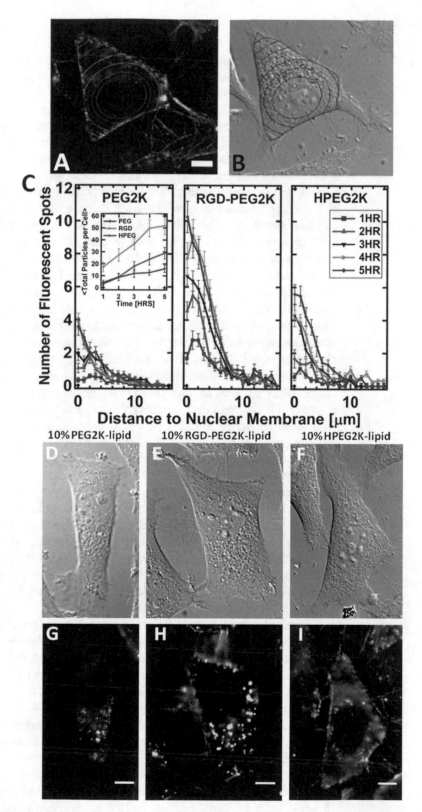

Fig. 6 Measuring intracellular localization and uptake with quantitative fluorescence microscopy. (**a** and **b**) A merged fluorescent micrograph (**a**) and DIC image (**b**) of a cell that has been incubated with fluorescent NPs. Overlaid on both images are the cell boundary (*blue*), locations of fluorescent spots (*red crosses*) and regions defined by distance to the nuclear membrane (*various colors*). (**c**) The average number of fluorescent spots at a given

ful when NPs cannot be effectively washed off the outside of the cell and methods such as flow cytometry would measure the total fluorescence intensity of cell-associated NPs as opposed to cell-internalized NPs. Although our software can also measure internalization by measuring net fluorescence, object-based colocalization (where individual NPs are counted) is preferable because it produces consistent results independent of fluorescent label density, camera settings or photobleaching.

Figure 6c presents intracellular localization data which shows the average number of particles found at a given distance to the nuclear membrane for PEGylated NPs, RGD-tagged NPs, and HPEGylated NPs. The results show that RGD-tagged NPs are taken up by cells more efficiently than PEGylated and HPEGylated NPs. When comparing HPEGylated NPs to PEGylated NPs, we see similar uptake at early time points ($t \leq 2$ h). However, as individual NPs escape the endosome (in the case of HPEGylated NPs), more NPs are spatially resolvable and counted. Figure 6d–i contains examples of the DIC and fluorescent micrographs used to generate the data shown in Fig. 6c. The TE of RGD-tagged and HPEGylated NPs are similar, but quantitative imaging shows significant differences [37, 44]. This implies that HPEGylation and RGD-tagging improve TE through distinct mechanisms. RGD NPs are internalized more efficiently than HPEGylated NPs. Thus, the image analysis suggests that RGD-tagging of NPs partially recovers TE relative to PEGylated NPs due to high uptake [37], while HPEGylated NPs partially recover TE due to efficient endosomal escape [44]. We see perinuclear accumulation in all three cases, indicating that the NPs are inside endosomes which are being trafficked by motor proteins. In the case of HPEGylated NPs, they are trafficked by early endosomes to the perinuclear region before the endosome matures and lowers its pH, allowing NPs to shed their PEG coat and escape endosomes. Quantitative fluorescent imaging thus allows discrimination between NP formulations which show low TE due to inefficient uptake or endosomal escape.

Another powerful application of quantitative image analysis is the study of colocalization, in particular for deciphering endocytic pathways. Escape from endosomes is a limiting step in transfection with CL–DNA complexes and is strongly affected by PEGylation [37, 44]. Thus, it is highly desirable to have a means for investigating the endosomal trafficking and escape properties of lipid-based NPs. Fluorescence imaging can be used to quantify colocalization of NPs and fluorescently tagged organelles, allowing unambiguous determination of the NP's intracellular pathway as well as measurement of intracellular targeting efficiency. One promising approach is direct labeling of various endocytic stages using the Rab family of enzymes [53–55]. Rab GTPases mediate budding, trafficking and fusion of membrane-bound organelles, with over 70 distinct Rab proteins in humans reported to date [56]. Each Rab GTPase associates with a

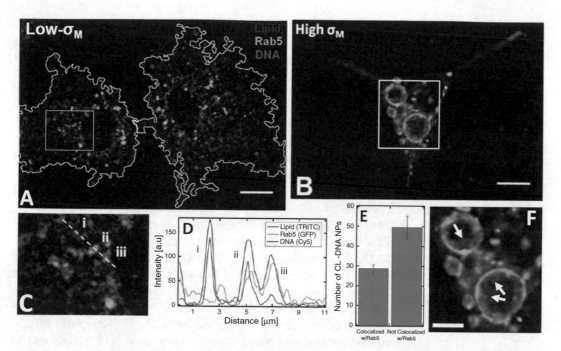

Fig. 7 NPs colocalize with wild type Rab5-GFP and mutant Rab5-Q79L-GFP (**a** and **b**) Fluorescent micrographs of L-cells expressing wild type (**a**) and mutant (**b**) Rab5-GFP that have been incubated with dual-fluorescently labeled RGD-tagged NPs for 60 min at 4 °C followed by 60 min at 37 °C. (**c**) A cropped region from (**a**) showing a NP lacking GFP colocalization (*i*), and 2 NPs colocalized with GFP-Rab5 (*ii* and *iii*). (**d**) Intensity profile of *dashed line* in (**c**). (**e**) Average number of NPs colocalized and not colocalized with GFP-Rab5 at 60 min of 37 °C incubation (*n* = 20 cells). (**f**) Cropped region from (**b**) showing giant early endosomes containing individual, resolvable nanoparticles (*arrows*). Scale bars in (**a** and **b**) and (**f**) are 10 and 5 μm, respectively. Adapted and reprinted with permission from ref. 53; copyright Elsevier

distinct stage of the endosomal pathway, allowing discrimination between NPs found in early, recycling or late endosomes.

Figure 7 features fluorescence micrographs and cropped regions of wild type Rab5-GFP (*see* Fig. 7a, c) and mutant Rab5-GFP-Q79L (*see* Fig. 7b, f) expressing mouse L-cells that have been incubated with dual-labeled NPs. In the case of wild type Rab5, early endosomes appear as small, diffraction-limited spots in the green channel (*see* Fig. 7a). The cropped region (*see* Fig. 7c) and corresponding intensity scan (*see* Fig. 7d) show two classes of fluorescent signal. The first signal (Fig. 7c, d (i)) is from a NP that lacks Rab5-GFP colocalization, while the other two objects (Fig. 7c, d (ii, iii)) are NPs colocalized with GFP-Rab5, implying that they are inside early endosomes [53]. We have developed a software routine that counts the fraction of total intracellular NPs inside fluorescently labeled endosomes. Our analysis uses an object-based colocalization algorithm that measures the number of NPs that are inside versus outside of GFP-labeled endosomes based on the distance between a NP and the closest endosome. Pixel-based colocalization methods (Pearson's coefficient, Mander's coefficient [57]) are useful measures for comparing colocalization of fluorescent proteins but our method provides nanoparticle statistics, which allows direct mapping of an NP's intracellular pathway. Much like the localization algorithm described above, object-based colocalization is insensitive to photobleaching, camera settings and variations in fluorescent label per NP. Figure 7e shows an example of the resulting data for the early endosome marker, Rab5, at an early time point (60 min). In the case of wild type Rab5, only a small fraction of NPs are found to be colocalized with early endosomes.

Figure 7b, f show a micrograph and cropped region of a cell expressing mutant Rab5-Q79L-GFP. In contrast to wildtype Rab5, cells expressing the mutant Rab5-Q79L show nearly all intracellular NPs within early endosomes or giant early endosomes (GEEs). The Q79L mutation of Rab5 inhibits GTP hydrolysis, increasing the early endosome's size and lifetime. The results with the mutant Rab5 show that the lack of colocalization of NPs with wildtype Rab5-GFP is due to the short lifetime of early endosomes and not indicative of escape from early endosomes; if NPs could escape early endosomes, we would expect to see more NPs outside of the GEEs that are present when the mutant Rab5-Q79L is used. The slow maturation and spatially resolvable size of the GEEs that form with the mutant Rab5 make it a powerful assay for measuring NP escape from early endosomes. Wildtype Rab5 is not an ideal marker for measuring escape from early endosomes because intracellular NPs that lack Rab5 colocalization could be in a later endosomal compartment (e.g., late or recycling endosomes).

Below we provide protocols for preparing fluorescent CL–DNA NPs and imaging the transfection of mammalian cells in vitro using optical microscopy. We also describe how to perform the analysis shown in Figs. 6 and 7 using our custom-developed software routines. All the routines were developed in Matlab and are provided as m-files at http://www.mrl.ucsb.edu/~safinyaweb/lab.htm. We encourage users to modify and implement the routines to their liking. A typical experiment takes 5 days (liposomes are prepared separately), with glass slide preparation (**3.2.1**) on day 1, seeding cells (**3.2.2**) on day 2, transfection with Rab-GFP (**3.2.3**) on day 3, media change and recovery on day 4, and cell imaging or fixation (**3.3**) on day 5.

2   Materials

2.1 Liposome Preparation

1. 9:1 (v:v) chloroform–methanol ($CHCl_3$–MeOH) mixture.
2. 15:13:2 (v:v:v) $CHCl_3$–MeOH–dH_2O mixture.
3. High-resistivity dH_2O.
4. Desired lipids to be used (e.g., DOTAP, MVL5, DOPC, PEG2K-DPSE) as solids (*see* **Note 1**).

5. Fluorescently tagged lipid (*see* **Note 2**).

6. 1.5 mL vials with Teflon-lined caps (*see* **Note 3**).

7. Oven at 37 °C.

8. Nitrogen (N_2) stream.

9. Rotary evaporator.

10. Tip sonicator.

2.2 Imaging Assays

1. Liposome solutions.

2. 100 µg/mL stock solution of NA (*see* **Note 4**).

3. Solution of fluorescently labeled NA (*see* **Note 5**).

4. Appropriate formation buffer for CL–DNA complexes (cell culture medium or water at desired salt concentration).

5. 1.5 mL polypropylene microcentrifuge tubes.

6. Tweezers.

7. 22 mm×22 mm No. 1.5 coverslips and 6-well plates or glass bottom dishes (GBDs) (*see* **Note 6**).

8. Poly-(l-lysine) solution (molecular weight (MW): 30,000–70,000 g/mol, 0.1% (wt/v) solution).

9. 7× cleaning solution

10. Ethanol (EtOH), 190 proof (100% EtOH).

11. 70:30 (v/v) EtOH–dH_2O mixture (70% EtOH).

12. Sterile plastic petri dishes.

13. Phosphate buffered saline (PBS).

14. Serum-free cell culture media (e.g., DMEM, RPMI).

15. Cell culture media supplemented with fetal bovine serum (complete medium).

16. Enzyme-free disassociation buffer (Thermo Fisher Scientific, Waltham, Massachusetts).

17. Hemocytometer.

18. Lipofectamine 2000 (L-2000) or alternative transfection reagent.

19. Rab-GFP pDNA (*see* **Note 7**).

20. Solution of "noncoding" DNA (e.g., calf thymus or salmon sperm DNA).

21. Refrigerator at 4 °C.

22. 50 U/mL heparin sulfate in PBS (*see* **Note 8**).

23. Microscope equipped for fluorescent imaging.

24. Mounting medium.

25. Mammalian cells (e.g., HeLa, PC-3, M-21)

2.3 Software

1. ImageJ (with PSF Generator and Iterative Deconvolve 3D plug-ins).
2. Matlab (with Image Processing Toolbox).

---

3 Methods

3.1 Liposome Preparation

Relevant Parameters (parameters marked with * are set by the user and can be varied):

Z_{CL}: Charge of the cationic lipid (e.g., MVL5: $Z_{CL} = 5$, DOTAP: $Z_{CL} = 1$).

MW_{CL}: MW of the cationic lipid.

MW_{NL}: MW of the neutral lipid.

MW_{FL}: MW of functional lipid (e.g., PEG2K-lipid, RGD-PEG2K-lipid).

Φ_{CL}: Mol fraction of cationic lipid (determines membrane charge density)*.

Φ_{FL}: Mol fraction of functionalized PEG-lipid (determines PEG coverage and conformation)*.

Φ_{NL}: Mol fraction of neutral lipid ($= 1 - \Phi_{FL} - \Phi_{CL}$).

C_S: Concentration of lipid stock solution (in mM/L)* (This can be optimized depending on m_{NA}, ρ, V_F, and number of experiments to be performed (*see* **Note 9**)).

V_S: Volume of lipid stock solution (in µL)* (*see* **Note 10**).

c_{NA}: Concentration of stock NA (in µg/mL).

ρ_{chg}: Desired lipid–NA charge ratio (ratio of positive charges (from cationic lipid) to negative charges (from NA))* (*see* **Note 11**).

m_{NA}: Desired mass of NA to be complexed (in µg) (*see* **Note 12**).

V_{TL}: The total volume of lipid suspension used to form CL–DNA NPs.

V_F: Total volume of buffer containing CL–DNA complexes* (*see* **Note 13**).

m_L: Total mass of lipid to be delivered (determined by m_{NA} and ρ).

Based on the chosen Φ_{CL}, Φ_{NL}, Φ_{FL}, V_S, and C_S, the user will form a stock solution of liposomes. Using the liposome stock solution, the user can prepare multiple samples of CL–NA complexes, where the desired m_{NA} and ρ will determine the volume of liposome stock solution required per sample.

3.1.1 Forming Stock Solutions of Lipids in Organic Solvents

1. Based on individual lipid stock solution volume (V_{CL}) and concentration (M_{CL}), determine how much lipid to weigh: e.g., $m_{CL} = M_{CL} \times V_{CL} \times MW_{CL}$ (*see* **Note 14**).
2. Weigh out the lipid into a glass vial (*see* **Note 15**).

3. Dissolve the lipid in the appropriate volume of organic solvent (e.g., V_{CL}) (*see* **Notes 16** and **17**).

4. Repeat **steps 1–3** for all lipids to be used in the formulation.

3.1.2 Liposome Formation

1. Calculate the required volume of lipid stock solutions (*see* Subheading 3.1.1) to combine:

$$V_{CL} = V_S \times (C_S / M_{CL}) \times \Phi_{CL}$$

2. Calculate the additional volume of solvent (V_{sol}) needed to achieve V_S, according to the following formula:

$$V_{sol} = V_S - (V_{CL} + V_{NL} + V_{FL})$$

3. Add V_{sol} of organic solvent to a new glass vial. Then pipette the calculated volumes of lipid stock solutions into the vial (*see* **Notes 17** and **18**).

4. Calculate the total weight of cationic and neutral lipids in V_S and add 0.2 wt% of fluorescent lipid to V_S (e.g., $m_{FL} = V_S \times C_S \times (\Phi_{CL} \times MW_{CL} + \Phi_{CNL} \times MW_{NL})$) (*see* **Notes 19** and **20**).

5. Use a N_2 stream (or rotary evaporator for large volumes) to evaporate the 9:1 (v:v) chloroform–methanol mixture and form a lipid film on the side of the vial (*see* **Note 21**).

6. To ensure complete removal of organic solvent, place the vial containing the dried lipid film in a vacuum desiccator for at least 8 h.

7. Add V_S of dH$_2$O or desired buffer to the vial containing the lipid film.

8. To ensure complete hydration of the lipid film, close the vial tightly, seal the lid with Parafilm, and incubate overnight in an oven at 37 °C (*see* **Note 22**).

9. Remove lipid solutions from the incubator and sonicate with a tip sonicator (*see* **Notes 23** and **24**).

10. After tip sonication, filter liposome solution (*see* **Notes 25** and **26**). Store at 4 °C until use.

3.2 Rab-GFP Expression in Mammalian Cells

3.2.1 Preparation of Coverslips or Glass Bottom Dishes

Glass bottom dishes are packaged as sterile and do not require the cleaning steps outlined below in **steps 1–10**.

1. Using clean tweezers, pick individual coverslips from their casing and drop them into a beaker containing a solution of soap (we recommend 7× cleaning solution) and dH$_2$O.

2. Sonicate in a bath sonicator for 15 min.

3. Discard soap–dH$_2$O mixture and rinse coverslips 3 times with dH$_2$O. Perform rinsing by discarding dH$_2$O, replacing with fresh dH$_2$O and swirling for 5–10 s.

4. Sonicate the coverslips in dH$_2$O.

5. Discard the dH$_2$O and rinse the coverslips 3 times with dH$_2$O.

6. Add 70% EtOH to the coverslips and sonicate them.

7. Discard 70% EtOH and rinse the coverslips once with 70% EtOH.

8. Add 100% EtOH to the beaker, cover the beaker with aluminum foil, and store it at room temperature (RT).

9. To dry the coverslips, place a clean piece of aluminum foil in an oven at 37 or 60 °C, remove individual coverslips from 100% EtOH, and place them on the aluminum foil for 10–15 min.

10. Using tweezers, remove the dried coverslips from the oven and place them in a plastic petri dish.

11. Apply 500 µL of poly-(l-lysine) solution to each coverslip (or GBD well). Spread the solution with the pipette tip to ensure full surface coverage of the poly-(l-lysine) solution (*see* **Note 27**).

12. Gently shake the petri dish for 15 min.

13. Aspirate excess poly-(l-lysine) solution and rinse coverslips (or GBD wells) by adding dH$_2$O and gently swirling.

14. Aspirate the dH$_2$O and repeat the rinsing step with PBS.

15. Aspirate the PBS and perform the rinsing step with dH$_2$O.

16. Place petri dish containing coverslips (or GBD wells) in an oven at 37 or 60 °C for 2 h to dry.

3.2.2 Cell Seeding

1. When using coverslips, remove coverslips from petri dish (*see* **Note 28**). Using tweezers, place single coverslips in the wells of a 6-well plate; ensure that the poly-(l-lysine) coated side is facing up.

2. Add 2 mL of serum free medium to each well containing a coverslip (or each GBD well) and then place 6-well plate (or GBD wells) in the incubator for 20 min.

3. Remove a cell culture flask containing cells at >80% confluency from the incubator and discard the medium.

4. Wash the cells 3 times with PBS, then aspirate and discard the PBS.

5. Add enzyme-free disassociation buffer (EFDB) to the cell culture flask and incubate for 3–5 min at 37 °C (*see* **Note 29**).

6. Aspirate EFDB and firmly tap the sides of the culture flask to dislodge the cells.

7. Resuspend the cells by thoroughly rinsing the bottom of the flask with complete medium. Visually inspect the flask to ensure all cells are detached and suspended in solution.

8. Measure cell density using a hemocytometer and prepare a stock suspension of cells at the appropriate density, typically between 1.8 and 2×10^5 cells/mL (*see* **Note 30**).

9. Take the 6-well plate (or GBD wells) from the incubator and discard the medium.

10. Apply 2 mL of cell suspension to each well and gently rock back and forth to ensure an even distribution of cells in each well (*see* **Note 31**).

11. Place the 6-well plate containing cells (or GBDs) in the incubator.

3.2.3 Cell Transfection
with Rab pDNAs

1. Add 250 μL of serum-free medium into polypropylene microcentrifuge tubes. Use two microcentrifuge tubes for each well that is to be transfected with a Rab pDNA.

2. In one polypropylene microcentrifuge tube, add the appropriate amount of L-2000. We found that 10 μL/well (or GBD) of L-2000 achieves reasonable expression without excessive toxicity (*see* **Note 32**).

3. To the other microcentrifuge tube, prepare the DNA mixture by adding 2 μg of "noncoding" DNA (e.g., calf thymus or salmon sperm DNA) followed by 2 μg of the pDNA. Gently pipette up and down to ensure homogenous mixing (*see* **Note 33**).

4. Add the L-2000 containing solution to the DNA mixture, and pipette up and down to promote mixing and complexation.

5. Incubate the L-2000–DNA mixture for 20 min at RT.

6. Remove cells from the incubator, aspirate the old medium, rinse with PBS, and add 2 mL of fresh serum-free medium.

7. Add the L-2000–DNA mixture to the wells (or GBDs) by gently dropping the suspension across various regions of each well (or GBD) and gently agitate to ensure a homogenous distribution of the NPs.

8. Incubate the 6-well plate (or GBDs) for 4–6 h at 37 °C.

9. Take the 6-well plate (or GBDs) out from the incubator, discard the old culture medium, rinse with PBS, and add fresh serum-free medium (*see* **Note 34**).

10. Incubate for additional 18–24 h.

3.3 Optical
Fluorescence
Microscopy

3.3.1 General Protocol
to Form Complexes
(See **Note** *35)*

1. Using the desired charge ratio (ρ) and mass of NA m_{NA}, calculate the volume of the master liposome stock solution required (*see* **Note 36**).

2. Calculate the desired m_{NA} and dilute the corresponding volume of NA stock solution in the desired buffer such that the final volume of DNA solution is 50 μL (*see* **Note 37**).

3. Dilute the desired amount of lipid solution in the appropriate buffer such that the final volume is 50 µL (*see* **Notes 36–38**).

4. Add 50 µL of the DNA solution to the liposome solution and gently pipette up and down.

5. Incubate the NP solution for 20 min at RT.

3.3.2 Single Pulse of Completely Labeled NPs

1. Prepare fluorescent NPs by mixing the appropriate amount of fluorescently labeled liposome suspension with fluorescently labeled DNA (*see* **Note 5**). Add 0.1 µg/well (or GBD) of labeled DNA, and calculate the lipid amount based on the desired ρ and membrane charge density (*see* **Note 36**).

2. Take the 6-well plates (or GBDs) out from incubator, discard the old medium, rinse with PBS, and add 2 mL/well of cold (4 °C) serum-free medium to the cells.

3. Add the NPs to cells by dropping solution across different regions of the well. Gently agitate the dish to ensure the NPs are homogeneously distributed throughout each well.

4. Place cells in a 4 °C refrigerator for 1 h (*see* **Note 35**).

5. Take the 6-well plates (or GBDs) out from the refrigerator and place them in the incubator for the desired time (typically 60 min).

3.3.3 Cell Fixation with Formaldehyde

1. Remove the 6-well plates (or GBDs) from incubator, discard the old medium and rinse the cells with PBS 3 times.

2. Incubate cells in a PBS solution containing 3.7% formaldehyde for 15 minutes at RT followed by washing the cells 3 times with PBS, and incubating them in 2 mL PBS for 3–5 min at RT.

3. Discard the PBS, add the mounting medium and mount the coverslips to microscope slides.

4. Place the samples on the microscope stage and take pictures of them.

3.3.4 Pulse-Chase with Labeled and Unlabeled NPs

1. Follow the protocol in Subheading 3.3.2.

2. In the meantime, prepare unlabeled NPs by mixing the appropriate amount of liposome suspension with unlabeled DNA. Add 3 µg/well (or GBD) of labeled DNA, and calculate the lipid amount based on the desired ρ and membrane charge density (*see* **Notes 36** and **37**).

3. After 60 min of incubation, take the 6-well plates (or GBDs) out from the incubator.

4. Wash the cells twice with ice-cold 50 U/mL heparin solution and once with PBS.

5. Add 2 mL/well of warm (37 °C) serum-free DMEM to the cells.

6. Add the unlabeled NPs to the cells and incubate them at 37 °C for the desired time (1–6 h).

7. Image live cells or fix cells at the desired time point.

3.3.5 Simultaneous Coadministration of Labeled and Unlabeled NPs

1. Prepare fluorescent NPs by mixing the appropriate amount of fluorescently labeled liposome suspension with fluorescently labeled DNA (*see* **Note 5**). The final amount of labeled DNA to add to each well is 0.1 μg, and the amount of lipid is calculated based on the desired ρ and membrane charge density (*see* **Note 36**).

2. Prepare unlabeled NPs by mixing the calculated amount of unlabeled liposome solution with unlabeled DNA. The total amount of unlabeled DNA to add to each well is 3 μg, and the lipid amount is calculated based on the desired ρ and membrane charge density (*see* **Notes 36** and **39**).

3. After incubating labeled and unlabeled NPs for 20 min, take the 6-well plates (or GBDs) out from the incubator, discard the old medium, wash the cells with PBS, and add 2 mL/well of warm serum-free media to them.

4. Mix labeled and unlabeled NPs by repeated pipetting up and down.

5. Add the mixed NPs to the cells and incubate at 37 °C for the desired time.

6. Image live or fixed cells.

3.4 Intracellular Localization Analysis

If 3D imaging is performed (using a spinning disk or laser confocal microscope), then image stacks should be processed via a deconvolution algorithm. Below we briefly describe one protocol for doing so, but numerous alternatives are available.

3.4.1 Deconvolution and Image Processing

1. Generate PSF: Download and install the ImageJ plugin "Generate PSF", run the plugin, and generate individual PSFs for each fluorescent channel that has been imaged (*see* **Note 40**).

2. Download and install the ImageJ plugin "Iterative Deconvolve 3D". Run the plugin and select the desired image stack and PSF to be used (*see* **Note 41**).

3.4.2 NP Localization

Localization requires a pair of 2D images for each cell to be analyzed. One should be an 8-bit TIFF file of the bright field image in which the edge of the cell and nuclear membrane are clearly visible. The second image should be an 8-bit TIFF file of the fluorescent image showing NPs as resolution-limited spots.

Our website (http://www.mrl.ucsb.edu/~safinyaweb/lab. htm) provides links to the 4 m-files necessary for performing localization analysis. The files pkfnd.m and cntrd.m are Matlab versions of the software developed by Eric Weeks which feature the original particle tracking routines written by Crocker and Grier [52]. The m-file fit_ellipse.m was developed by Ohad Gal and is available from the Mathworks website. The file Localizer.m is our code which contains numerous functions for executing the analysis. To run the software, type:

output = Localizer('brightfield_prefix', 'fluorescent_prefix', first_ file_number, last_file_number, interactive_logical, ellipse_spacing)

The six inputs are:

brightfield_prefix: The filename of the brightfield image without the file extension or file number (e.g., for a file named 'RPAR_bright_1.tif' the prefix would be 'RPAR_bright_').

fluorescent_prefix: The filename of the fluorescent image without the file extension or file number (e.g., for a file named 'RPAR_TRITC_1.tif' the prefix would be 'RPAR_TRITC_').

first_file_number: The number of the first file that the software is to analyze (e.g., first_file_number = 1 to start with 'RPAR_ bright_1.tif' and 'RPAR_TRITC_1.tif').

last_file_number: The number of the last file that the software should analyze. (e.g., last_file_number = 10 to end with 'RPAR_bright_10.tif' and 'RPAR_TRITC_10.tif').

interactive_logical: Set this to 1 if you want the software to write a TIFF file showing the results; set to 0 if you just want the results as a text file.

ellipse_spacing: This parameter sets how thick, in pixels, each cell region (distance between colored lines in Fig. 5b, c) should be. We recommend using a pixel value that corresponds to 2.5 μm.

To run the software using the test images from our website:

output = Localizer('RPAR_bright_', 'RPAR_TRITC_', 1, 2, 1, 10)

When the program is run it will take the user through five steps:

1. Clicking two opposing corners of an empty region of the image for determining the background fluorescence value (this number will be used to normalize the fluorescent results of each image).

2. Identifying the number of cells in a given image and cropping each of them by clicking on two opposing corners.

3. Identifying the boundary of a cell by clicking on points on each side of the cell and hitting enter after clicking a side.

4. Identifying the nuclear membrane by clicking around it.

5. Setting the parameters for identifying particles which include the intensity threshold (an 8-bit TIFF image will have intensity values between 0 and 255) for identifying a particle and the minimum distance between particles (in pixels). These parameters are direct inputs for Eric Week's pkfnd.m and cntrd.m. The structure *output* contains the following eight arrays, where each array element is a data point for a region of the cell:

output.average_NPs_region: The average number of NPs per region.

output.ERROR_NPs: The statistical error of the average number of NPs per region.

output.averge_F_region: The total fluorescence intensity of each region (averaged over the number of cells analyzed).

output.ERROR_F_in_region: The statistical error for the average fluorescence intensity each region.

Output.average_NP_perpix_region: The average number of NPs per region normalized by the average number of pixels per region.

output.ERROR_NP_perpix_region: The statistical error of NPs per region normalized by the average number of pixels per region.

output.average_F_perpix_region: The average fluorescence intensity value per pixel in each region.

output.ERROR_F_perpix_region: The statistical error of the average fluorescence intensity per pixel in each region.

The user has the choice of accessing the results in the Matlab command window by calling the output structure and desired array (e.g., type "*output.average_NPs_region*") or using the text file that the program will write upon completion. The text file is titled using "*fluorescent_prefix*". For example, the data above would result in a text file called *RPAR_TRITC_DATA*.*txt* being created.

3.4.3 Measuring NP-Endosomal Marker Colocalization

Colocalization analysis contains similar features to the localization pipeline but the raw data for the GFP channel can be used to automatically define cell boundaries. Furthermore, subtracting the NP image from the GFP image can generate an image whose boundary defines the intracellular environment, allowing the program to easily disregard any NPs which are not internalized. Our merged fluorescent micrographs contain the lipid signal in the first channel, the Rab signal in the second channel and the DNA signal in the third channel. We define objects as liposomes if they show fluorescence in the first channel but not the third. NPs are defined as objects which fluoresce in the first and third channel.

1. Generate relevant images for analysis using image processing. Image 1: A 3D stack of merged fluorescent images where the second channel is a marker for the organelle (e.g., Rab-GFP or Lysotracker) and the first and third channels are nanoparticle labels (*see* Fig. 6a for an example). Image 2: A 3D stack of the GFP channel that has had its contrast adjusted so that it is nearly a threshold binary image. Image 2 will be used to locate the boundary of the cell. The two sets of images should have the following naming convention:

   (a) Image 1: FirstHalf_1_merged.tif, FirstHalf_2_merged. tif,…

   (b) Image 2: FirstHalf_1_GFP.tif, FirstHalf_2_GFP.tif,…

2. Run the program by typing output = Colocalize(*'First_Half_FileName'*, *'Second_Half_Merged_Filename'*, *'Second_Half_GFP_Filename'*, *num_files*, *coloc_threshold*). The five input parameters are:

   First_Half_FileName: The first half of all filename; everything that comes before the file number.

   Second_Half_Merged_Filename: The second half of the merged images' filenames; everything that comes after the file number.

   Second_Half_GFP_Filename: The second half of the GFP images' filenames; everything that comes after the file number.

   num_files: The number of images that will be analyzed.

   coloc_threshold: The minimum distance between a nanoparticle and endosome for it to be considered colocalized (in pixels). We suggest using a pixel length that corresponds to a length of 500 nm.

3. Identify the number of cells in an image and crop individual cells in the image by clicking opposing corners of a region of interest.

4. Input the slice numbers that correspond to the bottom and top of the volume of interest.

5. Mask regions of the image by clicking around the region you would like to mask (forming a polygon) and then double-clicking in the center of the user-defined polygon.

6. Input relevant parameters for detecting cell boundary and confirm parameters for each slice of the stack. The program will prompt the user for two parameters *Threshold* and *Minsize*. *Threshold* refers to the minimum intensity value of a pixel that should be considered inside the cell. *Minsize* refers to the smallest fluorescent object that should be considered inside a cell. *Minsize* is useful for images that contain extracellular fluo-

rescent debris. One novel feature of the software is that it will subtract the image of the particles from the thresholded GFP image that is used to detect the cell boundary. By doing this, particles which are bound to the surface are excluded from the colocalization analysis.

7. Set threshold and minimum inter-particle distance for locating particles. Each channel can have its own particle location parameters defined.

8. The results are written to a text file that contains:

    (a) The average number and standard deviation of liposomes per cell.

    (b) The average number and standard deviation of liposomes colocalized with an endosomal marker per cell.

    (c) The average number and standard deviation of CL–DNA NPs per cell.

    (d) The average number and standard deviation of CL–DNA NPs colocalized with an endosomal marker per cell.

    (e) The text file also contains the results for each cell analyzed. A 2D TIFF showing the locations of all four signals is also written for each cell.

4   Notes

1. Avanti Polar Lipids sells lipids in powder form or as $CHCl_3$ solutions. If starting with lipids already dissolved in $CHCl_3$, then dilute to the appropriate concentration.

2. We typically use TRITC-DHPE or Texas Red-DHPE from Life Technologies. These dyes do not have spectral overlap with GFP or Cy5, which are used to label endosomes and DNA, respectively.

3. Teflon lining minimizes solvent evaporation. We recommend vials with conical bottoms to maximize the volume that can be recovered from the vials.

4. We have had success purchasing our pDNAs from addgene. org and propagating in *Escherichia coli* (*E. coli*) using the kits and protocol provided by Qiagen. Purification from *E. coli* is done using a Mega or Giga Kit from Qiagen. pDNAs in aqueous solution can be stored in the freezer for years. A suitable stock concentration is 250 μg/mL.

5. Labeling DNA is done using the Mirus Label IT Nucleic Acid Labeling Kit. We follow the manufacturer's protocol with the only modification being an extension of the 37 °C incubation to 2 h, thereby increasing the labeling efficiency.

6. Coverslips are eventually mounted to microscope slides and used for fixed cell imaging. Glass-bottom dishes (MatTek) are used for live cell imaging.

7. Over 70 types or Rab proteins have been identified in humans, we suggest starting with Rab 5 or Rab 7, which label early and late endosomes, respectively.

8. Heparin sulfate solution removes most extracellular NPs. Purchase Heparin Sulfate as a powder (Sigma-Aldrich) and form stock solutions at 2000 U/mL in dH$_2$O. Prepare a working solution of 50 U/mL in PBS the day of the experiment.

9. Before choosing a liposome concentration we suggest calculating formulations from Subheading 3.1 (*see* **Note 38**) to ensure that the liposome solution is at reasonable concentration for making complexes. For liposomes containing monovalent lipids at 50 mol%, a concentration of liposomes at 2 mM allows formation of NPs with reasonable volumes. Fluorescently labeled liposomes are used in much smaller quantities such that the stock solution of liposomes could be prepared at 500 μM.

10. If using a tip sonicator to generate small vesicles, there is typically a lower limit on V_S such that the sonicating tip can be sufficiently submerged. Otherwise the volume can be optimized depending on m_{NA}, ρ, V_F and number of experiments to be performed.

11. The molar charge ratio of CLs to anionic DNA sets the effective charge of the CL–DNA NPs. Above the isoelectric point ($\rho_{chg} \approx 1$), the NPs have a net positive charge. At high charge ratios ($\rho_{chg} > 1$), the NPs coexist with cationic liposomes at equilibrium.

12. When forming samples for imaging, each well (or GBD) uses 0.1 μg of labeled DNA and 3 μg of unlabeled DNA (*see* Subheading 3.3.3, 3.3.4 or 3.3.5).

13. The total volume of complexes depends on the size of the wells that the cells will be seeded in. For 6-well plates, add 2 mL/well of culture medium and then add 500 μL/well of complex solution. For 24-well plates, complexes are formed in 200 μL/well of culture medium and added to empty wells.

14. As an example, if the cationic lipid is MVL5 (MW$_{MVL5}$ = 1164.86 g/M) and you want a stock solution at 2 mM M_{CL} with 1 mL of V_{MVL5}, then m_{MVL5} = (2 mM)×(1 mL)×(1164.86 g/M) = 2.33 mg. If you do not have a scale with necessary precision to weigh such small amounts, a more concentrated stock solution can be made and diluted to yield the appropriate stock solution concentration.

15. Some lipids are hydroscopic and will stick to the spatula. We recommend using two spatulas; one to scoop lipid from the

container while the other is used to scrape lipid off the first spatula into the new vial.

16. Most cationic and neutral lipids readily dissolve in 9:1 (v/v) $CHCl_3$–MeOH. We have found that peptide-PEG-lipids dissolve more readily in mixtures of $CHCl_3$, MeOH and dH_2O, e.g., 65:23:2 (v/v/v) $CHCl_3$–MeOH–dH_2O.

17. We suggest filling and emptying the pipette tip once or twice before aspirating the desired volume. This prevents dripping of the organic solvent from the pipette tip due to its high vapor pressure.

18. When adding lipid solutions, pipette up and down so that the solvent added as V_{sol} can rinse off any lipid solution that adhered to the inside of the pipette tip.

19. When the stock solutions of fluorescent lipid are at 1 mg/mL, a typical volume of fluorescent lipid on the order of 1 µL is added to a V_S of 500 µL at 1 mM.

20. The weight fraction of fluorescent lipid has to be adjusted based on the sensitivity of the imaging system. We recommend using the least amount of fluorescent lipid that makes imaging feasible.

21. If drying via nitrogen stream use the fastest speed that does not splash solution out of the vial. Slow speeds result in thick films which are hard to dry and hydrate.

22. If using lipids that have a higher transition temperature, incubate in an oven at a temperature such that all lipids are in the liquid phase.

23. After incubation, the lipid solutions may appear cloudy or turbid due to the formation of large multilamellar vesicles (LMVs). Sonication promotes the formation of SUVs.

24. We strongly recommend a tip sonicator instead of an ultrasound bath sonicator, which in our experience is not powerful enough.

25. A 200 nm filter will remove metal debris deposited by the tip sonicator.

26. After a period of 2–4 weeks it is strongly suggested to resonicate the liposome suspension to ensure that the liposomes remain as small unilamellar vesicles (SUVs).

27. We strongly advise against coating with fibronectin or other proteins which contain RGD sequences when performing studies with RGD-tagged NPs. Variations in fibronectin concentration are hard to control and will affect the reproducibility.

28. Drying the coverslips can result in them adhering to the petri dish. Gentle deformation of the petri dish will help detach them, but take care not to fracture the coverslips in the process.

29. We do not recommend detaching cells with trypsin. Trypsin acts by cleaving integrins, and although cells do eventually replenish integrins, results are more easily reproducible with enzyme-free disassociation buffer from Life Technologies.

30. The number of cells plated per well should be adjusted depending on the cell line's growth rate. The optimal seeding density is one where cells are 80% confluent on the day they are imaged.

31. Avoid swirling the wells, as this causes cells to accumulate in the center. Avoid vigorous agitation, as this causes cells to be seeded underneath the coverslips.

32. Other transfection reagents can be used in place of L-2000. We recommend optimizing the transfection settings such that (1) minimal toxicity occurs (2) GFP-expression is not heterogenous and (3) cells are not over-expressing GFP-Rabs. To rule out over-expression, ensure that cells expressing GFP-Rab show similar uptake and particle localization as control cells that have not been transfected with GFP-Rab.

33. GFP-Rab pDNAs are diluted with "filler" DNA to prevent overexpression without significantly reducing the total number of cells that express GFP-Rab.

34. If cells are below 70% confluency, complete medium can be added instead of serum-free medium at this step. We prefer synchronizing our cells through serum starvation to minimize variations in cell volume. We strongly suggest not starting the imaging experiment on the day after transfection with GFP-Rab. Rather, allow an extra day for the cells to recover from L-2000 transfection.

35. We describe three strategies for labeling NPs and performing fluorescent imaging. Method 1 is recommended for observing initial endocytic events at early time points ($t < 1$ h). Method 2 allows users to track NPs that are in similar stages of the endocytic pathway by synchronizing their uptake into cells. In contrast to the first method, the second method ensures that cells are exposed to the same concentration of NPs as used in transfection experiments. Method 3 completely mimics a transfection experiment in terms of NP concentration but results in a steady stream of NPs being internalized during the 6 h incubation, which can obfuscate results by having individual fluorescent NPs internalize at any time point between 1 and 6 h. Methods 1 and 2 avoid the ambiguity of a distribution of NP-internalization times by cold-incubating the NPs with cells. In the case of PEGylated NPs with and without RGD-tagging, cold incubation allows NPs to settle and coat cells while endocytosis is inhibited. When NPs in solution are removed and

cells transferred to a 37 °C incubator, all cell-associated fluorescent NPs are on the outside of the plasma membrane.

36. For a typical imaging experiment we might use $m_{NA} = 100$ ng of DNA at $\rho = 10$. To calculate the volume of lipid required (V_{TL}):

$$V_{TL} = m_{NA} \times \left(MW_{CL} \times Z_{BP} / \left(MW_{BP} \times Z_{CL} \right) \right) \times \rho \times \left(100 / \Phi_{CL} \right) \times \left(1 / MW_{CL} \right) \times \left(1 / M_S \right)$$

where Z_{BP} and MW_{BP} the charge and MW of NA base pairs, respectively. $Z_{BP} = 2$ for DNA and $MW_{BP} = 660$ g/mol for long double-stranded DNA, but for short DNA (such as oligonucleotides, which are typically ~20 bps long) MW_{BP} must be calculated based on the sequence.

37. Forming NPs in dH_2O before transferring into cell culture media results in NPs with a larger number of layers than forming the NPs in culture media (*see* Subheading 1.2 or ref. 28 for more information).

38. Liposome suspensions are typically formed under the assumption they will be used for multiple experiments. For example, 10–50 µL out of 500 µL is typically used to form NPs for a single experiment. If lipid material is precious and must be conserved, reduce V_S or C_S (*see* **Note 9**).

39. pGFP can be used as a reporter gene.

40. To do this, imaging system specifications must be known (e.g., camera resolution, objective NA, and emission wavelength of each fluorescent channel).

41. We have developed an ImageJ script that automatically opens each image and the appropriate PSF file, performs deconvolution, and then saves the output. Our automated deconvolution script for ImageJ is available on the website. For displaying images we use a secondary processing step that includes the ImageJ commands "Background Subtraction" and "Smooth." This step removes noise and allows for easy discrimination of fluorescent NPs.

Acknowledgements

This work was supported by the National Institutes of Health (NIH) under grant number R01 GM59288 (transfection efficiency and colocalization studies with Rab GTPases) and the National Science Foundation (NSF) under grant number DMR-1401784 (nanoparticle imaging and automated image analysis). The Rab5-Q79L-GFP pDNA was a gift from the Weimbs laboratory at UC-Santa Barbara.

References

1. Seedon JM, Templer RM (1995) Polymorphism of lipid-water systems. In: Lipowsky R, Sackmann E (eds) Handbook of biological physics, vol 1. Wiley, New York

2. Feigenson GW (2006) Phase behavior of lipid mixtures. Nat Chem Biol 2:560–563

3. van Meer G, Voelker DR, Feigenson GW (2008) Membrane lipids: where they are and how they behave. Nat Rev Mol Cell Biol 9:112–114

4. Bangham AD, Horne RW (1964) Negative staining of phospholipids and their structural modification by surface-active agents as observed in the electron microscope. J Mol Biol 8:660–668

5. Gregoriadis G, Leathwood PD, Ryman BE (1971) Enzyme entrapment in liposomes. FEBS Lett 14:95–99

6. Greogriadis G, Ryman BB (1972) Fate of protein-containing liposomes injected into rats – approach to treatment of storage diseases. Eur J Biochem 23:485–491

7. Gregoriadis G (1976) Carrier potential of liposomes in biology and medicine. N Engl J Med 295:704–765

8. Pagano RE, Weinstein JN (1978) Interactions of liposomes with mammalian cells. Annu Rev Biophys Bioeng 7:435–568

9. Felgner PL, Gader TR, Holm M, Roman R, Chan HW, Wenz M, Northrop JP, Ringold GM, Danielsen M (1987) Lipofection: a highly efficient, lipid-mediated DNA transfection procedure. Proc Natl Acad Sci U S A 90:11307–11311

10. Lasic DD (1994) Liposomes in gene delivery. CRC Press, Boca Raton

11. Lasic DD, Martin FJ (eds) (1995) Stealth liposomes. CRC Press, Boca Raton

12. Klibanov AL, Maruyama K, Torchilin VP, Huang L (1990) Amphiphatic polyethyleneglycols effectively prolong the circulation of liposomes. FEBS Lett 268:235–237

13. Blume G, Cevc G (1990) Liposomes for the sustained drug release in vivo. Biochim Biophys Acta 1029:91–97

14. Abuchowski A, van Es T, Palczuk C, Davis FF (1977) Alteration of immunological properties of bovine serum albumin by covalent attachment of polyethylene glycol. J Biol Chem 252:1578–3581

15. Du H, Chandaroy P, Hui SW (1997) Grafted poly-(ethylene glycol) on lipid surfaces inhibits protein adsorption and cell adhesion. Biochim Biophys Acta 1326:236–248

16. Kuhl TL, Leckband DE, Lasic DD, Israelachvili JN (1994) Modulation of interaction forces between bilayers exposing short-chained ethylene oxide headgroups. Biophys J 66:1479–1488

17. Kenworthy AK, Hristov K, Needham D, McIntosh TH (1995) Range and magnitude of the steric pressure between bilayers containing phospholipids with covalently attached poly(ethylene glycol). Biophys J 68:1921–1936

18. Lasic DD (1993) Liposomes: from physics to applications. Elsevier, San Diego

19. Safinya CR, Ewert KK, Majzoub RN, Leal C (2014) Cationic liposome-nucleic acid complexes for gene delivery and gene silencing. New J Chem 38:5164–5172

20. Noble GT, Stefanick JF, Ashley JD, Kiziltepe T, Bilgicer B (2014) Ligand-targeted liposome design: challenges and fundamental considerations. Trends Biotechnol 32:32–45

21. Pearce TR, Shroff K, Kokkoli E (2012) Peptide targeted lipid nanoparticles for anticancer drug delivery. Adv Mater 24:3803–3822

22. Radler JO, Koltover I, Salditt T, Safinya CR (1997) Structure of DNA-cationic liposome complexes: DNA intercalation in multilamellar membranes in distinct interhelical packing regimes. Science 275:810–814

23. Koltover I, Salditt T, Radler JO, Safinya CR (1998) An inverted hexagonal phase of cationic liposome-DNA complexes related to DNA release and delivery. Science 281:78–81

24. Koltover I, Salditt T, Safinya CR (1999) Phase diagram, stability and overcharging of lamellar cationic lipid-DNA self-assembled complexes. Biophys J 77:915–924

25. Martin-Herranz A, Ahmad A, Evans HM, Ewert KK, Schulze U, Safinya CR (2004) Surface functionalized cationic lipid-DNA complexes for gene delivery: PEGylated lamellar complexes exhibit distinct DNA-DNA interaction regimes. Biophys J 96:1160–1168

26. Ewert KK, Evans HM, Zidovska A, Bouxsein NF, Ahmad A, Safinya CR (2006) A columnar phase of dendritic lipid-based cationic liposome-DNA complexes for gene delivery: hexagonally ordered cylindrical micelles embedded in a DNA honeycomb lattice. J Am Chem Soc 128:3998–4006

27. Shirazi RS, Ewert KK, Leal C, Majzoub RN, Bouxsein NF, Safinya CR (2011) Synthesis and characterization of degradable multivalent cationic lipids with disulfide-bond spacers for gene delivery. Biochim Biophys Acta 1808:2156–2166

28. Silva BFB, Majzoub RN, Chan C-L, Li Y, Olsson U, Safinya CR (2014) PEGylated cationic liposome-DNA complexation in brine is pathway dependent. Biochim Biophys Acta 1838:398–412

29. Helfrich W (1973) Elastic properties of lipid bilayers – theory and possible experiments. Z Naturforsch C C28:693–703

30. Seddon JM (1989) Structure of the inverted hexagonal phase and non-lamellar phase transitions of lipids. Biochim Biophys Acta 1031:1–69

31. Gruner SM (1989) Stability of lyotropic phases with curved interfaces. J Phys Chem 93:7562–7570

32. Israelachvili JN (1992) Intermolecular and surface forces, 2nd edn. Academic Press, London

33. Safinya CR, Sirota EB, Roux D, Smith GS (1989) Universality in interacting membranes: the effect of cosurfactants on the interfacial rigidity. Phys Rev Lett 62:1134–1137

34. Bouxsein NF, McAllister CS, Ewert KK, Samuel CE, Safinya CR (2007) Structure and gene silencing activities of monovalent and pentavalent cationic lipid vectors complexed with siRNA. Biochemistry 446:4786–4792

35. Leal C, Bouxsein NF, Ewert KK, Safinya CR (2010) Highly efficient gene silencing activity of siRNA embedded in a nanostructured gyroid cubic lipid matrix. J Am Chem Soc 132:16841–16847

36. Leal C, Ewert KK, Shirazi RS, Bouxsein NF, Safinya CR (2011) Nanogyroids incorporating multivalent lipids: enhanced membrane charge density and pore forming ability for gene silencing. Langmuir 27:7691–7697

37. Majzoub RN, Chan C-L, Ewert KK, Silva BFB, Liang KS, Jacovetty EL, Carragher B, Potter CS, Safinya CR (2014) Uptake and transfection efficiency of PEGylated cationic liposome-DNA complexes with and without RGD-tagging. Biomaterials 35:4996–5005

38. Majzoub RN, Ewert KK, Jacovetty EL, Carragher B, Potter CS, Li Y, Safinya CR (2015) Patterned threadlike micelles and DNA-tethered nanoparticles: a structural study of PEGylated cationic liposome–DNA assemblies. Langmuir 31:7073–7079

39. Lin AJ, Slack NL, Ahmad A, George CX, Samuel CE, Safinya CR (2003) Three-dimensional imaging of lipid gene carriers: membrane charge density controls universal transfection behavior in lamellar cationic liposome-DNA complexes. Biophys J 83:3307–3316

40. Ahmad A, Evans HM, Ewert KK, George CX, Samuel CE, Safinya CR (2005) New multivalent cationic lipids reveal bell curve for transfection efficiency versus membrane charge density: lipid–DNA complexes for gene delivery. J Gene Med 7:739–748

41. Ruoslahti E, Bhatia SN, Sailor MJ (2010) Targeting of drugs and nanoparticles to tumors. J Cell Biol 188:759–768

42. Ruoslahti E (1996) RGD and other recognition sequences for integrins. Annu Rev Cell Dev Biol 12:697–715

43. Temming K, Schiffelers RM, Molema G, Kok RJ (2005) RGD-based strategies for selective delivery of therapeutics and imaging agents to the tumor vasculature. Drug Resist Updat 8:381–402

44. Chan C-L, Majzoub RN, Shirazi RS, Ewert KK, Chen Y-J, Liang KS, Safinya CR (2012) Endosomal escape and transfection efficiency of PEGylated cationic liposome-DNA complexes prepared with and acid-labile PEG-lipid. Biomaterials 33:4928–4935

45. Rehman Z, Hoekstra D, Zuhorn IS (2013) Mechanism of polyplex- and lipoplex-mediated delivery of nucleic acids: real-time visualization of transient membrane destabilization without endosomal lysis. ACS Nano 7:3767–3777

46. Suh J, Wirtz D, Hanes J (2003) Efficient active transport of gene nanocarriers to the cell nucleus. Proc Natl Acad Sci U S A 100:3878–3882

47. Hama S, Akita H, Ito R, Mizuguchi H, Hayakawa T, Harashima H (2006) Quantitative comparison of intracellular trafficking and nuclear transcription between adenoviral and lipoplex systems. Mol Ther 13:786–794

48. Akita H, Ito R, Khalil IA, Futaki S, Harashima H (2004) Quantitative three-dimensional analysis of the intracellular trafficking of plasmid DNA transfected by a nonviral gene delivery system using confocal laser scanning microscopy. Mol Ther 9:443–451

49. Gilleron J, Querbes W, Zeigerer A, Borodvsky A, Marisco G, Schubert U, Manygoats K, Seifert S, Andree C, Stoter M, Epstein-Barash H, Zhang L, Koeliansky V, Fitzgerald K, Fava E, Bickle M, Kalaidzidis Y, Akinc A, Maier M, Zerial M (2013) Image-based analysis of lipid nanoparticle-mediated siRNA delivery, intracellular trafficking and endosomal escape. Nat Biotechnol 31:638 646

50. Sahay G, Querbes W, Alabi C, Eltoukhy A, Sarkar S, Zurenko C, Karagiannis E, Love K, Chen D, Zoncu R, Buganim Y, Schroeder A, Langer R, Anderson D (2013) Efficiency of siRNA delivery by lipid nanoparticles is limited by endocytic recycling. Nat Biotechnol 31:653–658

51. Adil MM, Erdman ZS, Kokkoli E (2014) Transfection mechanisms of polyplexes, lipoplexes, and stealth liposomes in α5β1 integrin bearing DLD-1 colorectal cancer cells. Langmuir 30.3802 3810

52. Crocker JR, Grier DG (1996) Methods of digital video microscopy for colloidal studies. J Colloid Interface Sci 179:298–310

53. Majzoub RN, Chan CL, Ewert KK, Silva BFB, Liang KS, Safinya CR (2015) Fluorescence

microscopy colocalization of lipid-nucleic acid nanoparticles with wildtype and mutant Rab5-GFP: a platform for investigating early endosomal events. Biochim Biophys Acta 1848:1308–1318

54. Rehman Z, Hoekstra D, Zuhorn IS (2011) Protein kinase A inhibition modulates the intracellular routing of gene delivery vehicles in HeLa cells, leading to productive transfection. J Control Release 156:76–84

55. Sharma VD, Lees J, Hoffman NE, Brailoiu E, Madesh M, Wunder SL, Ilies MA (2014) Modulation of pyridinium cationic lipid–DNA complex properties by pyridinium gemini surfactants and its impact on lipoplex transfection properties. Mol Pharm 11:545–599

56. Stenmark H (2009) Rab GTPases as coordinators of vesicle traffic. Nat Rev Mol Cell Biol 10:513–525

57. Costes SV, Daelemans D, Cho EH, Dobbin Z, Pavlakis G, Lockett S (2004) Automatic and quantitative measurement of protein-protein colocalization in live cells. Biophys J 86: 3993–4003

Targeted Delivery of Peptide-Tagged DNA Lipoplexes to Hepatocellular Carcinoma Cells

Mario Ariatti

Abstract

The application of homing peptides to direct DNA and RNA lipoplexes to target cells is a rapidly evolving area of study, which may find application in corrective gene therapy for the treatment of neoplasms and other disorders of a genetic origin. Here, a step-wise account of the assembly and characterization of hepatocellular carcinoma cell-specific DNA lipoplexes and their cytotoxicity assessment in and delivery to the human hepatocellular carcinoma cell line HepG2 is given.

Key words Lipoplex, Hepatocellular carcinoma, Homing-peptide, Targeting, Gene delivery

1 Introduction

Hepatocellular carcinoma (HCC) is one of the leading causes of cancer-related mortality worldwide [1] and its incidence is particularly high in East Asia and sub-Saharan Africa, where the occurrence of Hepatitis B is also elevated [2, 3]. Treatment modalities for this condition are limited and gene therapy approaches that introduce corrective nucleic acids into tumour cells may offer a promising new avenue, which could be considered alongside transplantation, surgical resection, and trans-catheter chemoembolization (TACE). Although the asialoglycoprotein receptor (ASGP-R), which is over-expressed on HCC cells, has been widely exploited to direct ligand-tagged liposome-DNA complexes (lipoplexes) to HCC cells in nonviral gene therapy approaches [4–6], this receptor is also expressed on normal hepatocytes. An alternative, more specific, approach involves the tagging of lipoplexes with peptide ligands that specifically recognize HCC cells and not healthy hepatocytes (Fig. 1). In this regard, biopanning of phage display libraries, and other techniques, have identified a hexapeptide (FQHPSF sequence) [7], a heptapeptide HCBP1 (FGHPSFI sequence) [8] and the dodecamers AM-2 (SLSLITMLKISR sequence) [9] and

Gabriele Candiani (ed.), *Non-Viral Gene Delivery Vectors: Methods and Protocols*, Methods in Molecular Biology, vol. 1445, DOI 10.1007/978-1-4939-3718-9_7, © Springer Science+Business Media New York 2016

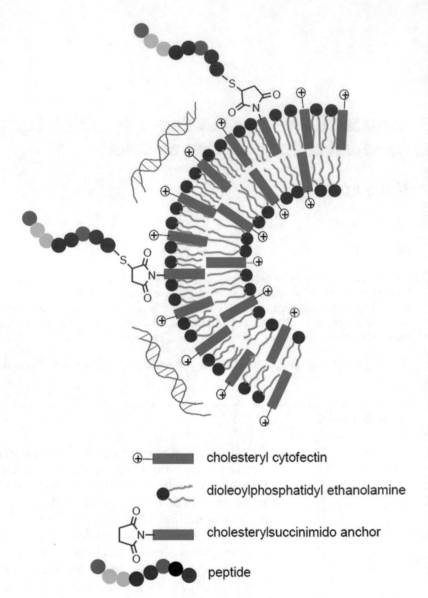

cholesteryl cytofectin

dioleoylphosphatidyl ethanolamine

cholesterylsuccinimido anchor

peptide

Fig. 1 Covalent attachment of homing peptide to unilamellar liposomal bilayer and electrostatic binding of cargo DNA. Drawing not to scale

SP94 (SFSIIHTPILPL sequence) [10]. HCBP1 has been tagged to cationic liposomes with and without a poly(ethylene glycol) spacer for gene delivery [11, 12] although no advantage was gained by inclusion of the polymer in the delivery of plasmid DNA (pDNA) to the human hepatoma HepG2 and human embryo kidney HEK293 cells in vitro [12]. Here the incorporation of HCBP1 into cationic liposomes containing the cytofectin 3β-[N-(N',N'-dimethylaminopropane)-carbamoyl]-cholesterol (Chol-T) [13], or its commercially available lower homologue 3β-[N-(N',N'-dimethylaminoethane)-carbamoyl]-cholesterol (DC-Chol) [14], and the neutral co-lipid dioleoylphosphatidylethanolamine (DOPE),

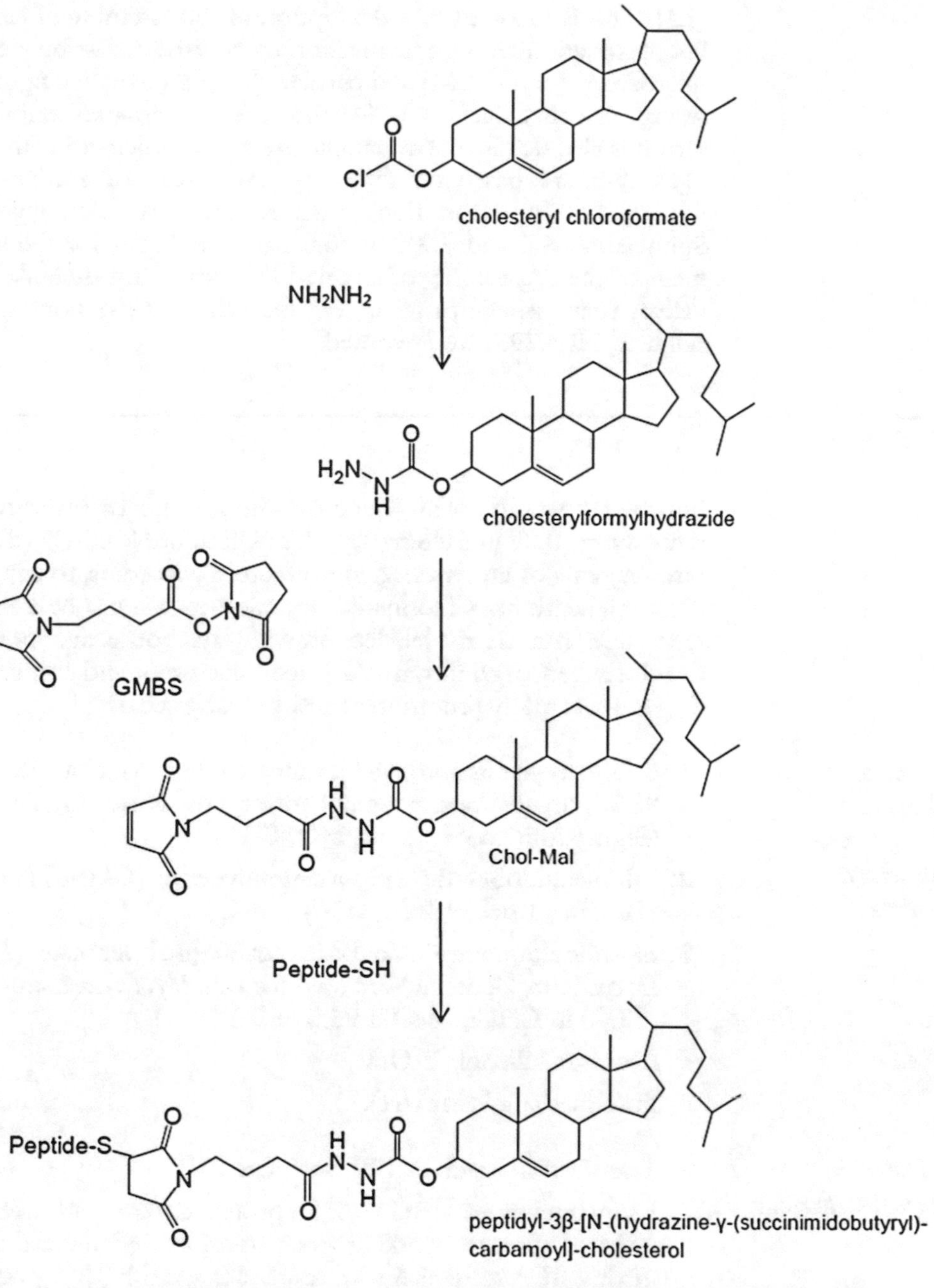

Fig. 2 Reaction scheme to illustrate the synthesis of Chol-Mal and its reaction with peptide HCBP1-Cys. GMBS: 4-maleimidobutyric acid succinimidyl ester; Chol-Mal: 3β-[-(hydrazine-γ-maleimidobutyryl)-carbamoyl]-cholesterol. Figure reprinted, with permission, from ref. 12. *Copyright© American Scientific Publishers*

is described. The procedure entails the reaction of the SH group from a cysteine residue, which has been attached to the C-terminal of HCBP1 (HCBP1-Cys), and a liposomal membrane-embedded maleimido moiety linked to a cholesteryl anchor (3β-[*N*-(hydrazine-γ-maleimidobutyryl)-carbamoyl]-cholesterol) (Chol-Mal) (Fig. 2)

[12]. This is followed by a description of the assembly of targeted lipoplexes and their characterization by cryo-transmission electron microscopy (cryo-TEM) and particle sizing by dynamic light scattering. A convenient assay for the study of lipoplex stability in serum is also detailed. Two simple methods, which are commonly used, but are based on different principles, for studying the liposome-DNA association process, are also described (*see* Subheading 3.5 and 3.7). In conclusion methods for the assessment of the cytotoxicity of targeted lipoplexes and their ability to deliver their genetic cargo to HepG2 cells and the non-targeted cell line, HEK293, are presented.

2   Materials

For the preparation of all aqueous solutions, use 18 MΩ-cm resistivity water (0.22 μm-filtered), such as Ultrapure Milli-Q® (dH₂O). Use reagents of analytical grade and store according to suppliers' recommendations. Chlorinated organic waste must be collected separately in a clearly labeled brown glass bottle and not with unchlorinated organic waste. All manufacturers and institutional disposal and safety procedures must be observed.

2.1   Reagents and Materials for the Synthesis of Cholesteryl Derivatives

1. 3-Dimethylaminopropyl-1-amine, cholesteryl chloroformate, 98% pure hydrazine monohydrate (*see* **Note 1**), DC-Chol (Sigma-Aldrich, St. Louis, MO, USA).

2. 4-Maleimidobutyric acid succinimidyl ester (GMBS) (Thermo Scientific, Rockford, IL, USA).

3. Flexible aluminum-backed silica gel 60 thin layer plates (Merck, Darmstadt, Germany) are used for thin layer chromatography (TLC) in CHCl₃:MeOH 95:5 or 9:1 (v/v).

4. Absolute ethanol (EtOH).

5. Pure methanol (MeOH).

2.2   Liposome and Lipoplex Reagents

1. Transfection grade DOPE (*see* **Note 2**).

2. Bicinchoninic acid (BCA) kit for protein determination (Sigma-Aldrich). Prepare working stock solution fresh before use by mixing BCA reagent A with reagent B in a 50:1 (v/v) ratio.

3. Peptide HCBP1-Cys (sequence FGHPSFIC) (GL Biochem, Shanghai, China) (*see* **Note 3**).

4. 3β-[*N*-(*N'*, *N'*-dimethylaminopropane)-carbamoyl]-cholesterol (Chol-T) (*see* **Note 4**).

5. 2-[-(2-hydroxyethyl)-piperazinyl]-ethanesulfonic acid (HEPES)—buffered saline (1× HBS): 20 mM HEPES pH 7.5, 150 mM NaCl. Dissolve 1.19 g of HEPES and 2.19 g of NaCl in 200 mL of dH₂O. Adjust pH to 7.5 by drop-wise addition of 4 M NaOH. Mix

and adjust volume to 250 mL with dH_2O (see **Note 5**). Sterilize solution by autoclaving. Store at 4 °C.

6. pCMV-luc pDNA (Plasmid Factory, Bielefeld, Germany) (see **Note 6**).

7. Vortex mixer.

8. Bath-type sonicator (ELMA transonic H/60, 35 kHz or similar).

2.3 Components for Characterization of Lipoplexes

1. UltraPure™ agarose (Life Technologies, Invitrogen, Carlsbad, CA, USA).

2. Negative stain for electron microscopy: 2 % (w/v) uranyl acetate. Weigh 100 mg of uranyl acetate in a 10 mL glass beaker and dissolve in 4 mL of dH_2O. Transfer to 5 mL volumetric flask and make up to volume (see **Notes 5** and **7**).

3. 6× gel loading buffer: 40 % (w/v) sucrose, 0.5 % (w/v) bromophenol blue. Weigh 4 g of sucrose and 50 mg of bromophenol blue in a 25 mL glass beaker. Dissolve in 8 mL of dH_2O and make up to 10 mL. Store the solution at 4 °C (see **Note 8**).

4. 10× electrophoresis buffer: 360 mM Tris(hydroxymethyl)-aminomethane hydrochloride (Tris–HCl), 300 mM of sodium phosphate (NaH_2PO_4), 100 mM of ethylenediaminetetraacetic acid (EDTA) disodium salt, pH 7.5. Weigh 14.18 g of Tris–HCl, 9.00 g of NaH_2PO_4, and 9.31 g of EDTA disodium dihydrate into a 500 mL beaker. Dissolve in 200 mL of dH_2O with gentle stirring (glass rod or magnetic stirrer). Check pH and adjust with diluted Tris base or Tris–HCl solutions, if necessary. Dilute up to 250 mL with dH_2O in volumetric flask (see **Note 5**). Store at 4 °C. The final concentrations of a 1× solution are: 36 mM Tris–HCl, 30 mM NaH_2PO_4, 10 mM EDTA, pH 7.5.

5. 10× EDTA solution: 100 mM EDTA, pH 8.0. Weigh 3.72 g EDTA disodium dihydrate into a 250 mL beaker and dissolve in 80 mL of dH_2O. Adjust pH to 8.0 with 1 M NaOH solution. Make up to 100 mL with dH_2O in a volumetric flask (see **Note 5**).

6. 10× sodium dodecyl sulfate solution (SDS): 5 % (w/v) SDS solution. Transfer 1.25 g of SDS into a 50 mL beaker. Dissolve in 20 mL of dH_2O (see **Note 9**). Transfer into a 25 mL volumetric flask and make up to volume (see **Note 5**).

7. Prepare a stock solution of ethidium bromide (EtBr) for inclusion in agarose gels by weighing 1 mg and dissolving in 1 mL of dH_2O (label container clearly with warning). To avoid weighing EtBr, a stock solution of 10 mg/mL may be purchased. The concentration of EtBr in the gel after addition of 20 µL of 1 mg/mL EtBr stock solution is 1 µg/µL (see **Note 30**).

8. Agarose gel: Suspend 0.2 g agarose powder in 18 mL water and heat to boiling point while stirring using a hot plate and magnetic stirrer. Continue boiling until all agarose has dissolved and a clear particle-free solution is obtained. Cool the solution to 75 °C. Add

2 mL of 10× electrophoresis buffer and 20 μL of 1 mg/mL EtBr solution. Mix thoroughly and pour into a gel-casting tray, taped at the open ends to contain the liquid agarose solution, and containing an 8-sample comb (*see* **Note 31**). Allow the gel to solidify and to cool to room temperature (RT) for about 45 min. Place the tray in the electrophoresis apparatus and gently add 1× electrophoresis buffer bringing the level of buffer to about 5 mm above the surface of the gel.

9. Use a Bio-Rad PowerPac™ (or similar) for electrophoresis.

10. View agarose gels in a Syngene G: Box Gel Documentation System (Syngene, Cambridge, UK).

11. Shimadzu RF-551 spectrofluorometric detector.

12. Leica Microsystems EM CPC Cryo workstation (Leica, Vienna, Austria).

13. Injector spring-loaded Gatan cryo-transfer system (Gatan Inc., Munich, Germany) for vitrification of sample.

14. Cryo-TEM (JEOL JEM-1010 electron microscope, Jeol, Tokyo, Japan).

15. MegaView III digital camera for capturing cryo-TEM images and processing using the Universal Imaging Platform software (Olympus, Münster, Germany).

16. Dynamic light scattering (DLS) analyser (Malvern ZetaSizer Nano-ZS instrument, Malvern Instruments, Worcestershire, UK) for determination of hydrodynamic size distribution and ζ-potential of nanoparticles. Data are recorded on ZetaSizer software (version 6.30).

2.4 Components for Cell Culture Studies

1. HEK293 cells (ATCC© CRL-1573™, *Homo sapiens*, embryonic kidney), HepG2 cells (ATCC© HB-8065™ *Homo sapiens*, hepatocellular carcinoma) (American Type Culture Collection, Manassas, VA, USA) (*see* **Note 10**).

2. Sterile disposable plasticware.

3. Phosphate-buffered saline (PBS) tablets. Dissolve one tablet in 1 L of dH_2O to a final concentration of 140 mM NaCl, 10 mM phosphate, and 3 mM KCl, pH 7.4, at 25 °C. Autoclave and store in 100–250 mL aliquots at 4 °C.

4. Cell culture medium: Eagle's Minimum Essential Medium (EMEM) supplemented with L-glutamine, Trypsin-Versene® (0.5 mg/mL of trypsin, 0.2 mg/mL of EDTA), 5000 I.U./mL potassium penicillin, 5 mg/mL of streptomycin sulfate. Store at 4 °C and warm to 37 °C prior to use.

5. Fetal Calf Serum (FCS) (Highveld Biological, Sandton, South Africa) (*see* **Notes 10** and **11**). Store at −20 °C.

6. Complete medium: Working in a biosafety hood, add 5.6 mL of penicillin-streptomycin stock solution and 28 mL of FCS to 250 mL EMEM and mix thoroughly. The complete medium, which contains 10% (v/v) FCS, 100 U/mL of penicillin, and 100 μg/mL of streptomycin, should be stored at 4 °C. Note that some laboratories work with half the above concentrations of antibiotics. The antimycotic agent Fungizone® is also often used at 0.25–2.5 μg/mL.

7. Freezing medium: Prepare by adding 0.1 mL of dimethylsulfoxide (DMSO) to 0.9 mL complete medium. Mix and equilibrate at 22 °C. Prepare fresh, prior to use.

8. 3-(4,5-dimethylthiazol-2-yl)-2,5-diphenyltetrazolium (MTT) bromide salt.

9. Sterile-filtered DMSO.

10. Luciferase assay kit (Promega Corporation, Madison, WI, USA).

11. 1× cell culture lysis reagent: 25 mM Tris-phosphate, pH 7.8, 2 mM dithiothreitol (DTT), 2 mM 1,2-diaminocyclohexane-N,N,N',N' tetraacetic acid, 10% glycerol, 1% Triton®X-100.

12. Microplate reader.

13. Orbital shaker.

14. Lumac Biocounter M1500.

3 Methods

3.1 Synthesis of Cholesteryl Derivatives

3.1.1 3β-[N-(N',N'-Dimethylaminopropane)-carbamoyl]-cholesterol (Chol-T)

The synthesis of this cholesteryl cytofectin is adapted from a procedure described elsewhere for its close relative DC-Chol [14].

1. Dissolve 2.29 mL (18.2 mmol) dimethylaminopropylamine in 3 mL of CHCl$_3$ (see **Note 12**) and chill to 0 °C. Add drop-wise to an ice-cold solution of 2.25 g (5 mmol) cholesteryl chloroformate in 5 mL of CHCl$_3$ over 5–10 min (see **Note 13**).

2. Stopper and store the reaction flask at RT in the dark for 1 h (see **Note 14**), after which the solvent has to be carefully removed by rotary evaporation under reduced pressure (see **Note 15**).

3. Redissolve the residue, which may appear as a viscous, straw colored oil, in 5 mL (or less) hot absolute EtOH and cool to 4 °C. Store for 24 h at 4 °C.

4. Isolate the crystalline product on a small Hirsch funnel, taking care to use a loose fitting paper disc (Whatman No. 1 or equivalent) (see **Note 16**). Wash the crystalline product in 1 or 2 mL of ice-cold absolute EtOH by pouring it over the product in the funnel, under suction.

5. Dry the product in a drying pistol (Büchi or similar) at 60 °C for 1 h and store it in a sample vial at −20 °C (see **Note 17**).

The synthesis of Chol-Mal is achieved in two reaction steps (Fig. 2). Cholesteryl chloroformate reacts with hydrazine in a dehydrohalogenation reaction to afford cholesterylformylhydrazide. The primary amino functionality in cholesterylformylhydrazide is then acylated by GMBS, which features a reactive N-hydroxysuccinimidyl ester, to give Chol-Mal.

1. Dissolve 1.13 g (2.5 mmol) cholesteryl chloroformate in 5 mL $CHCl_3$ and chill to 0 °C. Add this in a steady drop-wise manner to 380 µL (7.5 mmol) hydrazine monohydrate in 3 mL $CHCl_3$ and 1 mL of MeOH at 0 °C, while swirling. Stopper solution and allow warming to RT, while stirring using a magnetic bar.

2. Check for completion of reaction, after 30 min, by TLC (*see* **Note 14**). The product retardation factor (R_f) is about 0.6 ($CHCl_3$:MeOH = 9:1, v/v).

3. Remove solvent and excess of hydrazine hydrate by rotary evaporation (*see* **Note 15**).

4. Dissolve the white crystalline mass in 5–10 mL of $CHCl_3$ and extract hydrazine hydrochloride into 5–10 mL dH_2O by using a 25 mL separating funnel. Re-extract the $CHCl_3$ layer once more with 5–10 mL of dH_2O.

5. Dry the $CHCl_3$ layer over anhydrous Na_2SO_4 (*see* **Note 18**) and filter into a Quickfit® round-bottomed flask and evaporate the solvent by rotary evaporation (*see* **Notes 15**).

6. The crystalline product, cholesterylformylhydrazide, may be recrystallized from hot absolute EtOH containing a small amount of $CHCl_3$ (*see* **Note 19**).

7. Dissolve 14 mg (50 µmol) of GMBS in 200 µL of $CHCl_3$. Add 22.2 mg (50 µmol) of cholesterylformylhydrazide in a Quickfit® round-bottomed flask. Incubate overnight at RT in the dark. Evaporate the solvent by rotary evaporation (*see* **Note 15**).

8. Extract the product with 500 µL of dH_2O (repeat twice). The residual dH_2O is removed by rotary evaporation and Chol-Mal is obtained in a pure state by recrystallization from a minimal amount of hot absolute EtOH (*see* **Note 20**).

3.2 Preparation of Targeted Liposomes

1. Prepare stock solutions of 514.45 Da Chol-T, 744.03 Da DOPE, and 609.58 Da Chol-Mal in $CHCl_3$ (*see* **Notes 2** and **21**).

2. Dispense 1.03 mg (2 µmol) of Chol-T, 1.43 mg (1.92 µmol) of DOPE, and 49 µg (0.08 µmol) Chol-Mal (*see* **Note 21**) into a pyrex test tube fitted with a ground glass socket. Remove solvent by rotary evaporation under reduced pressure (*see* **Note 22**).

3. Place aluminum foil over socket and position tube in a pistol drier and heat at 40 °C overnight under vacuum to remove residual solvent, which is toxic to mammalian cells.

4. Add 1 mL of sterile HBS, seal and rotate tube manually to bring lipidic material into contact with buffer. Allow the film to hydrate overnight at 4 °C (*see* **Note 23**).

5. Vigorously agitate for 5 min in a manner that permits the suspension to remain at the bottom of the tube by using a vortex mixer. Sonicate the hazy suspension of multilamellar liposomes in a bath-type sonicator for 5 min at 22 °C (*see* **Note 24**). The unilamellar liposome suspension may be stored under N_2 in amber glass vials at 4 °C.

6. Add 313 μg (0.32 μmol, fourfold excess) of peptide HCBP1-Cys in 0.2 mL HBS to a 1 mL of liposome suspension. Stir gently and store overnight at RT in the dark. Dialyze against 300 mL of HBS at 4 °C with 3 changes over 48 h (*see* **Note 25**). Targeted liposomes are stored under N_2 at 4 °C.

7. Determine the peptide concentration in the liposome preparation in test tubes by the BCA method [16] (*see* **Note 26**).

3.3 Preparation of Lipoplexes

1. Prepare lipoplexes in 0.5 mL microcentrifuge tubes at 4 °C by adding 0.5 μg of pDNA in 2.0 μL of dH_2O to liposome suspensions of 0.0–18 μg lipid in 10 μL of HBS, to achieve DNA (–ve): cationic liposome (+ve) charge ratios in the range 1:0–1:7 (*see* **Note 27**).

2. Briefly vortex the mixtures and spin them in a microcentrifuge at $13,000 \times g$, to bring the entire sample to the bottom of the tube, and mature at RT for 30 min before use (*see* Subheading 3.9, **step 3**).

3.4 Liposome and Lipoplex Characterization

3.4.1 Cryo-TEM

1. Dilute 1:4 (v/v) liposome suspensions and lipoplexes at end-point ratios (*see* legend of Fig. 4) in HBS for cryo-TEM studies.

2. Apply 1 μL of the diluted suspensions to copper grids (coated with Formvar and a layer of carbon for added strength) and stain with 1 μL of 2 % uranyl acetate solution for 1 min. Remove excess liquid using a filter paper tip (Whatman No. 5).

3. Vitrify the sample by immersing the grid in liquid propane at –170 °C using an injector spring-loaded Leica Microsystems EM CPC Cryo workstation.

4. Transfer the grid using a Gatan cryo-transfer system in liquid N_2 and observe samples on a Cryo-TEM microscope operating at an accelerating voltage of 100 kV. Capture the images with a digital camera and process using the software (*see* **Note 28** and Fig. 3).

3.4.2 Zetasizing

1. Dilute 1:19 (v/v) liposome suspensions in HBS.

2. Dilute 1:100 (v/v) lipoplex preparations in HBS.

3. Transfer 1 mL of diluted samples in semi-micro disposable polystyrene cuvettes for sizing in a dynamic light scattering (DLS) apparatus at 25 °C (*see* **Note 29**). Take three measurements per sample.

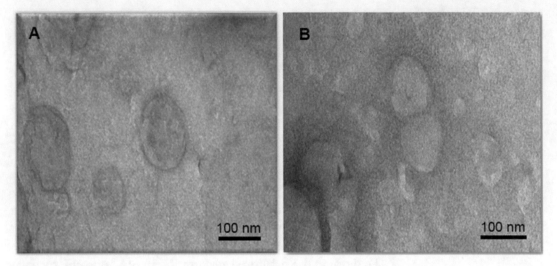

Fig. 3 Cryo-TEM images of (**a**) targeted liposomes and (**b**) targeted lipoplexes. (**a**) Reprinted, with permission, from ref. 12. *Copyright© American Scientific Publishers*

3.5 Liposome-DNA Gel Retardation Binding Assay

1. Assemble eight lipoplexes by varying pDNA:liposome ratios (*see* Subheading **3.3**, **steps 1** and **2**).

2. Add 2–3 μL of 6× gel loading buffer to each preparation and vortex briefly followed by $13,000 \times g$ centrifugation for 30 s, to collect the entire sample at the bottom of the microcentrifuge tube.

3. Load samples in the wells of agarose gel (*see* **Note 32**). Carry out electrophoresis (60–90 min) at 50 V.

4. Remove tray from apparatus and drain excess buffer from edge of tilted tray with paper towel or filter paper.

5. View gel under transillumination at $\lambda = 300$ nm (*see* **Note 33**).

3.6 Serum Nuclease Digestion Assay

1. Prepare lipoplexes at −ve/+ve charge ratios from below (1:1) to above (1:3) the end-point ratio (1:2) (Fig. 4, lane 3) using 1 μg of pCMV-luc as described in Subheading **3.3**.

2. Add FCS to a final concentration of 20 % (v/v). Mix by agitation, avoiding frothing, and incubate at 37 °C for 4 h.

3. Add 10× stock solutions of EDTA and SDS to achieve final concentrations of 10 mM and 0.5 % (w/v), respectively.

4. Vortex and spin ($13,000 \times g$, 30 s) at RT and incubate at 55 °C for 20 min.

5. Add 6× gel loading buffer to each lipoplex and subject to electrophoresis (*see* Subheading **3.5**, **steps 2** and **3**).

6. Include the following two controls: 1 μg of an untreated pDNA sample (Fig. 5, lane 1) and 1 μg of uncomplexed DNA,

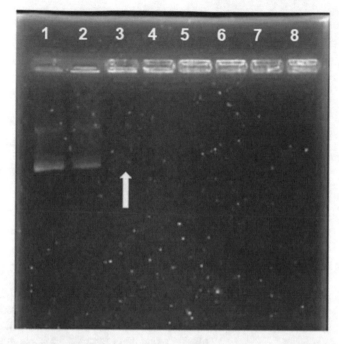

Fig. 4 Gel retardation assay. Incubation mixtures in HBS containing 0.5 µg of pCMV-luc pDNA and increasing amounts of liposome suspension to achieve −ve/+ve charge ratios of 1:1, 1:2, 1:3, 1:4, 1:5, 1:6, and 1:7 in *lanes 2–8,* respectively. *Lane 1* contained naked pDNA. *White arrow* indicates end-point ratio (1:2). Figure reprinted, with permission, from ref. 12. *Copyright© American Scientific Publishers*

which has been treated with 20 % FCS, as described (*see* Subheading 3.6, **steps 2–4**) (Fig. 5, lane 2) (*see* **Note 34**).

3.7 Ethidium Bromide (EtBr) Displacement Assay

1. Add 10 µL (1 µg) of EtBr solution (*see* **Note 35**), at 100 µg/mL, to 500 µL of HBS in a quartz cuvette with four polished sides.

2. Read fluorescence at $\lambda_{em} = 520$ nm and at $\lambda_{ex} = 600$ nm using a spectrofluorometric detector. Set this value to read 0 % relative fluorescence (RF).

3. Add 24 µL (6 µg) of a pCMV-luc DNA solution containing 0.25 µg/µL in dH_2O. Mix and read the fluorescence. Set this value to 100 % RF.

4. Add 2 µL of targeted liposome suspension at 2.5 µg/µL in HBS. Mix and allow 1 min for equilibration. Measure RF and repeat this process until a plateau in readings has been attained (*see* **Notes 35** and **36**).

5. Plot RF (%) against amount of liposome suspension added (expressed in µg of lipid) (*see* Fig. 6).

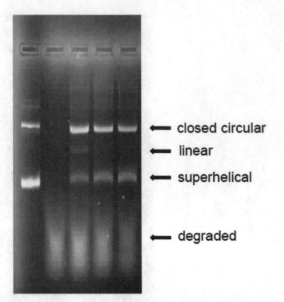

Fig. 5 Nuclease protection assay of DNA associated with lipoplexes, in the presence of 20 % FCS. Reaction mixtures contained 1 µg of pCMV-luc DNA and increasing amounts of targeted liposome suspension. *Lanes 3–5* (1:1, 1:2, 1:3 −ve/+ve charge ratios). *Lane 1*: untreated marker pCMV-luc DNA and *lane 2*: pDNA incubated with 20 % FCS. Figure reprinted, with permission, from ref. 12. *Copyright© American Scientific Publishers*

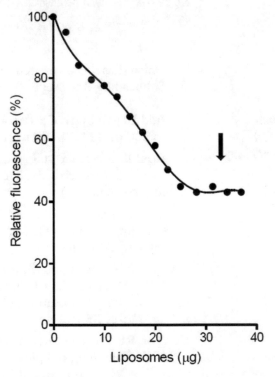

Fig. 6 Ethidium bromide (EtBr) displacement assay. pCMV-luc (6 µg) in 500 µL of HBS containing 1 µg of EtBr was treated with increasing amounts of targeted liposome suspension up to 40 µg. *Black arrow* indicates plateau region of curve

3.8 Maintenance, Storage, and Propagation of Cells

For requirements and guidelines relating to animal cell culture, *see* **Note 37**. Procedures for the thawing, maintenance and propagation, and cryopreservation of the mammalian cell lines used in cytotoxicity and transfection studies are detailed in **Notes 38–40** respectively.

3.9 Transfection Experiments

1. Seed cells at a density of $2.0–3.0 \times 10^4$ cells/cm^2 in a flat-bottomed 48-well cell culture plate in 250–300 μL of culture medium per well. Seal plate with adhesive film, apply lid, and incubate at 37 °C in an incubator for 24 h to permit full attachment of cells and to achieve at least 50% confluence (*see* **Note 38**).

2. After 24 h, remove old medium from wells by aspiration using a sterile narrow-tipped pipette and replace with 300 μL of serum-free medium (*see* **Note 42**). Tilt the plate slightly and apply the pipette tip at the edge of the well without disturbing the cell monolayer

3. Add to each well the desired amount of lipoplex suspension containing 1 μg of pCMV-luc and varying amounts of targeted liposome suspension in a final volume of 10 μL (*see* **Note 43**). Seal plate with a new adhesive film. Briefly rock the plate manually or mechanically on a shaker, at 30 revolutions/min, to ensure an even distribution of lipoplexes.

4. Incubate at 37 °C, 5% CO_2 in humidified atmosphere for 4 h, then aspirate the old medium from each well and replace with 250–300 μL of complete medium. Seal plate with adhesive film, close with lid, and incubate for 48 h at 37 °C.

3.10 Cell Viability Assay

The cell viability assay adopted here is based on the mitochondrial reduction of MTT (*see* **Note 44**). Follow Subheading 3.9 (**steps 1–4**).

1. Forty eight hours after transfection, remove the old medium from each well.

2. Add 200 μL/well of complete medium and 200 μL/well of MTT solution at 5 mg/mL in PBS. Seal the plate and briefly rock gently in a shaker. Thereafter incubate the plate at 37 °C for 4 h.

3. Remove the medium bathing the cells completely.

4. Add 200 μL/well of DMSO to dissolve the formazan which has formed in viable cells. Place the plate on a platform shaker, which has been set at 30 revolutions/min, for 1 h.

5. Read the absorbance at $\lambda = 575$ nm using a fluorescence microplate reader (*see* **Note 45**). Correlate cell viability (%) directly with absorbances (*see* Fig. 7). Calculate cell viability as:

$$\text{Percentage cell viability} = [\text{Abs}_{575nm}\text{treated cells}] / [\text{Abs}_{575nm}\text{untreated cells}] \times 100.$$

3.11 Transfection Studies Using the Luciferase Expression Assay

For points that must be considered in selecting a reporter gene assays, *see* **Note 47**.

3.11.1 Transfection Protocol

Forty eight hours after transfection (*see* Subheading 3.9, **steps 1–4**), remove old medium from each well and carry out protein determinations (*see* Subheading 3.11.3) and determine luciferase activity (*see* Subheading 3.11.4).

3.11.2 Peptide Competition Experiment

1. Dissolve 2.0 mg of HCBP1 in 200 μL HBS to afford a 10 mM solution of the peptide.

2. Seed cells in 48-well cell culture plate (*see* Subheading 3.9, **step 1**).

3. Add 300 μL/well of serum-free medium.

4. Add 15 μL/well of the peptide solution at least in triplicate. This will achieve a final concentration of 0.5 mM free peptide in each well.

5. Add the lipoplex suspensions and proceed as described in Subheading 3.9 (**steps 3** and **4**).

3.11.3 Bicinchoninic Acid Protein Assay

1. Forty eight hours after transfection, remove old medium from 48-well plates and rinse the cells with 250 μL PBS (repeat at least twice) (*see* **Note 46**).

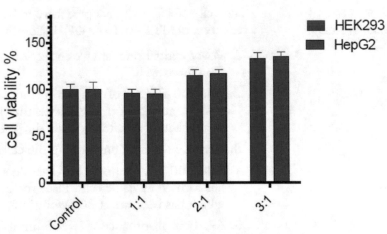

Fig. 7 Cell viability studies conducted with pCMV-luc pDNA-targeted liposome complexes (lipoplexes) on HepG2 and HEK293 cell lines. Incubation mixtures (300 μL) contained 1 μg of pDNA in lipoplex form at different −ve/+ve charge ratios as indicated. Control: untreated cells. Figure reprinted, with permission, from ref. 12. *Copyright© American Scientific Publishers*

2. Add 80 μL/well of 1× cell culture lysis reagent. Place the plate on a platform shaker operating at 30 revolutions/min for 15 min at RT.

3. Transfer cell lysates and debris into 500 μL microcentrifuge tubes and centrifuge at 12,000 rpm for 2 min at RT. Retain clear supernatants.

4. Prepare a set of bovine serum albumin (BSA) standards in 1.5 mL microcentrifuge tubes by dissolving BSA in dH$_2$O at different concentrations, covering the range 0–30 μg of proteins with increments of 5 μg/50 μL.

5. Dispense 50 μL of each standard and clear cell lysates into 1.5 mL microcentrifuge tubes.

6. Add 1 mL of BCA working stock solution to each sample.

7. Incubate all samples at 37 °C for 30 min.

8. After cooling to RT, dispense 200 μL of each sample into a 96-well plate.

9. Read the absorbance values at $\lambda = 540$ nm in a microplate reader.

10. Obtain the soluble protein content in the lysates by extrapolation from the standard curve.

3.11.4 Luciferase Assay

1. Pipette a 20 μL aliquot of each cell lysate supernatant (*see* Subheading 3.11.3, **step 3**) into a cuvette.

2. Add 100 μL/well of luciferase assay reagent (*see* **Note 48**). Vortex the sample for 10 s.

3. Insert cuvettes into a luminometer and record relative light units (RLUs) emitted for 10 s (*see* **Note 49**).

4. Normalize RLU value of each sample with the corresponding protein content to afford RLUs/mg protein.

3.12 Note on Experimental Design

Although the protocols described here have focussed on a hepatoma-targeting peptide, a parallel set of experiments must be conducted with liposomes tagged with a scrambled peptide sequence of the same length and composed of the same amino acids [11, 12].

4 Notes

1. Exercise extreme caution when handling hydrazine hydrate (a liquid). It is toxic if swallowed, causes severe skin burns and eye damage, and should be considered a potential human carcinogen. It is also very toxic to the environment. Only purchase amounts required. Dispense in a fume hood and wear a protective laboratory coat, gloves, and goggles. Avoid weigh-

ing in an open atmosphere. Rather use a micro-pipetting device or micro syringe. The volume to be dispensed may be calculated readily from its density (1.027).

2. Dissolve transfection grade DOPE in $CHCl_3$ to achieve a concentration of 10 mg/mL. Store under N_2 in 2 mL aliquots in 4 mL brown glass vials with screw tops fitted with septa in a desiccator at –20 °C. Handle $CHCl_3$ with caution throughout. Avoid contact with skin and inhalation. Work in a well-ventilated environment.

3. The manufacturers perform custom syntheses. Purchase about 15–20 mg, as this will suffice for the preparation of several 1 mL batches of tagged liposomes.

4. The preparation of Chol-T is described in Subheading 3.1.1. However, this cytofectin may be replaced in liposome formulations, in the same relative molar quantity, by DC-Chol, a lower homologue of Chol-T, which is readily available (Sigma-Aldrich; Avanti Polar Lipids Inc., Alabaster, AL, USA and elsewhere).

5. Once diluted to the mark in the volumetric flask, stopper and mix thoroughly by inversion.

6. pCMV-luc, a 5566 base pair (bp) pDNA, encodes the firefly (*Photinus pyralis*) luciferase gene, whose expression in animal cells is driven by the cytomegalovirus promoter. It is routinely dissolved in sterile dH_2O to a concentration of 0.25 μg/mL and stored in aliquots of 50 μL in 0.5 mL microcentrifuge tubes at –20 °C. This is to avoid repeated freeze-thaw cycles which may cause some shearing with resultant decrease in the relative amount of superhelical DNA in the sample. This, in turn, would negatively affect efficiencies in transfection experiments. It would be even better to store samples in a biofreezer (–80 °C).

7. Uranyl acetate solutions are weakly radioactive and light sensitive and toxic if ingested. The container should be wrapped in aluminum foil and the solution should be stored at 4 °C. Although stable for several months, filtration may be necessary from time to time.

8. Should last well over 1 year if stored at 4 °C.

9. Stir the mixture while warming gently to effect solution and to reduce frothing to a minimum. The final solution is stored at 4 °C but may require warming before use to redissolve any SDS precipitate, which may have formed on storage.

10. Some countries may impose restrictions on the importation of animal cells and animal by-products. Special permission and/or import licenses may be required.

11. This product has been Gamma-irradiated (2.8–3.2 Mrad) to inactivate all mycoplasma and most viruses without loss of biological efficacy.

12. Dimethylaminopropylamine is irritating to the eyes, skin, and mucous membranes and should be stored, dispensed, and used in a fume hood. The use of goggles, protective clothing, and impervious gloves is strongly advised.

13. The reaction is carried out conveniently in a 25 mL conical or round-bottomed Quickfit® flask with 14/23 or 19/26 ground glass socket, with gentle swirling during drop-wise addition.

14. The reaction may be monitored conveniently by silica gel thin layer chromatography (TLC) in the solvent system $CHCl_3$:MeOH = 9:1 (v/v) and is usually found to have reached completion within 1 h. The flexible aluminum-backed TLC plates may be cut into rectangles measuring 9×2 cm for this purpose. An empty spice jar will serve adequately as a chromatography chamber and will take about 5 mL of solvent. Ensure that the origin, where samples are applied on the plate, is above the level of the solvent. After development, the product and starting materials may be visualized by immersing the TLC plates in an iodine chamber (a few crystals of iodine in a 250 mL jar with ground glass lid) whereupon the cholesteryl-containing compounds will appear as brown spots. Alternatively, the plate may be sprayed lightly with dilute H_2SO_4 solution (approximately 5 N) in the fume hood and heated on a hot plate (in the fume hood). Cholesteryl compounds will appear as strong purple spots that darken on protracted heating. The product, Chol-T, will have a low R_f value (typically about 0.2).

15. The revolving flask is frequently lowered into a water bath at RT to avoid ice build-up on the exterior of the flask during evaporation. Caution should be exercised to avoid bumping. It is recommended that a vacuum pump (single stage or similar) be used as the vacuum source and that a solvent trap (e.g. −50 °C EtOH cold probe) be connected between the rotary evaporator and the vacuum pump.

16. The Hirsch funnel should be fitted to a small Büchner flask and a gentle vacuum applied during the filtration. This process should be rapid to avoid dissolution of the product in the mother liquor.

17. If a drying pistol is not available, the product may be placed in a small flask, attached to the rotary evaporator under slow rotation and immersed in a 60 °C glycerol bath. The vacuum should be 3 Torr or better. Chol-T may be stored at −20 °C for several years without decomposition. Chol-T analytical data: Typical yield: 82%. Melting point: 103–105 °C. ^{1}H NMR (300 MHz, $CDCl_3$): δ 0.65 (s, 3H, CCH_3), 0.83 (d, 6H, J = 5.2 Hz, CH(CH_3)$_2$), 0.89 (d, 3H, J = 6.5 Hz, CHCH_3), 2.19 (s, 6H, (CH_3)$_2$NCH$_2$CH$_2$), 2.3 (t, 2H, J = 6.6 Hz, (CH_3)$_2$NCH_2CH$_2$), 3.21 (q, 2H, J = 6.1 Hz, (CH_3)$_2$NCH$_2$CH$_2$CH_2NH), 4.46 (m, 1H, Chol H$_{3\alpha}$) 5.35 (d, 1H, J = 5.3 Hz, Chol H$_6$). M/z = 514.4490 [M$^+$] [$C_{33}H_{58}N_2O_2$ = 514.4498].

18. Add sufficient anhydrous Na_2SO_4 to achieve a clear $CHCl_3$ solution with free-flowing Na_2SO_4 crystals at the bottom of the container (no clumping).

19. The product obtained after rotary evaporation is already of high purity. Since large volumes of absolute EtOH are required for recrystallization, only recrystallize sufficient material for analytical purposes. The unrecrystallized product is sufficiently pure for the next step in the synthesis of Chol-Mal. Cholesterylformylhydrazide analytical data: Typical yield: 83%. Melting point: 225–227 °C. IR (film) 3416 (b, N-H), 2929 (st, C-H), 1731 (m, C=O), 1495 (m, C=C) cm^{-1}. ^{1}H NMR (300 MHz, DMSO d^6) δ 0.66 (s, 3H, C-CH_3), 0.86 (d, 6H, CH-CH_3), 0.91 (d, 3H, CH-CH_3), 0.99 (s, 3H, C-CH_3), 3.38 (bs, 2H, NH_2), 4.38 (m, 1H, Chol H$_{3\alpha}$), 5.33 (d, 1H, Chol H$_6$), 7.93 (s, 1H, NH). Ms, m/z, ES-TOF 445.44 [M+H$^+$], 467.39 [M+Na$^+$].

20. Chol-Mal is stored in an amber glass vial in a desiccator at 4 °C. Chol-Mal analytical data: Typical yield: 25 mg (85%).^{1}H NMR (300 MHz, CDCl$_3$): δ 0.67 (s, 3H, C-CH_3), 0.85 (d, 6H, J=5.1 Hz, 26-H, 27-H, CH-(CH_3)$_2$), 0.91(d, 3H, J=6.5, 21-H, CH-CH_3), 1.00 (s, 3H, 19-H, C-CH_3), 3.68 (t, 2H, J=6.2, CO-CH_2), 4.55 (m, 1H, Chol H$_{3\alpha}$), 5.37 (d, 1H, J=4.8, Chol H$_6$), 6.72 (s, 2H, maleimido $CH=CH$).

21. Accurately weigh a sample of Chol-T in excess of the amount required (>1.03 mg, 2 μmol) into a 1.5 mL microcentrifuge tube using a balance that reads to 5 decimal places in order to reduce errors. Measure into the tube, the correct volume of $CHCl_3$ required that will afford a stock solution of 10 μg/μL. This is best achieved using a glass microsyringe with Teflon-tipped plunger. The use of air displacement micropipettes is not advised, as the high vapor pressure of $CHCl_3$ may lead to significant errors in volumes dispensed. Place into a separate 0.5 mL microcentrifuge tube, a sample of Chol-Mal of the order of 1 mg and record its weight accurately (see above). Measure into the tube sufficient $CHCl_3$ to achieve a stock solution of 1 μg/μL (see above).

22. Tilt the angle of the tube on the rotary evaporator to about 130–150° from perpendicular. Rotate the tube while increasing the vacuum in stages by placing finger over air intake into the system to avoid bumping. If available, it is better to use dry N_2 for this purpose, and for pressure equilibration, as this minimizes oxidation of the double bond on the DOPE oleoyl moieties. When the system is stable, lower the tube into a water bath at 25 °C and continue until all visible solvent has been removed and the lipidic content has been deposited near the base of the tube. When held up to the light, clear rings of lipidic material should be visible to the naked eye.

23. After overnight storage, the lipidic material is visibly hydrated (swollen and opaque) and some may have already detached from the glass giving the HBS a turbid appearance.

24. The suspension, which takes on an opalescent appearance, typically contains unilamellar vesicles about 100 nm in diameter with a polydispersity index (PDI) < 0.3 (*see* **Note 29**). Lamellarity may be confirmed by transmission electron microscopy (TEM) (*see* Subheading 3.4). If measurements reveal vesicles to be much larger and more polydisperse (PDI > 0.3), sonication times may be increased, or the sample may be passed about ten times through a 200 nm polycarbonate filter followed by ten passes through a 100 nm filter at 22 °C. This may be performed manually using an extruder (Avanti Mini-Extruder or similar) comprised of two glass syringes of 1 mL fitted with metallic Teflon-tipped plungers, which are linked by a filter-housing assembly and mounted on a block which permits regulation of temperature. Generally the greater number of passes the preparation undergoes, the greater is the uniformity in size achieved and the lower the PDI value. PDIs > 0.5 generally suggest a low degree of uniformity.

25. Prepare the dialysis tubing (12,000 MWCO, 23 mm flat width, Sigma-Aldrich) according to the method described by Sambrook, Fritsch, and Maniatis [15]. Briefly, dialysis tubing is cut into 10 cm strips and after rinsing the tubing inside and out with dH_2O, it is boiled for 10 min in 250 mL of 2 % (w/v) sodium bicarbonate (NaH_2CO_3) containing 1 mM EDTA, pH 8.0. The tubing is allowed to cool and is then stored in 1 mM EDTA solution at 4 °C until use. Only handle tubing with gloves and rinse tubing with dH_2O before use.

26. Construct an HCBP1 peptide standard concentration curve for the BCA assay as follows: Dissolve 400 µg of peptide in 800 µL of dH_2O and dispense 50 µL (25 µg), 100 µL (50 µg), and 200 µL (100 µg) into three separate test tubes in triplicate. Adjust volumes to 300 µL with dH_2O and add 30 µL of 1 M NaOH containing 10 % (w/v) SDS to each tube. Heat tubes at 90 °C for 5 min and then cool at RT. Add 3 mL of BCA standard working stock solution to each tube. Incubate tubes at 37 °C for 30 min and cool to RT. Finally determine absorbance of solutions at $\lambda = 570$ nm in standard 1 cm glass cuvettes in a UV/visible spectrophotometer. Set the spectrophotometer against a 300 µL blank of dH_2O treated as described for the standard curve. At the same time, treat four separate aliquots (300 µL) of targeted liposome suspension as described for the standard curve. Correct for any absorbance attributed to the lipidic component of the liposomes by including 250 µL suspensions of untargeted liposomes in the assay. Concentrations of the HCBP1 peptide in the targeted liposome suspension are found to be 29–35 nmol/mL.

27. To calculate –ve/+ve charge ratios of lipoplexes, assume the following: each DNA nucleotide has an average MW of 330 Da and carries one negative charge at the inter-nucleotidic phosphodiester at pH 7.5. It is also assumed that the liposome cationic charge resides in the Chol-T head group (or DC-Chol head group, if using this cytofectin) and that its dimethylamino function is fully protonated at pH 7.5 (one positive charge per molecule of Chol-T). The volume of liposome suspension required to achieve –ve/+ve charge ratios of 1:1–1:3 is extremely small. Consider making an appropriate dilution of the liposome suspension in sterile HBS (such as 1:4) to increase pipetting volumes for these ratios. In cell culture studies, the quantity of DNA is doubled.

28. Liposome and lipoplex suspensions are diluted for cryo-TEM studies to improve fluidity of samples. Cryo-TEM offers a direct visualization of liposomes and liposome complexes, as the preparation procedure preserves their natural state. The liposome and lipoplex dispersions are spread across the holes of a supporting perforated carbon film, then rapidly vitrified, and observed without dehydration. Using this technique, vesicular structures remain undistorted and a number-weighted size distribution may be obtained, which is in general agreement with results obtained by DLS (Fig. 3a, b) [17–19]. However, if samples are aggregated, DLS size estimates will be considerably greater than those obtained by cryo-TEM.

29. Particle size distribution and hydrodynamic diameter are expressed as PDI and intensity-weighted means (Z-average ± SD), respectively. Assume viscosity and refractive index of dispersant to be 0.887 and 1.33, respectively and take readings at a detection angle of 173°.

30. Extreme caution must be exercised when handling EtBr, which is a powerful mutagen. Do not inhale powder dust and avoid all contact with skin and eyes (see **Note 1**). However, EtBr may be replaced altogether by safer DNA intercalators such as SYBR™ Safe (Life technologies, Carlsbad, CA, USA). Cast the gel on a level surface to ensure uniform thickness of the gel. Dispose of agarose gels and EtBr-contaminated solid waste by incineration and EtBr solutions must be disposed as hazardous waste (see refs. 15, 20 for typical protocols).

31. Ensure that the adjustable comb is placed at least 1 cm from one of the taped edges of the tray, and parallel to it. Make sure that there is a uniform clearance of 0.5–1 mm between the base of the teeth on the comb and the casting tray surface. This will generate a well volume of about 12 μL.

32. Care should be taken to lower the micropipette tip (or microsyringe needle) to a position just inside the well, before releas-

ing the sample (blue) slowly. Placement of the electrophoresis apparatus on an opaque white surface may render the process of well loading more visible and therefore easier to control. The high density of the sample will ensure deposition of an even layer of solution from the bottom of the well, revealing a clear interface with the electrophoresis buffer. Do not overfill wells. Ensure that the tray is positioned to permit DNA migration toward the anode.

33. Gel trays are normally UV-transparent so may be placed directly on the viewing surface of the gel documentation system. However, better results are often obtained by gently sliding the gel directly onto the UV-transparent viewing surface of the instrument. Do not place paper on gel as residues will appear as white specs on the gel when viewed (Fig. 4). It is important to clean the viewing surface immediately after use and to dispose of paper as EtBr solid waste. Liposome-bound DNA will appear as pink fluorescent material in the wells. Capture images at 1–2 s exposure times. Liposome: DNA ratio is reached when all of the plasmid DNA is liposome-bound and the lipoplex is said to be electroneutral (Fig. 4, lane 3). At higher liposome:DNA ratios electropositive complexes are formed, which remain in the wells but gather at the cathodic wall as they are too large to enter the gel (Fig. 4, lanes 5–8).

34. In Fig. 5, lane 1 discloses the relative amounts of relaxed closed circular (nicked) and superhelical conformers of the pDNA used in the study, while lane two shows the degradation of naked pDNA by FCS treatment. Lanes 3–5 reveal some nicking of the superhelical form of lipoplex-associated pDNA and a relative increase in the amount of nicked form of the pDNA. At the infra end-point ratio (1:1), some linearized pDNA is also evident (lane 3). Lanes 2–5 show overlapping fragments of degraded low MW DNA (smear). Results obtained in this assay may vary considerably from batch to batch of FCS and with products from different suppliers. However, it is normally unrealistic to expect no signs of DNA degradation. Nevertheless, improved protection against the action of serum nucleases is observed with higher +ve/−ve charge ratios.

35. EtBr is an aromatic fluorophore whose emission intensity in aqueous solutions increases tenfold upon intercalation between successive DNA base pairs in double helical DNA [21, 22]. The binding and condensation of DNA by cationic liposomes, as they are gradually introduced, is accompanied by the displacement of DNA-intercalated EtBr [23, 24]. The associated decay in fluorescence may be measured and correlated with the progress of lipoplex formation. The method described hereunder is adapted from that described by Tros de Ilarduya et al. [25] and uses a Shimadzu RF-551 spectrofluorometric detector, which is

limited to measurements on one sample at a time. A steady decrease in RF values will be observed during the course of the experiment. The point at which the plateau region begins represents the liposome:DNA ratio at which the liposomes have maximally displaced the EtBr and the DNA is maximally bound and condensed (*see* arrow in Fig. 6). There is usually a good correlation between the DNA (−ve)/liposome (+ve) ratio at this point and the end-point ratio observed in gel retardation analyses.

36. If intending to follow DNA binding to multiple liposome formulations simultaneously, then the procedure should be adapted for execution in a 96-well flat-bottomed black plate employing a microplate reader operating at 25 °C [26]. Briefly place 100 μL of HBS in multiplate wells and to them add 2 μL/well of stock EtBr solutions at 100 μg/mL. Record the baseline EtBr fluorescences (F_o) at $\lambda_{ex} = 525$ nm and $\lambda_{em} = 580$ nm. Introduce pDNA solutions (5 μL/well) containing 1.25 μg of pCMV-luc, and record the fluorescence intensities (F_{max}). These will reflect 100 % RF. Add 1 μL aliquots of liposome suspensions at approximately 2.5 μg/μL (depending on composition), in a step-wise manner while recording fluorescence intensities (F_i) after a 30 s shaking period (performed by the instrument) between additions. Continue until a plateau in readings has been obtained for each liposome preparation. The smaller quantities used in this assay will permit triplicate determinations for each liposome preparation. Calculate RF $(\%) = (F_i - F_o)/(F_{max} - F_o) \times 100$: Plot RF(%) against amount of liposome (μg).

37. All cell culture procedures should be carried out in a dedicated cell culture facility, which operates under positive HEPA (high-efficiency particulate air) filtered air pressure, and is equipped with a class II biosafety cabinet, an incubator that provides a humidified atmosphere containing 5 % CO_2, an inverted phase contrast microscope and a biofreezer (−80 °C). Always wear protective clothing, goggles, and face mask and observe all institutional and product safety guidelines. All operations involving the treatment and dispensing of cells must be conducted in the biosafety cabinet. It is recommended that newcomers to cell culture familiarize themselves with the standard requirements of a cell culture facility and the operating procedures to be observed when working in a cell culture environment. Several books are available to assist professional workers in this process [27].

38. Thawing frozen cell lines: Place the 2 mL cryogenic vial containing frozen cells in a 37 °C water bath. Allow to thaw as quickly as possible (<1 min). Wipe ampoule with 70 % EtOH and place in a safety cabinet. Open and transfer contents into a sterile disposable centrifuge tube (15 mL). Spin at $200 \times g$ for 5 min. Remove clear supernatant comprised of complete medium con-

taining 10 % FCS and 10 % DMSO as cryo-protectant. Resuspend pelleted cells gently in 5 mL of complete medium, using a wide-tip sterile disposable pipette, and transfer into a disposable plastic 25 cm² vented cap flask. Place in the incubator at 37 °C. HepG2 and HEK293 are adherent cell lines. Overnight incubation will ensure that viable cells become anchored to the flask assuming characteristic morphologies and begin to divide, while nonviable cells remain rounded in appearance and mainly in suspension. Residual DMSO in the thawed cell pellet will also be diluted in the growth medium. Replacement of medium after overnight incubation should eliminate the cryo-protectant completely. Spent medium will usually take on a more orange appearance (phenol red indicator in the medium), as it becomes more acidic, and must be replaced with fresh medium to avoid cell damage and loss of viability. Cells in culture flasks should be viewed routinely on an inverted microscope for signs of contamination by microorganisms and to estimate the degree of confluence of the monolayer. HepG2 cells tend to grow at a slower rate and in a more clustered manner than HEK293 cells, which will reach a semi-confluent state sooner. If left too long at 100 % confluence, cells begin to die and lift off the flask.

39. Cell maintenance and propagation: Once cells have formed a monolayer (100 % confluence), passage or split the cells into new 25 cm² vented cap flasks. Aspirate spent medium and wash cells with 2 mL of PBS. Introduce the PBS slowly so as not to dislodge adherent cells, rock the flask gently to ensure removal of all residual medium. Tilt culture flask and insert pipette tip in one of the bottom corners of the flask when aspirating, taking care not to slide the tip over the cells. Failure to do this may lead to difficulties in trypsinization, as FCS contains proteins that inhibit trypsin activity. Add 1 mL of Trypsin—Versene® solution. Rock the flask to spread the solution evenly over the cell layer and observe the cells under inverted microscopy. Cells will visibly round-off and begin to lift into the medium. This process is accelerated by gently tapping the flask against the palm of the hand. Complete suspension will normally be achieved in 30–60 s. However times differ greatly between cell lines and may be affected by residual medium, which had not been removed in the washing step. Once cells have completely detached, immediately pipette the cell suspension into 2 mL complete medium to arrest the action of trypsin. Draw and expel the cell suspension in and out of a disposable plastic pipette gently, to ensure that the suspension contains individual cells and not clusters. Seed approximately 5–8 × 10⁵ cells into 25 cm² flasks containing 5 mL of fresh complete medium to achieve the desired split. HepG2 cells should be split in a manner that achieves a

high seeding density as they tend to be slow growing. Thus 1 mL of the cell suspension should be introduced into new flasks to achieve a 1:3 split. Hence three new sub-cultures may be obtained from the trypsinization of one flask of cells. HEK293 may be split at lower density (1:4). Cells may take up to 4 days to reach confluence. Times may vary.

40. Cryo-preservation ensures that the cell line is maintained in the laboratory for future use without continual passaging, which may otherwise lead to genetic drift. It also minimizes the risk of introducing chemical impurities and biological contaminants such as viruses, bacteria, and yeasts into the line. Trypsinize semi-confluent cells as described (*see* **Note 39**) and perform a cell count. This may be performed relatively quickly on a glass Bright-Line haemocytometer (Sigma-Aldrich), with some practice. Take great care to follow the instructions for correct use of the apparatus and in calculating the cell concentration. Cover slip and haemocytometer must be washed with EtOH to ensure that they are grease-free. Apply the cell suspension by placing the pipette tip in the depression in the haemocytometer, at the edge of the coverslip. Allow the suspension to run into the 0.1 mm space between the cover slip and the haemocytometer. Observe the cells on an inverted microscope at 100× magnification. To ensure that the small volume of cell suspension, which is applied to the haemocytometer, is representative, work quickly to prevent cells from settling out in the pipette. Count cells in the large corner squares (1 mm^2) including those cells lying on two contiguous lines defining the square, but excluding cells on the other two. If the cell count per square is >50–70, then consider diluting the cell suspension and repeating the cell count. The apparatus may also be used to measure live and dead cells with the aid of a vital stain such as Trypan blue (0.4% solution in equal parts with a sample of the cell suspension). Viable cells will be colorless and have excluded the dye, while dead cells will be stained. Alternatively one may use one of several automated cell counters available commercially. Centrifuge (200×g, 5 min) to obtain a cell pellet. Resuspend cells in "freezing medium." Transfer to a cryogenic vial and cool the sample to −80 °C (at a temperature drop rate of 1–2 °C/min) (*see* **Note 41**). Store at this temperature in the biofreezer. Do not add DMSO directly to a cell suspension in complete medium to achieve the desired 10% (v/v) concentration, as the process is exothermic and detrimental to the cells thus affecting viability. Some laboratories prefer to use glycerol as cryo-protectant, which is considered to be less toxic although various saccharides are also in use. There is also much interest in the possibility that the use of DMSO may cause genetic and epigenetic changes in eukaryotic cells [28].

41. In the past, we have used an immersion cooler fitted with ramping temperature controller and EtOH bath, to take cryogenic vials sealed in polythene jackets to –50 °C initially. These were then transferred directly to a biofreezer (–80 °C). Although cell viability after resuscitation was satisfactory, we now place cryogenic vials in a freezing container (Nalgene® Mr Frosty, Sigma-Aldrich) into which isopropanol is poured at RT. This is placed directly into the biofreezer and the following day vials are removed and placed into racks for storage. It is good practice to label the vials with the cell type, passage number, and date. Some laboratories also record the cell number. Cells stored in this manner remain viable for several months. It is also suggested that batches of cells be stored in liquid N_2 vapor at <–150 °C for long-term storage. Although immersion into liquid N_2 will guarantee a lower temperature (–196 °C), there remain the possibilities of cross contamination and entry of liquid N_2 into the vial. The latter event may result in an explosion during the quick thawing of cells.

42. If the effect of serum on transfection is to be studied, then incubate in the presence of medium supplemented with FCS. The relative amount of FCS in the complete medium, used throughout, may be varied as desired.

43. Remember to form lipoplexes at least 30 min before applying to cells to permit maturation of complexes at RT to take place. At least three replicates per each liposome-DNA ratio are suggested. Control wells of untreated cells should also be included.

44. The cytotoxicity of lipoplexes to cells in culture under transfection conditions may be estimated conveniently using the MTT assay [29]. It is held that MTT (yellow) is reduced by mitochondrial NAD(P)H oxidoreductases, in viable cells, to a purple insoluble formazan [30] although the precise cellular mechanism is not fully understood [31]. In essence, the colorimetric assay is used here to determine viable adherent cells without resorting to cell counting. Thus the number of viable treated cells may be expressed as a percentage of viable untreated cells. Other commonly used viability assays include the MTS, AlamarBlue®, and ATP detection assays. Although the last of these is most sensitive, for the present application, tetrazolium- or resazurin-based assays are adequate.

45. The absorbance of the formazan solutions is monitored in the range $\lambda = 550–600$ nm. Expect to see variations in the choice of wavelength in the literature. Moreover a reference $\lambda = 630$ nm may be used, though for most applications this is not necessary [31].

46. Introduce the PBS gently in order to avoid cell detachment from the well surface. Rock the plate briefly before complete aspiration of the rinse PBS.

47. The directed uptake and expression of exogenous genes by mammalian cells is conveniently measured by monitoring the expression of a model transgene, which meets certain criteria. Thus the protein product of transgene expression must be alien to the cells being transfected and be manifest in quantities proportional to the amount of transcribed mRNA. Moreover, the protein must be readily identified and quantified in a sensitive and straightforward assay [32, 33]. The luciferase gene from *Photinus pyralis* fulfills these requirements and is widely adopted in reporter gene assays. In the form described here, the luminescence, arising from the action of luciferase on its substrate luciferin, in the presence of ATP, is measured. Results are normally presented as relative light units (RLUs) per mg soluble protein (*see* Fig. 8).

48. The luciferase assay reagent is prepared beforehand by adding luciferase assay buffer to the vials containing the luciferase assay substrate. The quantities depend on which kit has been purchased and will be given clearly in the accompanying instruction sheet. The premixed luciferase assay reagent may also be purchased; however, it may be better to mix the reagents in your own laboratory, and then split the solution and store aliquots in the biofreezer until use. Avoid repeated freeze-thaw cycles as this will result in some loss in activity. All reagents must be equilibrated to RT before mixing and measuring.

49. This instrument is portable and measures RLUs of one sample at a time. It is small enough to fit into a Biosafety hood if desired or required. There are several other similar instruments manufactured by other suppliers. However, if high throughput

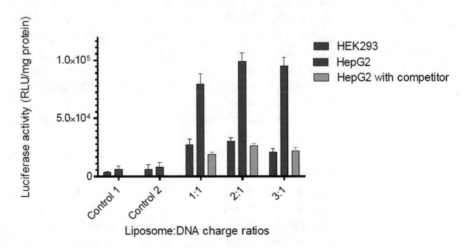

Fig. 8 Transfection studies of liposome-pCMV-luc complexes in HepG2 and HEK293 cells. Incubation mixtures contained cells in medium (300 μL) and lipoplexes (1 μg DNA) at different charge ratios. ***$p < 0.001$ versus unchallenged HepG2 cells. Data are presented as means ± S.D. ($n = 3$). Control 1: untreated cells; control 2: cells treated with naked plasmid DNA. Figure reprinted, with permission, from ref. 12. *Copyright© American Scientific Publishers*

is required, consider using a 96-well plate for samples, and a luminometer capable of reading all wells simultaneously, such as the GloMax®-Multi Detection System (Promega Biosystems, Sunnyvale, CA, USA). In this case, add 50 µL of Promega luciferase assay reagent to 20 µL of clear cell lysate in each well, and work as quickly as possible. Vortex the plate and fit with a microplate sample tray cover to minimize cross-talk signal from neighboring wells. Then place into the luminometer, whose photomultiplier tube (PMT) has been pre-warmed for at least 5 min. Record the RLUs in the $\lambda = 350$–650 nm range.

References

1. Shaw JJ, Shah SA (2011) Rising incidence and demographics of hepatocellular carcinoma in the USA: what does it mean? Expert Rev Gastroenterol Hepatol 5(3):365–370

2. Parkin DM, Bray F, Ferley J, Pisani P (2001) Estimating the world cancer burden: Globocan 2000. Int J Cancer 94(2):153–156

3. Michielsen PP, Francque SM, van Dongen JL (2005) Viral hepatitis and hepatocellular carcinoma. World J Surg Oncol 3:27. doi:10.1186/1477-7819-3-27

4. Shigeta K, Kawakami S, Higuchi Y, Okuda T, Yagi H, Yamashita F, Hashida M (2007) Novel histidine-conjugated galactosylated cationic liposomes for efficient hepatocyte-selective gene transfer in human hepatoma HepG2 cells. J Control Release 118(2):262–270

5. Habib S, Singh M, Ariatti M (2013) Glycosylated liposomes with proton sponge capacity: novel hepatocyte-specific gene carriers. Curr Drug Deliv 10(6):685–695

6. Farinha D, Pedroso de Lima MC, Faneca H (2014) Specific and efficient gene delivery mediated by an asialofetuin-associated nanosystem. Int J Pharm 473(1–2):366–374

7. Zhao QQ, Hu YL, Zhou Y, Li N, Han M, Tang GP, Qiu F, Tabata Y, Gao GQ (2012) Gene-carried hepatoma targeting complex induced high gene transfection efficiency with low toxicity and significant antitumor activity. Int J Nanomed 7:3191–3202

8. Zhang B, Zhang Y, Wang J, Zhang Y, Chen J, Pan Y, Ren L, Hu Z, Zhao J, Liao M, Wang S (2007) Screening and identification of a targeting peptide to hepatocarcinoma from a phage display peptide library. Mol Med 13(5–6):246–254

9. Zhao H, Feng X, Han W, Diao Y, Han D, Tian X, Gao Y, Liu S, Zhu S, Yao C, Gu J, Sun C, Lei L (2013) Enhanced binding to and killing of hepatocellular carcinoma cells *in vitro* by melittin when linked with a novel targeting peptide screened from phage display. J Pept Sci 19(10):639–650

10. Lo A, Lin CT, Wu HC (2008) Hepatocellular carcinoma cell-specific peptide ligand for targeted drug delivery. Mol Cancer Ther 7(3): 579–589

11. Ying T, Kim JS (2010) Selective gene transfer to hepatocellular carcinoma using homing peptide-grafted cationic liposomes. J Microbiol Biotechnol 20(4):821–827

12. Govender J, Singh M, Ariatti M (2014) Effect of poly(ethylene glycol) spacer on peptide-decorated hepatocellular carcinoma-targeted lipoplexes *in vitro*. J Nanosci Nanotechnol 15(6):4734–4742

13. Singh M, Kisoon N, Ariatti M (2001) Receptor-mediated gene delivery to HepG2 cells by ternary assemblies containing cationic liposomes and cationized asialoorosomucoid. Drug Deliv 8(1):29–34

14. Gao X, Huang L (1991) A novel cationic liposome reagent for efficient transfection of mammalian cells. Biochem Biophys Res Commun 179(1):280–285

15. Sambrook J, Fritsch EF, Maniatis T (1989) Molecular cloning: a laboratory manual. Cold Spring Harbor Laboratory press, New York

16. Kapoor KN, Barry DT, Rees RC, Dodi IA, McArdle SE, Creaser CS, Bonner PL (2009) Estimation of peptide concentration by a modified bicinchoninic acid assay. Anal Biochem 393(1):138–140

17. Egelhaaf SU, Werhli E, Müller M, Adrian M, Schurtenberger P (1996) Determination of size distribution of lecithin liposomes: a comparative study using freeze fracture cryo electron microscopy and dynamic light scattering. J Microsc 184(3):214–228

18. Johnsson M, Edwards K (2003) Liposomes, disks and spherical micelles: aggregate structure in mixtures of gel phase phosphatidyl

cholines and poly(ethylene glycol)-phospho-lipids. Biophys J 85(6):3839–3847

19. Govender D, Islam RU, De Koning CB, van Otterlo WA, Arbuthnot P, Ariatti M, Singh M (2015) Stealth lipoplex decorated with triazole-tethered galactosyl moieties: a strong hepatotropic gene vector. Biotechnol Lett 37(3):567–575

20. University of Kentucky-Knoxville: Guidelines for ethidium bromide waste management & disposal. http://web.utk.edu/~ehss/pdf/ebd. pdf. Accessed 14 Jun 2015

21. Lakowicz JR (1999) Principles of fluorescence spectroscopy, 2nd edn. Plenum Press, New York

22. Lepecq JB, Paoletti J (1967) A fluorescent complex between ethidium bromide and nucleic acids. J Mol Biol 27(1):87–106

23. Geall AJ, Blagbrough IS (2000) Rapid and sensitive ethidium bromide fluorescence quenching assay of polyamine conjugate-DNA interactions for the analysis of lipoplex formation in gene therapy. J Pharm Biomed Anal 22(5):849–859

24. Xu Y, Hui SW, Frederik P, Szoka FC Jr (1999) Physicochemical characterization and purification of cationic liposomes. Biochem J 77(1):341–353

25. Tros de Ilarduya C, Arangoa MA, Moreno-Aliaga MJ, Düzgüneş N (2002) Enhanced gene delivery *in vitro* and *in vivo* by improved transferrin-lipoplexes. Biochim Biophys Acta 1561(2):209–221

26. Gorle S, Ariatti M, Singh M (2014) Novel serum-tolerant lipoplexes target the folate receptor efficiently. Eur J Pharm Sci 59:83–93

27. Mather JP, Roberts PE (1998) Introduction to cell and tissue culture: theory and technique. Plenum Press, New York

28. Riesco M, Robles V (2013) Cryopreservation causes genetic and epigenetic changes in Zebrafish genital ridges. PLoS One. doi:10.1371/journal. pone0067614

29. Mosmann T (1983) Rapid colorimetric assay for cellular growth and survival: application to proliferation and cytotoxicity assays. J Immunol Methods 65(1–2):55–63

30. Berridge M, Tan A, McCoy K, Wang R (1996) The biochemical and cellular basis of cell proliferation assays that use tetrazolium salts. Biochemica 4:14–19

31. Riss TL, Moravec RA, Niles AL, Benink HA, Worzella TJ, Minor L, Storts D, Reid Y (2013) Cell viability assays. In: Sittampalam GS, Coussens NP, Nelson H et al (eds) Assay guidance manual. National Library of Medicine and National Center for Advancing Translation Sciences, Bethesda, MD, http://ncbi.nlm.nih. gov/books/NBK144065/. Accessed 17 Jun 2015

32. Bronstein I, Martin CS, Fortin JJ, Olesen CE, Voyta JC (1996) Chemiluminescence: sensitive detection technology for reporter gene assays. Clin Chem 42(9):1542–1546

33. Habib S (2012) Galactosylated liposomes with proton sponge capacity: a novel hepatocyte—specific gene transfer system. Dissertation, University of KwaZulu-Natal. http://hdl.han-dle.net/10413/9862. Accessed 20 Jul 2015

Chapter 8

Lipoplexes Strengthened by Anionic Polymers: Easy Preparation of Highly Effective siRNA Vectors Based on Cationic Lipids and Anionic Polymers

Danielle Campiol Arruda, Anne Schlegel, Pascal Bigey, and Virginie Escriou

Abstract

RNA interference is an invaluable tool in biology to specifically silence a given gene. Synthetic duplexes of RNA oligonucleotides are widely used to induce mRNA degradation in cultured cells or in whole organisms. They have to be vectorized to reach their target site. Here, we describe the preparation of highly efficient siRNA vectors based on cationic liposomes and polyanionic polymers and their application in cultured cells to silence reporter and/or endogenous genes.

Key words RNA interference, siRNA delivery, Lipoplexes, Cationic lipid, Anionic polymer

1 Introduction

Since the discovery of RNA interference (RNAi) by Fire and Mello [1] in 1998, small interfering RNAs, or siRNAs, have become indisputable tools to specifically silence a target gene. In addition, synthetic siRNAs are emerging as an exciting and highly promising new class of therapeutics to treat a variety of diseases. The main obstacle for the development of siRNA as an efficient drug is to deliver it to target tissues in a whole organism and across the cell membrane. Indeed, the RNAi machinery that triggers the sequence-specific mRNA degradation is localized in the cytoplasm. In the absence of transfection reagents or physical treatments that may transiently damage the cellular membrane, most cells do not spontaneously take up siRNAs. Several cationic lipid-based siRNA delivery systems, also called lipoplexes, have been reported so far [2]. They promote the increase of the stability of siRNA in biological medium and its cellular uptake. Recently, we developed efficient cationic lipid-based siRNA vectors whose characteristic is to also contain anionic polymers [3]. We previously reported that the

Gabriele Candiani (ed.), *Non-Viral Gene Delivery Vectors: Methods and Protocols*, Methods in Molecular Biology, vol. 1445,
DOI 10.1007/978-1-4939-3718-9_8, © Springer Science+Business Media New York 2016

incorporation of anionic polymers in siRNA lipoplexes increases the gene silencing efficiency of the vectors in cultured cells, decreases their cellular toxicity at higher siRNA doses, and increases siRNA recovery from organs after intravenous administration of the vectors [4]. In addition, these vectors were able to efficiently deliver therapeutic siRNA in transgenic mice expressing hepatitis B virus [5]. The polymers used to design these siRNA vectors are biodegradable and FDA-approved for use in humans. Hence they can be used to enhance the efficiency of several cationic lipid-based siRNA delivery vectors. Here we show how to easily prepare and use anionic polymer-containing cationic lipid-based siRNA delivery vectors to efficiently silence target genes in cultured cells.

2 Materials

2.1 Cell Culture

1. B16 mouse melanoma (B16-F0) (American Type Culture Collection (ATCC), LGC Promochem, Molsheim, France).
2. B16 cells modified to constitutively express luciferase (*see* **Note 1**).
3. Dulbecco's Modified Eagle's Medium (DMEM).
4. Glutamax.
5. Fetal calf serum (FCS).
6. Penicillin.
7. Streptomycin.
8. Complete cell-culture medium: DMEM supplemented with Glutamax, 10 % (v/v) FCS, 100 U/mL penicillin, and 100 µg/mL streptomycin.
9. OptiMEM (*see* **Note 2**).
10. Phosphate buffered saline (PBS).

2.2 siRNA and Anionic Polymer

1. Synthetic unmodified siRNA (Eurogentec, Seraing, Belgium) (*see* **Note 3**).
2. Poly-L-glutamate sodium salt.
3. Anionic polymer (*see* **Note 4**).
4. DNase RNase-free water.

2.3 Cationic Lipids and Liposomes (See Note 5)

1. 2-{3-[Bis-(3-amino-propyl)-amino]-propylamino}-*N*-ditetradecyl carbamoyl methyl-acetamide (DMAPAP).
2. 1,2-Dioleoyl-sn-Glycero-3-Phosphoethanolamine (DOPE) (Coger, Paris, France).
3. Lipofectamine™ (Fisher Scientific, Illkirch, France).
4. DMRIE-C reagent (Fisher Scientific, Illkirch, France). DMRIE-C is a 1:1 (M/M) liposome formulation of the cationic lipid 1,2-dimyristyloxypropyl-3-dimethyl-hydroxy ethyl ammonium bromide (DMRIE) and cholesterol in membrane filtered water.

5. Chloroform ($CHCl_3$).

6. Rotary evaporator.

7. Bath sonicator.

8. 1.5 mL polypropylene microcentrifuge tubes.

2.4 Luminometry

1. 5× Luciferase Cell-Culture Lysis reagent (Promega, Charbonnière, France).

2. Luciferase Assay System (Promega, Charbonnière, France).

3. Bicinchoninic Acid (BCA) Protein Assay Kit (Fisher Scientific, Illkirch, France).

4. Microplate reader equipped for luminescence and absorbance.

5. White and clear polystyrene flat bottom 96-microwell plates.

6. PBS.

2.5 qPCR

1. Trypsin-ethylenediaminetetraacetic acid (EDTA).

2. PBS.

3. 26G needles.

4. RNAble reagent (Eurobio Abcys, Courtaboeuf, France).

5. $CHCl_3$.

6. Isopropanol.

7. 70% (v/v) ethanol (EtOH) in deionized water (dH_2O).

8. RNAse DNase-free water.

9. Quant-iT™ RiboGreen® RNA and Quant-iT™ OliGreen® ssDNA Assay Kits (Fisher Scientific, Illkirch, France).

10. SuperScript II Reverse Transcriptase, 5× First Strand Buffer, 0.1 M DTT, 2.5 mM dNTPs, random primers (hexamers), and RNAseOUT Recombinant Ribonuclease Inhibitor (Fisher Scientific, Illkirch, France).

11. Thermocycler.

12. Oligonucleotide primers.

13. 2× Power SYBR Green Mastermix (Fisher Scientific, Illkirch, France).

14. Real-Time PCR thermocycler.

15. Clear optical 384-microwell plates with optical adhesive covers (Fisher Scientific, Illkirch, France).

3 Methods

3.1 Liposome Preparation

1. Dissolve 17 mg of DMAPAP and 15 mg of DOPE in 2 mL of $CHCl_3$, then mix.

2. Allow the organic solvent to evaporate under vacuum at 20 °C using a rotary evaporator to form a thin film.

3. Hydrate the dried film with 1 mL of 0.2 µm filtered dH_2O for 24 h at 20 °C to produce large multilamellar vesicles (LMVs).

4. Sonicate the suspension at 115 V, 80 W, 50–60 Hz, with a sonicator to obtain a homogeneous suspension of liposomes (20mM) with a diameter of 80–100 nm.

3.2 Cells Preparation (See Note 6)

1. Seed B16 or B16-Luc cells at a density of 2×10^4 cell/cm^2 in a 24-well cell culture plate in 1 mL of complete cell-culture medium per well.

2. Grow overnight until they reach 70% confluence.

3.3 siRNA Lipoplexes Preparation

For siRNA lipoplexes preparation (*see* **Note 7**), all the volumes are given for three wells of a 24-well plate.

1. Solubilize synthetic unmodified siRNA in DNase RNase-free water to reach the final concentration of 100 µM (stock solution). Aliquot can be stored at –80 °C.

2. Prepare a 20 µM working solution in DNase RNase-free water from the stock solution. Store for no longer than 3 weeks at –20 °C. Specific sequences are given in Table 1.

3. Solubilize poly-L-glutamate sodium salt at 0.3 µg/µL in RNase-free water. Aliquot can be stored at –20 °C.

4. In a 1.5 mL polypropylene microcentrifuge tube, prepare master mix 1 by diluting 3 µL of 20 µM working stock (60 pmol) of siRNA and 0.9 µg of anionic polymer in 150 µL of 150 mM NaCl for transfection with DMAPAP/DOPE (*see* **Note 8**) or in 150 µL of OptiMEM for transfection with Lipofectamine™ or DMRIE-C. Mix gently.

5. In a 1.5 mL polypropylene microcentrifuge tube, prepare master mix 2 by adding 5.8 µL of 2 mM DMAPAP/DOPE to 150 µL of 150 mM NaCl, or 6 µL of Lipofectamine™ or 15 µL of 2 µg/µL DMRIE-C to 150 µL OptiMEM. Mix gently.

6. Combine equal volume of master mixes 1 and 2, mix vigorously, and incubate for 30 min at room temperature (RT).

3.4 Cell Transfection

1. Transfer 300 µL of siRNA lipoplexes suspension in a 15 mL conical tube.

2. Add 3 mL of complete cell-culture medium (*see* **Note 9**) for transfection with DMAPAP/DOPE or 3 mL of OptiMEM for transfection with Lipofectamine™ or DMRIE-C. Mix gently (*see* **Note 10**).

3. Remove old medium from the 24-well culture plate and add 1 mL of the siRNA lipoplexes suspension in culture medium obtained at **step 2** to each well (in triplicate).

Table 1
Sequences of siRNAs directed against various genes. siRNAs are composed of two complementary strands, 19 unmodified RNA bases plus 2 × 3′-DNA(d) overhang bases, usually dTdT

siRNA		Sequence (5′-3′)
Control	Sense	UUC UCC GAA CGU GUC ACG UdTdT
	Antisense	ACG UGA CAC GUU CGG AGA AdTdT
Firefly luciferase	Sense	CUU ACG CUG AGU ACU UCG AdTdT
GL3	Antisense	UCG AAG UAC UCA GCG UAA GdTdT
RIP	Sense	GCA GAG AGC UCG UGA GAA UdTdT
	Antisense	AUU CUC ACG AGC UCU CUG CdTdT
VEGF	Sense	CGA UGA AGC CCU GGA GUG CdTdT
	Antisense	GCU ACU UCG GGA CCU CAC GdTdT
cMyc	Sense	GAA CAU CAU CAU CCA GGA CdTdT
	Antisense	GUC CUG GAU GAU GAU GUU CdTdT
MDM2	Sense	GCU UCG GAA CAA GAG ACU CdTdT
	Antisense	UAA GCG UAA GCA GUG UUG GdTdT
STAT3	sense	GGA CGA CUU UGA UUU CAA CdTdT
	Antisense	GUU GAA AUC AAA GUC GUC CdTdT
Survivin	Sense	Unknown
(SantaCruz sc-29500)	Antisense	Unknown

4. For transfection with Lipofectamine™ or DMRIE-C, add 100 µL of FCS to each well, 4–6 h after the addition of transfection medium.

5. Incubate the cells for 24 h in a 5 % CO_2 at 37 °C.

6. Replace transfection medium with fresh complete cell-culture medium and incubate the cells for an additional 24 h (*see* **Note 11**).

3.5 Analysis of Luciferase Activity: Luciferase Silencing in Luciferase Expressing Cells

1. Wash transfected cells twice with 1 mL/well of PBS.

2. Add 200 μL of 1× Luciferase Cell-Culture Lysis reagent to each well, and then incubate for 15 min at RT.

3. Transfer the cell lysate into a 1.5 mL polypropylene microcentrifuge tube and centrifuge at $10,000 \times g$ for 10 min at 4 °C.

4. Transfer 10 μL of sample supernatants into a 96-well white plate.

5. Measure light emission due to luciferase using a microplate reader equipped for luminescence and automatic injector (injection of 50 μL Luciferase Substrate).

6. Determine total protein concentration using the BCA Protein Assay Kit according to manufacturer instructions on 96-well clear plate.

7. Normalize the luciferase activity obtained in cps (count per sec) (**step 5**) to the total protein concentration of each sample (**step 6**) and expressed relative to nontransfected control cells (Fig. 1) (*see* **Note 12**).

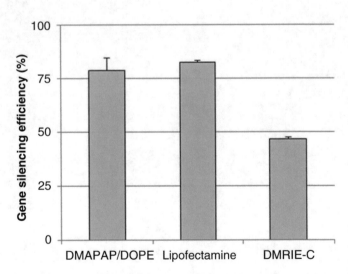

Fig. 1 Gene silencing efficiency obtained with polyglutamate-containing siRNA lipoplexes. B16-Luc cells were transfected for 24 h with siRNA lipoplexes (20 nM siRNA Luciferase) prepared with DMAPAP/DOPE liposome, Lipofectamine™ or DMRIE-C and addition of polyglutamate, in complete cell-culture medium (transfection with DMAPAP/DOPE) or OptiMEM (transfection with Lipofectamine™ or DMRIE-C). Luciferase activity was measured at 48 h. Inhibition of luciferase activity was expressed as a percentage of luciferase activity in nontransfected cells. Mean ± SD, $n = 3$

3.6 qPCR:
Endogenous Gene
Silencing in Any Cell
Line

3.6.1 RNA Isolation

1. Remove old medium from cells.

2. Rinse cells with 1 mL/well of PBS.

3. Add 500 µL of trypsin-EDTA and incubate for 5 min at 37 °C.

4. After incubation, add 500 µL of complete cell-culture medium.

5. Transfer the detached cells to a 1.5 mL polypropylene microcentrifuge tube, and centrifuge at $400 \times g$ for 5 min.

6. Remove supernatant, add 500 µL of PBS, mix gently, and centrifuge at $400 \times g$ for 5 min.

7. Remove supernatant and add 500 µL of RNAble to the pelleted cells.

8. Pass through a 26G needle thrice to homogenize, leave for 5 min at RT.

9. Add 100 µL of $CHCl_3$, shake vigorously for 15 s, and centrifuge at $12,000 \times g$ for 15 min at 4 °C.

10. Transfer the aqueous phase (*see* **Note 13**) to a fresh 1.5 mL microfuge tube.

11. Add 200 µL of isopropanol, invert to mix, and then allow it to stand for 5–10 min at RT.

12. Centrifuge at $12,000 \times g$ for 15 min at 4 °C (*see* **Note 14**).

13. Remove supernatant and wash the pellet by adding 1 mL of 70 % EtOH.

14. Vortex sample and centrifuge at $7500 \times g$ for 5 min at 4 °C.

15. Briefly dry the RNA pellet for 5–10 min by air-drying or under vacuum.

16. Add 20 µL of RNase-free water to RNA pellet. Mix by pipetting.

17. Quantify the RNA with the Quant-iT™ RiboGreen® RNA Assay Kit.

3.6.2 Reverse
Transcription

1. Perform reverse transcription of 1 µg of total RNA in a final volume of 20 µL containing 4 µL of 5× First strand buffer, 0.5 µL of 40 U/µL RNaseOUT Recombinant Ribonuclease inhibitor, 2 µL of 0.1 M DTT, 1 µL of 2.5 mM dNTPs, and 1 µL random hexamers.

2. Incubate for 10 min at 25 °C.

3. Add 0.5 µL of 200 U/µL Superscript II RNase H-reverse transcriptase.

4. Incubate in a thermocycler for 30 min at 42 °C, then for 5 min at 99 °C.

3.6.3 cDNA
Quantification
*(See **Note 15**)*

1. Mix 2 μL of the cDNA solution obtained as described in Subheading 3.6 with 3 μL of Quant-iT™ OliGreen® ssDNA Reagent 200-fold diluted in DNase-free TE in a well of a clear 384-well optical reaction plate and transfer to the qPCR machine.

2. Read fluorescence continuously at 80 °C for 1 min.

3.6.4 Quantitative
Real-Time PCR

1. Solubilize oligonucleotide primers at 100 μM in RNase DNase-free water (Table 2, *see* **Note 16**).

2. Mix 2 μL of the cDNA solution obtained in the previous step and 3 μL of a homemade target-specific mix composed of 5/6 2× Power SYBR Green Master Mix and 1/6 of 100 μM primers solution in a well of a clear 384-well plate, then transfer to the qPCR machine.

3. Perform a standard amplification by carrying out cycle of 10 min at 95 °C, followed by 45 cycles of 15 s at 95 °C and of 1 min at 60 °C.

4. Obtain cycle threshold values (Ct) from the qPCR machine software.

5. Calculate the relative expression level of the gene as $2^{(-Ct)}$ and normalized with the fluorescence value obtained in Subheading 3.6.3 (Figs. 2 and 3).

Table 2
Sequences of the primers used for qPCR assay

Gene	PCR fragment (bp)	Primer	Sequence 5′-3′	Position
MDM2	167	Sense	AGTCCACAGAGACGCCCTCGC	887
		Antisense	TGAGAGCTCGTGCCCTTCGTC	1053
cMyc	175	Sense	CCCTGAGCCCCTAGTGCTGC	1325
		Antisense	GTGCGGAGGTTTGCTGTGGC	1499
VEGF	139	Sense	GGTGCACTGGACCCTGGCTT	1042
		Antisense	CGGACGGCAGTAGCTTCGCT	1180
STAT3	83	Sense	CCAGGAGCACCCCGAAGCC	2352
		Antisense	TGCTGCAGGTCGTTGGTGTCA	2434
Survivin	160	Sense	AGAGCGAATGGCGGAGGCTG	219
		Antisense	AGTGAGGAAGGCGCAGCCAG	378
RIP	248	Sense	GCTACTGGGCATCATCATAGA	367
		Antisense	CCACACCAAGATCGGCTAT	614

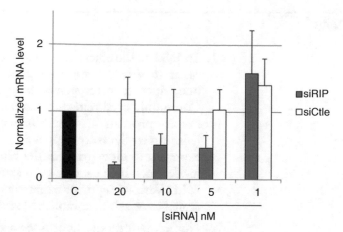

Fig. 2 RIP gene silencing efficiency of siRNA lipoplexes prepared with polygluta-mate and DMAPAP/DOPE liposome. B16 cells were transfected with decreasing concentrations (from 20 to 1 nM) siRNA anti-RIP or Ctle. Two days post-transfection, mRNA level was assayed using RTqPCR. Results were normalized relative to the mRNA level found in nontransfected cells. Mean ± SD, $n = 3$

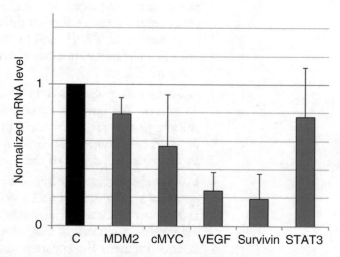

Fig. 3 Endogenous genes silencing. Levels of various mRNA in B16 cells trans-fected with siRNA lipoplexes prepared with polyglutamate and DMAPAP/DOPE liposome and specific siRNA (MDM2, cMYC, VEGF, Survivin, and STAT3), mea-sured by RTqPCR. Histograms represent means ± SD with control group (non-transfected cells, *black*) arbitrarily taken as 1 ($n = 4$ per group). B16 cells were transfected with 20 nM siRNA. Two days post-transfection, total RNA was extracted and specific mRNA was assayed by RTqPCR

4   Notes

1. To validate the efficiency of a siRNA delivery vector, it is usually easier to silence a reporter gene rather than an endogenous one, since reporter genes code for a protein easy to assay. Commonly used reporter genes encode fluorescent and luminescent proteins. Examples include the gene that encodes jellyfish green fluorescent protein (GFP), which causes cells that express it to glow green under blue light, or the firefly enzyme luciferase, which catalyzes a reaction with luciferin to produce light. Various reporter-expressing cell lines are commercially available or can be established as described [6, 7].

2. Numerous cationic liposomes are known to be inefficient of delivering nucleic acids (pDNA or siRNA) to cultured cells in the presence of serum. OptiMEM is a commonly used medium for transfection with that kind of liposomes. It can be complemented with antibiotics and used to dilute siRNA lipoplexes.

3. Annealed unmodified siRNAs are composed of two complementary strands, 19 unmodified RNA bases plus $2 \times 3'$-DNA overhang bases, usually dTdT. Specific sequences are given in Table 1. Regarding the design of sequences for siRNA, numerous reviews have been written, and the reader is referred to other recent texts for further discussion [8]. Many companies have developed siRNA design tools, and some of them also offer prevalidated sequences where the efficacy has been tested using qPCR.

4. Other anionic polymers can also be used to strengthen siRNA lipoplexes. We have reported efficiency with seven different anionic polymers [3], namely polyglutamate, alginate, hyaluronate, carboxymethyl cellulose, polyacrylate, dextran sulfate, and heparan sulfate, all of them sodium salts.

5. Commonly used cationic lipid-based vectors are liposomes, composed of a cationic lipid and a zwitterionic or neutral lipid like DOPE or Cholesterol. Liposomes are artificially-prepared spherical vesicles composed of a lamellar phase lipid bilayer separating an aqueous internal compartment from the bulk aqueous phase. Cationic lipids prepared as micelles can also be used to deliver siRNA and their efficiency is also enhanced by the addition of anionic polymer (unpublished data). Micelles are closed lipid monolayers with a fatty acid core and polar surface.

6. Typical experiments use duplicate or triplicate samples from each condition. We routinely include nontransfected control samples and samples from cells transfected with a non-targeting or control siRNA (see Table 1 for sequence of siRNA control).

7. The colloidal properties of the lipoplexes are principally determined by the $+/-$ charge ratio, defined as the molar ratio between

the positive charges brought by cationic lipid and the negative charges brought by nucleic acid. Here the addition of anionic polymer also brings negative charges and these charges have to be taken into account. We previously reported the amount of negative charges exhibited by each anionic polymer we assayed in siRNA lipoplexes [3]. In order to determine the optimal charge ratio for a given lipoplex, characterized by its composition (siRNA/anionic polymer/cationic lipid or liposome), you just have to prepare lipoplexes with a fixed amount of siRNA + anionic polymer and increase the amount or volume of cationic lipid or liposome, and assay them on cells.

8. Lipoplexes can be prepared in various buffers or aqueous solutions like saline (150 mM NaCl), 5 % (w/v) glucose in dH_2O, HEPES, or serum-free culture medium (OptiMEM).

9. Most cationic lipids or liposomes are more efficient to transfect cells in serum-free medium. Some of them, like Lipofectamine™, are even completely inhibited by the presence of serum in the cell-culture medium. Few of them are able to efficiently transfect cells in the presence of serum, like DMAPAP/DOPE. For fragile cell types, the ability to transfect in the presence of serum is clearly a benefit.

10. Lipoplexes suspensions are diluted in cell-culture medium in a separate tube before removing cell-culture medium from wells and adding the suspension of lipoplexes in culture medium. This step allows better homogenization of lipoplexes than dropwise addition to wells.

11. Luciferase assay is performed 48 h after the start of the transfection. We determined that 48 h is the necessary time to obtain the optimal gene silencing of luciferase. This time may vary according to cell types and/or targeted gene.

12. Results obtained with luciferase assay only give a global value of the extent of gene silencing. In order to obtain a value cell by cell, GFP (green fluorescent protein) should be chosen as reporter gene to silence. Then the analysis of the transfection efficiency should be done using flow cytometry.

13. The samples separate into two phases: the lower, organic phase contains proteins, lipids, and DNA; and the upper, aqueous phase contains the RNA.

14. The RNA precipitate forms a pellet on the side and bottom of the tube.

15. We normalized qPCR results with the amount of cDNA precisely determined using a single-step OliGreen fluorescence measurement protocol performed on a real-time PCR thermocycler in post-RT solution as described [9]. We have shown previously that this assay is based on the preferential affinity of OliGreen to ssDNA compared to ssRNA, by working

in adapted thermal conditions. This permits observing only ssDNA-based fluorescence even in the presence of RNA.

16. Oligonucleotide primers are required for the amplification. These can be designed using the free online Primer-BLAST (NCBI, http://www.ncbi.nlm.nih.gov/tools/primer-blast/) with the following parameters: Entry of refseq record for the target gene, PCR product size between 80 and 180 bp, Primer melting temperatures Min/Max 57/61 °C, Max Tm difference 2 °C, and Primer pair must be separated by at least one intron on the corresponding genomic DNA.

Acknowledgement

This work was supported by ANRT, Oséo Innovation and ANR.

References

1. Fire A, Xu S, Montgomery MK, Kostas SA, Driver SE, Mello CC (1998) Potent and specific genetic interference by double-stranded RNA in Caenorhabditis elegans. Nature 391: 806–811

2. Hope MJ (2014) Enhancing siRNA delivery by employing lipid nanoparticles. Ther Deliv 5:663–673

3. Schlegel A, Largeau C, Bigey P, Bessodes M, Lebozec K, Scherman D, Escriou V (2011) Anionic polymers for decreased toxicity and enhanced in vivo delivery of siRNA complexed with cationic liposomes. J Control Release 152:393–401

4. Schlegel A, Bigey P, Dhotel H, Scherman D, Escriou V (2013) Reduced in vitro and in vivo toxicity of siRNA-lipoplexes with addition of polyglutamate. J Control Release 165:1–8

5. Marimani MD, Ely A, Buff MC, Bernhardt S, Engels JW, Scherman D, Escriou V, Arbuthnot P (2015) Inhibition of replication of hepatitis B virus in transgenic mice following administration of hepatotropic lipoplexes containing guanidinopropyl-modified siRNAs. J Control Release 209:198–206

6. Rhinn H, Largeau C, Bigey P, Kuen RL, Richard M, Scherman D, Escriou V (2009) How to make siRNA lipoplexes efficient? Add a DNA cargo. Biochim Biophys Acta 1790:219–230

7. Miller VJ, McKinnon CM, Mellor H, Stephens DJ (2013) RNA interference approaches to examine Golgi function in animal cell culture. Methods Cell Biol 118:15–34

8. Petri S, Meister G (2013) siRNA design principles and off-target effects. Methods Mol Biol 986:59–71

9. Rhinn H, Scherman D, Escriou V (2008) One-step quantification of single-stranded DNA in the presence of RNA using Oligreen in a real-time polymerase chain reaction thermocycler. Anal Biochem 372:116–118

Chapter 9

Polymer Based Gene Silencing: In Vitro Delivery of SiRNA

Margarida I. Simão Carlos, Andreas Schätzlein, and Ijeoma Uchegbu

Abstract

Gene silencing may be achieved by harnessing the RNA interference mechanism to effect down-regulation of protein expression. The therapeutic use of siRNA is dependent on its delivery to the intracellular space. This chapter describes the delivery of siRNA by N-(2-ethylamino)-6-O-glycolchitosan (EAGC). EAGC is a chitosan-based polymer, which binds to siRNA to form nanoparticles (NPs). The steps necessary to determine the delivery capacity of a polymer are presented in this chapter using EAGC as an example. The steps include: the transfection of cells with EAGC-siRNA polyplexes and protein detection by a Western Blotting assay.

Key words Gene delivery, siRNA, Cationic polymer, Western Blotting, Transfection, Down-regulation, N-(2-ethylamino)-6-O-glycolchitosan (EAGC)

1 Introduction

Gene silencing is the inhibition of protein expression by genes and this normally occurs at the messenger ribonucleic acid (mRNA) level, stopping the expression of proteins at the post-transcriptional level. Gene silencing may be achieved by the ribonucleic acid interference (RNAi) mechanism. An important prerequisite for small interfering ribonucleic acid (siRNA) to be used as a therapeutic, is its successful delivery to the cells and subsequent release in the intracellular space [1]. In therapeutic applications, a delivery system is required not only to protect the siRNA from enzymatic degradation but also to enhance siRNA delivery to the target organ, facilitate cellular uptake, and finally release the siRNA in the cell cytoplasm in order for the siRNA to be incorporated in the RNAi machinery [2]. In vivo cationic polymers are useful as siRNA delivery systems, ultimately improving the pharmacokinetics and pharmacodynamics of siRNA [3]. Cationic polymers are efficient siRNA cell transfer (transfection) agents due to their ability to bind and condense the nucleic acids (NAs) into stabilized nanoparticles (NPs) [4]. They have also demonstrated cellular uptake through

Gabriele Candiani (ed.), *Non-Viral Gene Delivery Vectors: Methods and Protocols*, Methods in Molecular Biology, vol. 1445,
DOI 10.1007/978-1-4939-3718-9_9, © Springer Science+Business Media New York 2016

nonspecific endocytosis and endosomal escape [1]. Prior to their in vivo use, there is a need to evaluate the transfection ability of such polymers in vitro.

This chapter describes in vitro gene silencing with a model polymer, *N*-(2-ethylamino)-6-*O*-glycolchitosan (EAGC), as the siRNA carrier. EAGC is a new chitosan-based polymer soluble at physiological pH with primary, secondary, and tertiary amines that are normally required for good buffering, proper binding, and release of NAs.

Western blotting is one of the techniques available to determine the success of the in vitro gene silencing. Western blotting is a protein analysis technique that identifies proteins bound to the surface of a membrane, using specific antibodies. Firstly, the proteins are separated according to their size by gel electrophoresis. These are then transferred to a membrane that is subsequently blocked to prevent nonspecific binding of the antibodies. The proteins in the membrane are detected by specific antibodies and are revealed through different detection methods, such as e.g., chemiluminescence. Western blotting is a qualitative technique but is sometimes used as a semi-quantitative technique, where the intensity of the signal is correlated with the amount of adsorbed protein [5, 6].

2   Materials

2.1 NPs Preparation

1. Sterile 5 % (w/v) dextrose solution: 5 g of dextrose in 100 mL of distilled water (dH$_2$O).

2. 0.22 μm pore-size polycarbonate filters.

3. siRNA/scrambled siRNA, insiMAX universal buffer (Eurofins mwg/operon, London, UK) (*see* **Note 1**).

4. 6 μg/μL of EAGC stock solution in 5 % (w/v) dextrose solution (UCL—School of Pharmacy, London, UK).

5. Polypropylene microcentrifuge tubes.

2.2 In Vitro Transfection

1. A431, epidermoid carcinoma cell line (ATCC, Teddington, UK).

2. Complete cell-culture medium: Minimum Essential Medium (MEM) supplemented with 10 % Fetal Bovine Serum (FBS), 1 % (w/v) L-glutamine, and 1 % (w/v) nonessential amino acids (*see* **Note 2**).

3. Dulbecco's phosphate-buffered saline (PBS).

4. 6-well polystyrene culture plates.

2.3 Protein Extraction

1. Trypsin—0.25 % (w/v) ethylenediaminetetraacetic acid (EDTA), phenol red.

2. 1 mL of lysis buffer or Radio-Immunoprecipitation Assay (RIPA) buffer: 50 mM Tris–HCl, pH 8.0, with 150 mM sodium chloride (NaCl), 1.0 % Igepal CA-630 (NP-40), 0.5 % sodium deoxycholate, and 0.1 % sodium dodecyl sulfate (SDS), 10 μL of 100× protease inhibitor (Life Technologies, Paisley, UK), 10 μL of 100× phosphatase inhibitor (Life Technologies). Store at 4 °C until use.

2.4 Determination of Protein Concentration

1. 50 μL/well of working reagent (number of unknown protein samples + 9 BCA protein samples) × 3 replicates (*see* **Note 3**).

2. 96-well polystyrene plates.

3. Microplate reader ELX 808 (BioTek, Swindon, UK).

2.5 Protein Electrophoresis

1. 4× NuPAGE® Lithium Dodecyl Sulfate sample (LDS) (Life Technologies).

2. 1 M dithiothreitol (DTT) in dH$_2$O.

3. NuPAGE® Bis-Tris 4–12 % polyacrylamide gel (Life Technologies).

4. Molecular weight (MW) marker.

5. NuPAGE® Antioxidant (Life Technologies).

6. Running buffer: 50 mL of NuPAGE® (Life Technologies) in 950 mL of dH$_2$O.

2.6 Western Blotting

1. Nitrocellulose membrane and filter papers.

2. Stock solution of transfer buffer: 0.75 g of EDTA, 13.1 g of Bis-Tris free base, pH 7.5, 10.2 g of bicine in 100 mL of dH$_2$O. Make up to a volume of 125 mL with dH$_2$O. Store at 4 °C until use.

3. Transfer buffer: 50 mL of transfer buffer stock, 100 mL of methanol (MeOH) in 850 mL of dH$_2$O. Store at 4 °C until use.

4. Blocking solution: 5 g of dried skimmed milk in 100 mL of 1 % (v/v) Tween 20 in 10 % PBS, pH = 7.4. Store at 4 °C until use.

5. XCell SureLock® Mini-Cell (Life Technologies).

2.7 Labeling with Antibodies

1. 1 L of washing buffer: 100 mL of PBS, pH = 7.4, and 900 mL of dH$_2$O.

2. 1 % (v/v) Tween 20 in washing buffer: 500 μL of Tween 20 in 500 mL of washing buffer.

3. Anti-ITCH antibody (BD Bioscience, San Jose, CA), used at a working dilution of 1:500 (v/v) in 1 % (v/v) Tween 20 dissolved in washing buffer.

4. Anti-actin antibody (Abcam, Cambridge, UK), used at a working dilution of 1:2500 (v/v) in 1 % (v/v) Tween 20 in washing buffer.

5. Horseradish peroxidase (HRP) (Invitrogen), used at a working dilution of 1:1000 (v/v) in washing buffer.

6. Chemiluminescent solution: SuperSignal West Pico Chemiluminescent Substrate (Thermo Scientific, Waltham, MA).

7. ChemiDoc™ XRS+ System (Bio Rad, Hemel, UK) and Image Lab software (BioRad).

3   Methods

3.1   NPs Preparation

The formation of the NPs occurs between the cationic EAGC polymer and the anionic NA siRNA.

1. Prepare a 6 µg/µL of EAGC stock solution dissolving the polymer in 5 % (w/v) dextrose in dH_2O.

2. Prepare a 0.1 µg/µL of siRNA/scrambled siRNA stock solution in insiMAX universal buffer (*see* **Note 1**).

3. From the polymer stock solution prepare polymer solutions at different concentrations (6, 3 and 1 µg/µL).

4. Prepare the complexes to a final siRNA/scrambled siRNA dose of 533 nM. In a polypropylene microcentrifuge tube, add equal volumes of siRNA/scrambled siRNA solution and EAGC solutions with different concentrations in order to obtain increasing EAGC, siRNA/scramble siRNA mass ratios (*see* **Notes 4** and **5**).

5. Incubate the NPs at room temperature (RT) for 1 h (*see* **Note 6**).

3.2   In Vitro Transfection

1. Seed cells at a density of 5×10^4 cells/cm^2 in a 6-well plate, add 5 mL/well of complete cell-culture medium and incubate overnight at 37 °C in a humidified atmosphere with 5 % CO_2.

2. After 24 h, rinse the cells with 2 mL of PBS and then add 750 µL/well of MEM.

3. Add 750 µL/well of 533 nM EAGC-siRNA/scrambled siRNA complexes to the cells (*see* **Note 7**).

4. Incubate for 6 h at 37 °C in a humidified atmosphere with 5 % CO_2 (*see* **Note 8**).

5. Rinse the cells with 2 mL of PBS and then add 4 mL of fresh complete cell-culture medium. Incubate the cells for a further 48 h at 37 °C in a humidified atmosphere with 5 % CO_2.

3.3   Protein Extraction

1. After 48 h, discard the medium and wash the cells with 2 mL of PBS.

2. Add 1 mL/well of trypsin and incubate for 3 min at 37 °C in humidified atmosphere, 5 % CO_2.

3. After incubation, add 4 mL/well of complete cell-culture medium.

4. Transfer the trypsinized cells to 15 mL polypropylene centrifuge tubes. Spin at $2500 \times g$ for 10 min at 4 °C (*see* **Note 9**).

5. Remove supernatant, resuspend the cell pellet in 1 mL of PBS and transfer to a microcentrifuge tube (*see* **Note 10**).

6. Spin at $2500 \times g$ for 10 min at 4 °C.

7. Remove supernatant as much as possible, then add 20 μL of lysis buffer and incubate for 1 or 2 h at 4 °C or 30 min on ice.

8. Spin at $14,400 \times g$ for 15 min at 4 °C.

9. Transfer the supernatant into a new microcentrifuge tube. Store the supernatant on ice or in a freezer at –50 °C until use (*see* **Note 11**).

3.4 Determination of Protein Concentration

Determine protein concentration for each unknown sample with the BCA assay using BSA standards.

1. Prepare the BSA standards (*see* **Note 12**).

2. In a 96-well plate pipette 25 μL of the BSA standards (three replicates) and 25 μL of each unknown protein sample (three replicates).

3. Add 50 μL of working reagent in each well.

4. Incubate for 20 min at 37 °C in a humidified atmosphere with 5 % CO_2.

5. Measure absorbance at $\lambda = 540$–590 nm by means of a microplate reader.

6. Build the standard curve by plotting the average absorbance measurement for each BSA standard vs. its concentration in mg/mL (*see* **Note 13**).

7. Use the standard curve to determine the protein concentration for each unknown sample.

8. Calculate the volume corresponding to 20 μg of protein for each unknown sample from the protein concentration.

3.5 Protein Electrophoresis

1. Prepare 20 μL of the unknown protein samples to be loaded in the gel by mixing 5 μL of LDS sample buffer, 2 μL of DTT buffer, a volume correspondent to 20 μg of protein from the unknown samples and dH_2O.

2. Heat each sample in a dry heat block for 15 min at 95 °C.

3. Prepare the Bis-Tris gel for electrophoresis by cutting the gel out of the package, removing the comb carefully, rinsing inside the wells with running buffer with a plastic Pasteur pipette, removing the electrical strip of the gel.

4. Assemble the gel in the apparatus, fill the internal and the external chamber with running buffer.

5. Add 500 μL of NuPAGE® Antioxidant to the internal chamber.

6. Load 5 µL of the MW marker in the first well, then load 20 µL of the unknown protein samples.

7. Run the gel for 50 min at a constant 200 V (*see* **Note 14**).

3.6 Western Blotting

1. Soak the membrane and the filter paper in transfer buffer.

2. Remove the gel from cassette. Separate the bonded sides of the gel cassette by inserting the gel knife into the gap between the cassette plates.

3. Make a sandwich of blotting pad, filter paper, gel, membrane, filter paper, and blotting pad (Fig. 1).

4. Place the sandwich on the blot module such that the gel is closest to the cathode plate (Fig. 1). Use a roller to remove any air bubbles between the gel and the membrane.

5. Mount the blot module inside the apparatus.

6. Fill the blot module with transfer buffer and the external chamber with dH$_2$O. Run for 1 h at 30 V (*see* **Note 14**).

7. When the run is over, open the blot module and transfer the membrane to a small plastic container.

8. Rinse and shake the membrane twice with washing buffer, 5 min each time.

9. Leave the membrane in blocking buffer overnight at 4 °C.

3.7 Labeling with Antibodies

1. Discard the blocking buffer.

2. Rinse and shake the membrane thrice with 1% Tween 20 in washing buffer for 5 min each time, followed by two washes with washing buffer for 5 min each time.

3. Incubate the membrane with anti-ITCH antibody and anti-actin antibody at RT for 2 h (*see* **Notes 15–17**).

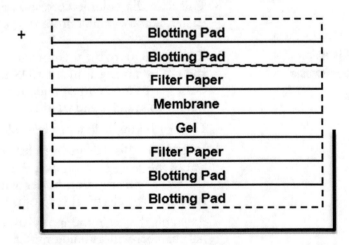

Fig. 1 Sandwich of blotting pad, filter paper, and gel and membrane for gel membrane transfer

4. Rinse and shake thrice with 1 % Tween 20 in washing buffer for 5 min each time, followed by two washes with washing buffer for 5 min each time.

5. Incubate the membrane with HRP secondary antibody for 1 h at RT.

6. Rinse and shake thrice with 1 % Tween 20 in washing buffer for 5 min each time, followed by two washes with washing buffer for 5 min each time.

7. Incubate the membrane with 5 mL of SuperSignal West Pico Chemiluminescent Substrate for 5 min at RT in the dark.

8. Detect the chemiluminescent signal.

9. Analyze the band intensity on the membrane using appropriate imaging software.

4   Notes

1. Scrambled siRNA presents as a sequence that does not target any particular gene. It is used as negative control to distinguish nonspecific effects from specific gene knockdown effects [7].

2. The medium composition depends on the chosen cell line. This medium is for A431 cells.

3. Preparation of working reagent: 50 % (v/v) of Reagent A + 48 % (v/v) reagent B + 2 % (v/v) reagent C.

4. EAGC, siRNA solutions (Table 1).

5. The polymer/siRNA mass ratios to be used depend on the polymer's ability to retain the siRNA. A study should be performed in order to understand ideal polymer/siRNA mass ratios. A balance between the stability of the polyplexes in the presence of biological challenges (e.g., serum and salt) and the release of NA should be obtained.

Table 1
Preparation of EAGC, siRNA solutions

Mass ratio	Concentration siRNA (μg/μL)	Volume siRNA (μL)	Concentration polymer (μg/ μL)	Volume polymer (μL)	Volume dextrose (μL)	Total volume of complexes (μL)	siRNA final concentration in the complexes solution (nM)
60	0.1	106.8	6	106.8	536.4	750	533
30	0.1	106.8	3	106.8	536.4	750	533
10	0.1	106.8	1	106.8	536.4	750	533

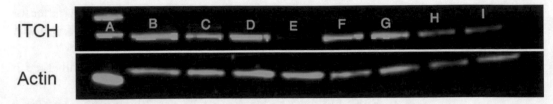

Fig. 2 Western Blotting analysis of ITCH down-regulation in the presence of different doses of siRNA (233 and 533 nM). The study was performed with A431 cells, with polyplexes in contact with the cells for 6 h. Anti-ITCH was the siRNA delivered, β-Actin was used as internal control, and Lipofectamine as positive control. *A*—Molecular weight marker, *B*—Untreated Cells, *C*—Polymer alone, *D*—Naked ITCH siRNA *E*—Lipofectamine + ITCH siRNA (133 nM siRNA), *F*—EAGC30, ITCH siRNA (60:1, 267 nM siRNA), *G*—EAGC30, ITCH siRNA (80:1, 267 nM siRNA), *H*—EAGC30, ITCH siRNA (60:1, 533 nM siRNA), and *I*—EAGC30, ITCH siRNA (80:1, 533 nM siRNA)

6. The time of incubation depends on the binding capability of the polymers with the siRNA. Normally the incubation time varies between 30 min to 1 h. An agarose gel should be run with the complexes at different times of incubation to confirm that there is no release of NA.

7. The dose of siRNA might vary from polymer to polymer depending of the transfection capacity of the transfection agent. A study with different doses of siRNA should be performed in order to identify the dose of siRNA with the highest gene silencing capacity and minimum toxicity to the cells (Fig. 2).

8. The transfection time varies depending on the kind of cells and toxicity of the transfection agent. Consider performing a study to determine the optimal time of incubation of the complexes with cells. A balance between detectable expression and limited toxicity should be achieved.

9. The tubes should be marked with the sample name. Since several tubes will be used, special care should be taken with the labeling of the tubes.

10. The microcentrifuge tubes should not have a flat bottom in order to easily visualize the difference between the pellet and the supernatant.

11. This is a suitable point to take a break in the protocol and carry on in the following day.

12. Please note that the preparation of the BSA standards for the determination of the protein concentration is based on the manufacturer's instructions for use of the BCA assay (Table 2).

13. For each absorbance measurement, subtract the average absorbance measurement of the blank standard from the absorbance measurements of all other individual standards and unknown sample replicates.

14. The time and voltage indicated are specific for the XCell SureLock® Mini-Cell. Adapt each parameter for different apparatus.

Table 2
Preparation of BSA standards

Vial	Volume of DPBS (μL)	Volume of BSA solution (μL)	Final BSA concentration (mg/mL)
A	0	300	2
B	125	375	1.5
C	325	325	1
D	175	175 of B	0.75
E	325	325 of C	0.5
F	325	325 of E	0.35
G	325	325 of E	0.125
H	400	100 of G	0.025
I	400	0	0

15. The dilutions of the antibodies vary with the different antibodies and manufacturers. Follow the instructions provided with the antibodies.

16. β-actin is the housekeeping gene chosen as the "internal" control. Housekeeping genes encode proteins that are essential for maintenance of cell function. β-actin allowed the assay to be controlled for cell toxicity and death.

17. The incubation time with the antibodies can vary between a few h and overnight and is dependent on the binding affinity of the antibody for the protein and the abundance of protein.

References

1. Liang W, Lam JKW (2012) Endosomal escape pathways for non-viral nucleic acid delivery systems. In: Ceresa B (ed) Molecular regulation of endocytosis. InTech, Croatia
2. Ragelle H, Vandermeulen G, Preat V (2013) Chitosan-based siRNA delivery systems. J Control Release 172(1):207–218
3. Buyens K, Meyer M, Wagner E, Demeester J, De Smedt SC, Sanders NN (2010) Monitoring the disassembly of siRNA polyplexes in serum is crucial for predicting their biological efficacy. J Control Release 141(1):38–41
4. Whitehead KA, Langer R, Anderson DG (2009) Knocking down barriers: advances in siRNA delivery. Nat Rev Drug Discov 8(2):129–138
5. Abcam (2014) Western Blotting—a beginner's guide. http://wolfson.huji.ac.il/purification/PDF/PAGE_SDS/Western/ABCAM_WB_BeginnerGuide.pdf. Accessed 17 Jul 2015
6. Thermo Scientific (2014) Western Blotting handbook and troubleshooting tools. https://tools.lifetechnologies.com/content/sfs/brochures/1602761-Western-Blotting-Handbook.pdf. Accessed 17 Jul 2015
7. Invitrogen - Life Technologies (2010) RNAi and epigenetics source book. https://http://www.lifetechnologies.com/content/dam/LifeTech/global/life-sciences/RNAi/PDFs/rnai sourcebook final.pdf. Accessed 17 Jul 2015

Chapter 10

Polyallylamine Derivatives: Novel NonToxic Transfection Agents

Magdalena Wytrwal and Chantal Pichon

Abstract

Cationic polymers have shown great potential for the delivery of proteins, nucleic acids forming complexes, called polyplexes. The most important issue in the context of using cationic polymers as carriers is the balance between the high transfection efficiency and low cytotoxicity. In this chapter, we report the preparation of polyallylamine derivatives mainly based on substitution of amino groups by glycidyltrimethylammonium chloride. The resulting polyplexes enhance the transfection of HeLa cell line without cytotoxic effects. Here, we describe methods for preparation and characterization of polyplexes using dynamic light scattering, ζ-potential measurements, gel retardation assay, and atomic force microscopy. Moreover, we provide protocols for the transfection of HeLa cell line by polyplexes, determination of their cytotoxicity, cell uptake, and intracellular trafficking.

Key words Polymer, Plasmid, Polyplexes, Transfection, Gene delivery, Nanocondensation, Carriers

1 Introduction

The interactions of negatively charged macromolecules, e.g., nucleic acids with positively charged polymers have attracted a great interest not only because of its direct biological implications, but also for a number of applications concerning separation, purification, and transfection of genetic materials [1]. Such electrostatic interactions and entropy change lead to self-assembly formation nanometric-size, stable complexes, called polyplexes (Fig. 1a) [2]. Polyplexes are fabricated either with natural or synthetic polymers. Polypeptides (poly-L-lysine) [3], cationic polysaccharides (chitosan) [4, 5], dendrimers (poly(amidoamines)) [6], poly(β-amino esters) [7], polyamines (polyethyleneimine, polyallylamine) [8–10], and lots of their chemical modifications are the most common polymers used. In designing polycations for gene delivery application, the most crucial issue is their chemical structure, architecture (liner, branch), molecular weight (MW), density of charge, low cytotoxicity, cost-effectiveness, etc [11].

Gabriele Candiani (ed.), *Non-Viral Gene Delivery Vectors: Methods and Protocols*, Methods in Molecular Biology, vol. 1445, DOI 10.1007/978-1-4939-3718-9_10, © Springer Science+Business Media New York 2016

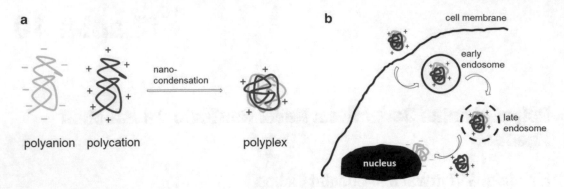

Fig. 1 (**a**) Polyplex formation; (**b**) Scheme of the polyplex trafficking into nucleus

It is considered that at least five major obstacles have to be overcome for the successful gene delivery: in vivo stability, cellular uptake, endosome escape, cytosolic transport, and nuclear delivery [12, 13]. Polyplexes offer possibilities for overcoming cellular barriers by escaping endosomal trafficking followed by cellular internalization and finally enhancing the efficacy of nucleic acids delivery to targeted cells (Fig. 1b) [5]. The mechanisms of endocytosis, including clathrin-mediated endocytosis, caveolae-mediated endocytosis, and macropinocytosis, have been proposed as the main pathway of polyplex internalization into cells [14, 15]. Due to the fact that most of cationic polymers contain generally protonable amines, their acid–base properties depend on the presence of different order amino groups in their structure [16]. The standard titration of polymer solution by strong acid or base is used to determine the buffer capacity of polymers. Cationic polymers induce endosomal escape due to the capture of protons by basic amino groups, when the pH in the endosome decreases from 7.4 to 5.1 [12]. This buffering effect (called proton sponge effect) induces an extensive inflow of water, hydrogen ions, and chloride ions into the endosomal environment which subsequently leads to rupture of the endosomal membrane and release of the entrapped components [17]. The structure and physicochemical properties of these polymers are directly associated with the structure and properties of appropriate polyplexes. The most important aspects in the designing of polycations are the balance between their ability to protect nucleic acids against nuclease degradation, DNA condensation to stable polyplexes, overcoming extra- and intracellular barriers, and finally effective transfection of the cells [13, 18]. However, if the polyplexes are not stable enough, premature dissociation will occur before delivery of the genetic material at the desired place, resulting in low transfection efficiency; on the other hand, a complex that is too stable will not release the DNA, also resulting in low gene expression [18]. The technique generally used to determine these properties are gel shift assay to evaluate either the DNA/polymer complexation or the strength of the affinity between the polymer and DNA in the presence of polyanion. ζ-potential measurements are performed to determine the global surface charge of polyplexes. Typically, the ζ-potential value of the objects above +30 mV and below −30 mV is considered to be stable [19]. The dynamic light scattering is used to determine the efficiency of DNA condensation by measuring the hydrodynamic diameter of the polyplexes. Using atomic force microscopy (AFM), the morphology and size of polyplexes can be examined. The DNA-to-polymer weight ratio, pH, and ionic strength of the solution, in which polyplexes are prepared, are also important factors in the outcome of complexation [20]. The complexes can undergo dissociation either in endosomes, the cytosol, or the nucleus [15, 21]. Cytometry-based methods are commonly used to determine the kinetics of cellular uptake, intracellular trafficking of polyplexes. The qualification of DNA distribution of in the cytosol, endosomes/lysosomes, and nucleus is determined using images captured by confocal laser scanning microscopy (CLSM) [12]. The polyplexes uptake by cells is generally performed by fluorescence-activated cell sorting (FACS analysis) using flow cytometry [12].

Understanding the effect of the cationic polymers' structure on the cytotoxicity, intercellular uptake and transfection let assists in optimal design of more effective carriers for DNA. Polyamines are extensively used as nucleic acids carriers even though some of them are known to be cytotoxic [22, 23]. There are many literature reports that researchers try to decrease the polymers toxicity and increase their transfection efficiency [24]. Based on these, here we present preparation of the novel cationic derivatives of poly(allylamine hydrochloride) (PAH). PAH was modified with glycidyltrimethylammonium chloride (GTMAC) to PG polymer (Fig. 2). This modification significantly improves the biological properties of the PAH in vitro assays [25]. The other synthetic approach was used to decrease the amount of strong quaternary ammonium groups in PAH derivatives' structure. Hence, in the first part of the reaction, the primary amino groups of PAH were partially methylated by CH_3I to PM (~49% of primary, ~24% of secondary, ~27% of tertiary amino groups). Such modifications led to the reduction of toxicity of the polymer and strengthen its capability to complex DNA. Moreover, it improved its buffer capacity [10]. Subsequently, PM was modified with GTMAC at two different degree to PMGG (~49% of mers) and PMG (~21% of mers). Our results indicate that these derivatives show great complexation efficacy of DNA, resulting in reduction of the polymer amount in DNA-to-polymer weight ratio in polyplexes. This has an indirect impact on the decline of the toxic side effects, maintaining the great transfection efficiency [25].

In this chapter, we present the general protocols that can be used for the preparation of polymeric transfection agents based on polyallylamine. Next, we provide typical procedures to analyze the physicochemical properties of polyplexes composed from our

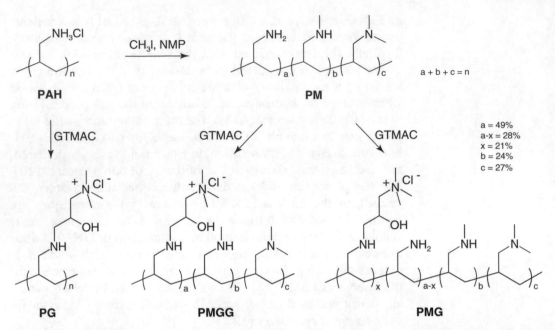

Fig. 2 Scheme of the PAH modifications with the percentage of selected mers. PAH was completely substituted by glycidyltrimethylammonium chloride (GTMAC) to PG or partially methylated by CH_3I to PM. In the second step, PM was substituted at different degree by GTMAC to PMGG (all primary amino groups of PM, ~49%) and PMG (~21% of primary amino groups of PM)

derivatives such as determination of their hydrodynamic diameter, surface ζ-potential, morphology, and ability to complex plasmid DNA (pDNA). The strictly retaining physicochemical properties of polymers and polyplexes offer unique possibilities for overcoming cellular barriers by escaping endosomal trafficking followed by cellular internalization and, consequently, enhancing the transfection efficacy of the pDNA delivery to targeted c ells. Hence, we also provide the standard transfection protocol with or without the endosomotropic agent (chloroquine) and how we investigated pDNA intracellular trafficking and localization.

2 Materials

2.1 Modification of Poly(Allylamine Hydrochloride)

1. Poly(allylamine hydrochloride) (PAH, average MW of ~15,000).

2. 99% pure *N*-methyl-2-pyrrolidone (NMP, spectrophotometric grade).

3. 99% pure iodomethane (CH_3I).

4. Sodium iodide (NaI).

5. 15% (w/v) sodium hydroxide (NaOH) in deionized water (dH_2O).

6. Glycidyltrimethylammonium chloride (GTMAC).

7. Acetic acid (CH₃COOH).

7. Acetic acid (CH_3COOH).

8. Dimethyl sulfoxide-d_6 (DMSO-d_6, 99.9 atom% D).

9. D_2O (99.9 atom% D).

10. NMP tubes.

11. 99% pure sodium chloride (NaCl).

12. 0.1 M hydrochloric acid (HCl) in dH_2O.

13. 1 M NaOH in dH_2O.

14. Benzoylated dialysis tubing (2000 g/mol MW cutoff).

15. Magnetic stirrer.

16. Reflux condenser.

17. Millipore-quality water.

18. Freeze-dryer.

19. Nuclear magnetic spectrometer.

20. Elemental analyzer.

21. Titrator.

2.2 Plasmid DNA (pDNA)

All reactions are prepared with endonuclease-free water.

1. pCMV-luc (pTG11033, 9514 bp, Transgene S.A., Strasbourg, France) encoding the firefly luciferase (luc) gene under the control of the human cytomegalovirus (CMV) promoter.

2. Isolate supercoiled DNA from *Escherichia coli* DH5α super competent bacteria (Invitrogen) by alkali lysis and purify with Mega Kit Endotoxin free Plasmid (Qiagen).

3. Label pDNA with cyanine 3 (Cy3-pDNA) or fluorescein (F-pDNA) using the Label IT nucleic acid labeling kit (MIRUS) at a 1:3 reagent/pDNA weight ratio according to the manufacturer instructions. Purify Cy3-pDNA and F-pDNA by precipitation from ethanol (EtOH). Labeling density should be set as recommended by the manufacturer's protocol (1 cyanine/80 bp).

4. Incubator at 37 °C.

5. Nanodrop.

2.3 Polyplexes

2.3.1 Preparation

1. Linear polyethyleneimine (lPEI, average MW of ~25 kDa).

2. PTG1 (lPEI grafted with 16% histidine residues, His-lPEI; average MW of ~ 34.5 kDa; Polytheragene, France) [26].

3. Synthesize polymers as aqueous solutions.

4. 10 mM HEPES buffer, pH 7.4, in endonuclease-free water: 238.3 mg of HEPES in 100 mL of sterile endonuclease-free water adjusted to pH 7.4 with a 10 N NaOH and passed through a 0.22 µm sterile syringe filter.

5. Vortex mixer.

2.3.2 Size and ζ-Potential Measurements

1. Malvern Nano ZS light-scattering apparatus (Malvern Instrument Ltd.).

2. Endonuclease-free water.

3. DTS 5050 standard beads of −50 mV (Malvern).

4. Disposable folded capillary cells.

2.3.3 Atomic Force Microscopy (AFM)

1. Dimension FastScan Bio AFM (Bruker).

2. FastScan-Dx Probe (nominal tip radius: 8 nm, spring constant: 0.25 N/m).

3. Endonuclease-free water.

4. Silicon wafers.

5. Piranha solution (3:1, v/v, H_2SO_4/H_2O_2) straight away to clean silicon wafers after preparation (*see* **Note 1**).

2.3.4 Gel Retardation Assay

1. Sub-Cell® GT electrophoresis cell for submerged horizontal gels.

2. Power supply.

3. Agarose.

4. 10× TAE running buffer: 400 mM Trizma® base, 200 mM CH_3COOH, 10 mM ethylenediaminetetraacetic acid (EDTA), pH 8.4.

5. 10 μg/mL ethidium bromide (EtBr) in dH_2O.

6. Dextran sulfate sodium salt (DS, average MW of 9000–20,000).

7. 10× gel loading dye: 50% (v/v) glycerol, 0.25% (w/v) bromophenol blue in 1× TAE.

8. Endonuclease-free water.

9. UV light box.

2.4 Cell and Cell Culture

1. Human cervical carcinoma cells (HeLa cells; CRL1772, C2C12, Rockville, MD, USA).

2. HeLa cells stably expressing Rab5-EGFP or Rab7-EGFP [27].

3. Phosphate-buffered saline (PBS).

4. 0.5 M EDTA in dH_2O, pH 7.2.

5. Trypsin/EDTA solution: dilute 10 mL trypsin/EDTA solution in 100 mL PBS.

6. Complete cell culture medium: Minimum Essential Medium (MEM) containing 10% heat-inactivated fetal bovine serum (FBS), 100 U/mL penicillin, 100 U/mL streptomycin, 1% w/v nonessential amino acids and 1% (w/v) GlutaMAX™. For Rab5-EGFP and Rab7-EGFP cells, MEM is supplemented with 100 μg/mL of G418.

2.5   In Vitro Transfection

1. 24-Well culture plates.

2. Trypsin/EDTA solution. Dilute 10 mL of trypsin/EDTA solution in 100 mL of PBS.

3. Freshly prepared polyplexes.

4. 5 mg/mL chloroquine in dH$_2$O.

5. Polypropylene microcentrifuge tubes.

6. PBS buffer.

7. Luciferase Assay System with Reporter Lysis Buffer kit.

8. Ice.

9. Chilled benchtop centrifuge.

10. Luminometer (Titertek-Berthold).

2.6   Cytotoxicity

1. Cell proliferation kit (XTT).

2. 24-Well culture plates.

3. Polymers and freshly prepared polyplexes.

4. Complete cell culture medium.

5. PBS buffer.

6. Microplate spectrophotometer.

2.7   Flow Cytometry Experiments (FACS)

1. HeLa cells.

2. 24-Well culture plates.

3. Freshly prepared polyplexes using F-pDNA.

4. PBS buffer.

5. Trypsin/EDTA solution.

6. Ice.

7. 12× 75-mm FACS Tube Acquisition.

8. 0.4 % (w/v) trypan blue in dH$_2$O.

9. Monensin sodium salt.

10. Chilled benchtop centrifuge.

11. Flow cytometer (LSR1, Becton Dickinson).

2.8   Confocal Laser Scanning Microscopy (CLSM)

1. Freshly prepared polyplexes using Cy3-pDNA.

2. 4-Well Lab-Tek chambered coverglass.

3. PBS buffer.

4. 5 µM DRAQ5™ in PBS.

5. 4 % (w/v) p-formaldehyde in dH$_2$O.

6. Fluoromount-G® (Catalog number 0100 01, Southern Biotechnology).

7. Glass coverslips.

8. Confocal inverted fluorescence microscope.

3   Methods

3.1   Polymer Synthesis

3.1.1   PG

1. Dissolve 2 g (21.4 mmol) of PAH in 70 mL of dH_2O.

2. Add 0.86 g (2.14 mmol) of NaOH and adjust pH to 7.0 using 10% HCl.

3. Add 0.38 mL of 0.5% CH_3COOH as a catalyst.

4. Stir the mixture for 30 min at RT.

5. Dropwise 20 mL (sixfold excess to the amino groups) of GTMAC with continuous stirring.

6. Stir mixture for 6 h at 60 °C and then for 12 h at 50 °C.

7. Put the reaction mixture to the dialysis tubing and dialyze against dH_2O for 7 day.

8. Evaporate dH_2O in a freeze dryer.

9. Solubilize 20 mg of polymer (PG) powder in 1 mL of 1:3 (v/v)D_2O/DMSO-d_6 mixture, put the solution into an NMR tube, and record the ^1H NMR spectrum at 80 °C (300 MHz). Use a DMSO-d_6 residual peak as internal standard.

10. Perform elemental analysis.

11. Determine the degree of substitution by integrating the methyl group signals in NMR spectrum (*see* **Note 2**). Correlate obtained results with elemental analysis data.

3.1.2   PM

1. Dissolve 1 g (10.7 mmol) of PAH in 3 mL of dH_2O and 10 mL of 15% solution of NaOH (*see* **Note 3**).

2. Add 40 mL of NMP. Keep the mixture for 0.5 h at RT.

3. Add 1.5 g of NaI and 1.06 mL (7.49 mmol) of CH_3I. Keep stirring for 12 h at 50 °C under reflux (*see* **Note 4**).

4. Put the reaction mixture to the dialysis tubing and dialyze against dH_2O for 7 day (*see* **Note 5**).

5. Evaporate dH_2O in a freeze dryer.

6. Solubilize 20 mg of polymer (PM) powder in 1 mL of 1:3 v/v D_2O/DMSO-d_6 mixture, put the solution into an NMR tube and record the ^1H NMR spectrum at 80 °C (300 MHz). Use a DMSO-d_6 residual peak as internal standard.

7. Perform elemental analysis.

8. Determine the degree of substitution by integrating the methyl group signals in NMR spectrum (*see* **Note 6**). Correlate obtained results with elemental analysis data.

3.1.3   PMG

1. Dissolve 0.3 g (4.4 mmol) of PM in 12 mL of dH_2O.

2. Apply the same procedure as described in Subheading 3.1.1, **steps 3–11**. Add dropwise 67 μL of GTMAC (5.72 mmol) for PMGG or 15.5 μL (1.32 mmol) for PMG.

3.2 Buffering Capacity of Polymers

1. Prepare 0.5 mg/mL PG, PMG, and PMGG solutions in 150 mM NaCl.

2. Adjust the pH of polymer solutions to pH ~11 with 1 M NaOH.

3. Titrate polymer solutions with 20 μL aliquots of 0.1 M HCl using a titrator with continuous stirring.

4. Measure pH after addition of each portion of acid.

5. Finish titration then the pH reached ~2.

3.3 Polyplexes Preparation

1. Add 2.5 μL of 1 mg/mL pDNA to a 1.5 mL polypropylene microcentrifuge tube containing appropriate volume of endonuclease-free water. Add a proper volume of 1 mg/mL polymer solutions to obtain desired DNA-to-polymer weight ratios (w/w) (e.g. 1:0.5, 1:1, 1:2, 1:3). The final volume of aqueous solutions at the each tube should be fixed.

2. Use as a control 2.5 μg of pDNA in 70 mL of 10 mM HEPES buffer, pH 7.4, mixed with lPEI or 15 μg of PTG1 in 30 mL of 10 mM HEPES buffer, pH 7.4.

3. Vortex gently the solutions of polyplexes.

4. To perform transfection in the presence of chloroquine, add to the polyplexes solutions of 10 μL at 5 mg/mL. The final concentration of chloroquine in polyplexes solutions should be fixed at 100 μM (*see* **Note 7**).

5. Incubate polyplexes for 30 min at RT.

6. Adjust the final volume of polyplexes to 500 μL using complete cell culture medium.

3.4 Polyplexes Size and ζ-Potential Measurements

1. Set the following parameters on the ZetaSizer: viscosity, 0.887 cP; dielectric constant, 79; temperature, 25 °C; F(κa), 1.50 (Smoluchowski); maximum voltage of the current, 15 V.

2. To calibrate the size measurement, put 200 ± 5 nm polystyrene polymer into a polystyrene cuvette in dH_2O and insert the cuvette in the size measurement place of the apparatus.

3. Measure the size ten times under the automatic mode.

4. To calibrate the ζ-potential measurement, put 0.7 mL of DTS 5050 standard beads of -50 ± 5 mV into a polystyrene cuvette and insert it in the aqueous dip cell of the apparatus and the electrodes on the dip cell.

5. Measure the ζ-potential ten times with the zero field correction.

6. Prepare aqueous solution of pDNA and solution of polyplexes, at the same pDNA concentration, as described in Subheading 3.3.

7. Put 0.7 mL of solutions into the disposable folded capillary cell.

8. Measure the hydrodynamic diameter of the objects at least ten times under the automatic mode and ζ-potential ten times with the zero field correction.

3.5   AFM Observation

1. Prepare polyplex suspensions (*see* Subheading 3.3).

2. The freshly cleaned silicon wafers in piranha solution put for 15 min into the 5 mL of aqueous polyplex solution (C_{DNA} = 0.2 µg/mL).

3. Gently wash with dH_2O the silicon wafers with deposited polyplexes.

4. Measure the topography of samples at 110 kHz resonant frequency of the probe in dH_2O. Obtain the images in tapping mode at a typical line frequency of 10 Hz.

3.6   Electrophoretic Mobility Shift Assay

1. Check the quality of pDNA and polyplexes by electrophoresis (Fig. 3) (*see* **Note 8**).

2. Prepare a 0.9% agarose gel. For 60 mL of gel, dissolve 0.54 g of agarose in 60 mL of 1× TAE buffer in a microwave device.

3. Cool the solution to about 60 °C.

4. Add 2 µL of 10 mg/mL solution of EtBr.

5. Remove any bubbles and allow it to set. Remove the comb and place the gel in the gel tank. Cover with 1× TAE running buffer.

6. Prepare polyplex samples by mixing 2 µL of Load Dye in 1× TAE, 1 µL of pDNA at 0.5 mg/mL, appropriate volume of aqueous polymer solutions to prepare polyplexes at different weight ratios (1:0.5, 1:1, 1:2, 1:3 pDNA-to-polymer) and 1:6 pDNA/PTG1. Finally, add endonuclease-free water to obtain 10 µL of the final volume of each sample. Incubate polyplexes for 30 min.

7. Use free pDNA as a control.

8. Load the samples onto the wells.

9. Run the gel in 1× TAE buffer for 1 h at 70 V until the bromophenol blue dye is near the bottom of the gel.

10. Examine the gel on an UV light box (*see* **Note 9**).

11. Check the stability of polyplexes using DS sodium salt solution. Add DS to polyplex solutions at 1:1 weight ratio of pDNA/DS. Incubate polyplexes for 1 h with DS. Load mixtures onto 0.9% agarose gel and perform experiment as describe above.

3.7   HeLa Cells Transfection

1. Cell growth: Seed 1×10^6 cells in a 75 cm^2 culture flask with 20 mL of complete cell culture medium and incubate at 37 °C in a humidified 5% CO_2 atmosphere (*see* **Note 10**).

2. Harvest the cells at confluence: Aspirate medium, wash cells with 10 mL of PBS, treat for 10 min at 37 °C with 10 mL trypsin/EDTA solution, add 10 mL complete cell culture medium to block trypsin, collect cell suspension, and spin in a 50 mL sterile centrifuge tube for 15 min at $300 \times g$ in a chilled benchtop centrifuge.

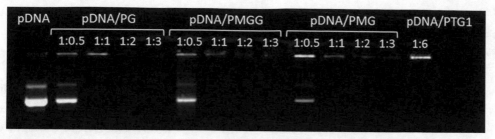

Fig. 3 Electrophoretic mobility shift assay of free pDNA and condense as polyplexes at different polymer-to-weight ratio (0.5 µg of pDNA). Samples are loaded in a 0.9% agarose gel and electrophoresis is run for 1 h at 60 V in TAE buffer. pDNA is stained with EtBr

3. Seed 5×10^4 cells per well in 500 µL of suspension in complete cell culture medium.

4. Prepare solutions of polyplexes at different DNA-to-polymer weight ratios in endonuclease-free water or in 10 mM HEPES buffer as described in Subheading 3.3.

5. Replace the culture medium with medium containing polyplexes suspension.

6. Incubate the cells with polyplexes solution for 4 h at 37 °C.

7. Remove medium and replace it with the fresh complete cell culture medium.

8. After 48 h of transfection, remove the culture medium and wash the cells once with PBS.

9. Determine expression of the luciferase gene using the Luciferase Assay System with Reporter Lysis Buffer kit following the manufacturer's recommendations. Briefly, wash the cell monolayer with PBS, dry completely before adding 100 µL of cell culture lysis reagent (CCLR). Scrape carefully the cell monolayer using a cell scraper. The resulting cell lysate is incubated on ice for 10 min and centrifuge at $6000 \times g$ for 5 min. Transfer an aliquot of 20 µL of cell supernatant to a luminometer tube and add 100 µL of Luciferase Assay Reagent containing the luciferin substrate to the tube using an automatic luminometer. Record the light emitted from the catalyzed luciferin product for a 2-s integration time. Read each sample in duplicate to ensure accurate and reproducible results.

10. Use a 10 µL aliquot of pre-cleared lysate to determine the protein content in sample using the standardized BCA method. Normalize relative Luciferase activities (RLU) to protein content and express data as RLU/mg of proteins. Represent the final data as fold of luciferase induction relative to control cells.

3.8 Polymers and Polyplexes Cytotoxic Activity on HeLa Cells

1. Prepare cells for transfection assay using polymers alone and in the form of polyplexes (*see* Subheading 3.7).

2. Prepare XTT reagent mixture by mixing 5 mL of XTT Labeling Reagent and 100 µL of Electron-coupling Reagent.

3. Dilute mixture for three times with complete cell culture medium.

4. After 48 h of transfection, remove medium, wash cells with PBS, and add 500 µL of complete cell culture medium containing XTT reagent.

5. Incubate cells with XTT for 18 h at 37 °C (*see* **Note 11**).

6. Measure the absorbance of each well at $\lambda = 560$ nm with the microplate spectrophotometer.

7. Calculate the cells' viability as a percentage of control (untreated cells).

3.9 Measurements of Polyplexes Uptake by HeLa Cells

1. Seed 5×10^4 cells per well in 500 µL of suspension in culture medium.

2. Prepare solutions of polyplexes at different DNA-to-polymer weight ratios in endonuclease-free water, e.g. F-pDNA/PG (1:2) or F-pDNA/PMG (1:1).

3. Replace the culture medium with medium containing polyplexes.

4. Incubate cells with polyplexes for 1, 2, and 4 h at 37 °C.

5. Remove culture medium, wash cells two times with ice-cold PBS, harvest them by 200 µL of trypsin, centrifuge at $400 \times g$ for 5 min at 4 °C, suspend in 300 µL of PBS, and put them to the special FACS tubes on ice.

6. Measure the cell fluorescence intensity by flow cytometry. As a blank measure cells not treated with polyplexes.

7. Add to the tubes 5 µL of 1.2 mg/mL trypan blue solution [28]. Measure the cell fluorescence intensity by flow cytometry (*see* **Note 12**).

8. Prepare monensin solution: Dissolve 17.7 mg of monensin in 1 mL of EtOH. Add 40 mL of alcohol solution of monensin to 10 mL of PBS [29, 30].

9. Add to the tubes 300 µL of 50 µM monensin (a Na^+/H^+ ionophore) and incubate them for 30 min at 4 °C [31]. Measure the cell fluorescence intensity by flow cytometry performing each measurement with 1×10^4 cells at $\lambda_{em} = 520$ nm upon excitation at $\lambda_{ex} = 488$ nm (*see* **Note 13**).

3.10 Determination of Polyplexes Intracellular Routing

1. Two days before the experiment, seed Rab5-EGFP and Rab7-EGFP HeLa cells at a density of 1.4×10^4 cells/well in a 4-well Lab-Tek chambered coverglass.

2. Incubate cells at 37 °C for 30 min, 3 h, and 6 h with 1:1 Cy3-pDNA/PMG polyplexes.

3. Wash cells two times for 5 min with PBS, incubate cells for 5 min with 5 μM DRAQ5™ to stain nucleus, wash two times for 5 min with PBS, fix cells with 4% *p*-formaldehyde for 20 min, wash twice for 5 min with PBS.

4. Remove one slide at a time from aqueous buffer, add one drop of Fluoromount-G® directly to cell sample.

5. Mount coverslip and press gently to remove excess mounting medium and to seal the coverslip.

6. Allow mounted samples to air dry for 5 min before examination.

7. Perform confocal microscopy analysis using inverted microscope. Obtain images after multiple excitations at $\lambda_{ex} = 488$ nm (EGFP), $\lambda_{ex} = 568$ nm (Cy3), and $\lambda_{ex} = 687$ nm (DRAQ5™).

4 Notes

1. Before used, silicon wafers hold in piranha solution for 1 h, wash twice with deionized water, and dry under the inert gas.

2. The degree of substitution of PAH amino groups by GTMAC is determined from the ^{1}H NMR spectrum in 1:3 (v/v) D_2O/DMSO-d_6 mixture. Select the signals from PAH structure: 3H in the range of 0.45–2.00 ppm corresponds to hydrocarbon backbone. The best separated signal present in the range of 4.04–4.41 ppm comes from methine group (isopropanol spacer linker). If the integration value of this signal is 1H, the degree of substitution by GTMAC moiety is 100%. The rest signals in the spectrum come from methylene groups between PAH amino groups (in the range of 2.15–2.86 ppm), methylene groups from GTMAC moiety (in the range of 3.19–3.53 ppm), and methyl quaternized amino groups (in the range of 2.96–3.19 ppm).

3. This step is crucial to remove hydrochloride from PAH structure and obtain free primary amino groups.

4. With the time of reaction the mixture, change color from colorless to yellow, due to iodide release.

5. With the time of dialysis, the solution inside dialysis tubing will be discolored.

6. The percentage of amino order (degree of methylation) is determined from the ^{1}H NMR spectrum (recorded in 1:3 (v/v) D_2O/DMSO-d_6 mixture). Select the signals from PAH structure: 3H in the range of 0.85–1.81 ppm corresponds to hydrocarbon backbone and 2H in the range of 2.41–3.00 ppm corresponds to methylene groups bonded to amino groups. Extra signals present in the spectrum come from methyl groups

substituted to PAH amino groups. In the range of 1.90–2.30 ppm, methyl groups are substituted to tertiary amino groups, while in the range of 2.30–2.53 ppm methyl groups are substituted to secondary amino groups. Calculate the degree of methylation to tertiary or secondary amino groups by dividing integration value by 6 or 3 protons from two or one methyl group, respectively.

7. Chloroquine is a lysosomotropic agent that prevents endosomal acidification [32]. It accumulates inside the acidic parts of the cell, including endosomes and lysosomes. Chloroquine enhances gene transfer frequency by preventing the degradation of DNA in the lysosomes or lysosomal-like compartments and thus increases the delivery of more intact genes from the cytoplasm to the nucleus for gene expression [33].

8. pDNA, that was used in all experiments, migrates as two bands. That could be explain as a presence of two conformational forms of its structure (Fig. 3).

9. Starting from 1:1 DNA-to-polymer weight ratio, pDNA is completely condensed with PG, PMGG, and PMG. There are no free pDNAs, as in the control 1:6 polyplex pDNA/PTG1. Using 1:0.5 (w/w) DNA/polymer, not all amount of pDNA was complexed. There are extra bands from free pDNA which migrate in the gel.

10. Check cells for mycoplasma presence using the Mycoplasma Detection Kit.

11. In contrast to MTT, the cleavage product of XTT is soluble in dH_2O; therefore, a solubilization step of formazan is not required. This technique requires neither washing nor harvesting of cells.

12. The trypan blue is used to quench the fluorescence associated with the polyplexes bound on the surface of the cells. The ability to distinguish between extra- and intracellular particles/polyplexes is achieved by performing quenching experiments with trypan blue. This dye cannot permeate the cell membrane and it quenches the fluorescence of Cy3. Addition of trypan blue to cells incubated with Cy3-labeled polyplexes results in fluorescence quenching of extracellular particles whereas internalized particles remain fluorescent. Polyplexes can be quenched only once and do not recover their fluorescence. Therefore, one quenching experiment represents one single-cell measurement. In order to analyze trajectories in relation to the extra- or intracellular presence of the particles, streams with different time points of quenching should be recorded [34].

13. The monensin treatment restores the fluorescein fluorescence that is partially quenched in acidic vesicles (endosomes and lysosomes) [35].

Acknowledgment

This work was supported by the National Science Centre (NCN) Poland (Grant No. 2012/05/N/ST5/00809).

References

1. Miguel MG, Pais AACC, Dias RS, Leal C, Rosa M, Lindman B (2003) DNA-cationic amphiphile interactions. Colloid Surface A 228(1-3):43–55

2. Yang J, Liu HM, Zhang X (2014) Design, preparation and application of nucleic acid delivery carriers. Biotechnol Adv 32(4):804–817

3. Kwoh DY, Coffin CC, Lollo CP, Jovenal J, Banaszczyk MG, Mullen P, Phillips A, Amini A, Fabrycki J, Bartholomew RM, Brostoff SW, Carlo DJ (1999) Stabilization of poly-L-lysine/DNA polyplexes for in vivo gene delivery to the liver. Biochim Biophys Acta 1444(2):171–190

4. Agirre M, Zarate J, Ojeda E, Puras G, Desbrieres J, Pedraz JL (2014) Low molecular weight chitosan (LMWC)-based polyplexes for pDNA delivery: from bench to bedside. Polymers 6(6):1727–1755

5. Singh D, Han SS, Shin EJ (2014) Polysaccharides as nanocarriers for therapeutic applications. J Biomed Nanotechnol 10(9):2149–2172

6. Pourianazar NT, Mutlu P, Gunduz U (2014) Bioapplications of poly(amidoamine) (PAMAM) dendrimers in nanomedicine. J Nanopart Res 16 (4):2342 1-38.

7. Bishop CJ, Ketola TM, Tzeng SY, Sunshine JC, Urtti A, Lemmetyinen H, Vuorimaa-Laukkanen E, Yliperttula M, Green JJ (2013) The effect and role of carbon atoms in poly(beta-amino ester)s for DNA binding and gene delivery. J Am Chem Soc 135(18):6951–6957

8. Godbey WT, Wu KK, Mikos AG (1999) Poly(ethylenimine) and its role in gene delivery. J Control Release 60(2-3):149–160

9. Lungwitz U, Breunig M, Blunk T, Gopferich A (2005) Polyethylenimine-based non-viral gene delivery systems. Eur J Pharm Biopharm 60(2):247–266

10. Wytrwal M, Leduc C, Sarna M, Goncalves C, Kepczynski M, Midoux P, Nowakowska M, Pichon C (2015) Gene delivery efficiency and intracellular trafficking of novel poly(allylamine) derivatives. Int J Pharm 478(1):372–382

11. Tang MX, Szoka FC (1997) The influence of polymer structure on the interactions of cationic polymers with DNA and morphology of the resulting complexes. Gene Ther 4(8):823–832

12. Khalil IA, Kogure K, Akita H, Harashima H (2006) Uptake pathways and subsequent intracellular trafficking in nonviral gene delivery. Pharmacol Rev 58(1):32–45

13. Pathak A, Patnaik S, Gupta KC (2009) Recent trends in non-viral vector-mediated gene delivery. Biotechnol J 4(11):1559–1572

14. Pichon C, Billiet L, Midoux P (2010) Chemical vectors for gene delivery: uptake and intracellular trafficking. Curr Opin Biotechnol 21(5):640–645

15. Parhamifar L, Larsen AK, Hunter AC, Andresen TL, Moghimi SM (2010) Polycation cytotoxicity: a delicate matter for nucleic acid therapy-focus on polyethylenimine. Soft Matter 6(17):4001–4009

16. De Smedt SC, Demeester J, Hennink WE (2000) Cationic polymer based gene delivery systems. Pharm Res 17(2):113–126

17. Varkouhi AK, Scholte M, Storm G, Haisma HJ (2011) Endosomal escape pathways for delivery of biologicals. J Control Release 151(3):220–228

18. Bertin A (2014) Polyelectrolyte complexes of DNA and polycations as gene delivery vectors. Adv Polym Sci 256:103–195

19. Wytrwal M, Bednar J, Nowakowska M, Wydro P, Kepczynski M (2014) Interactions of serum with polyelectrolyte-stabilized liposomes: Cryo-TEM studies. Colloid Surface B 120:152–159

20. de Ilarduya CT, Sun Y, Duezguencs N (2010) Gene delivery by lipoplexes and polyplexes. Eur J Pharm Sci 40(3):159–170

21. Cho YW, Kim JD, Park K (2003) Polycation gene delivery systems: escape from endosomes to cytosol. J Pharm Pharmacol 55(6):721–734

22. Pegg AE (2013) Toxicity of polyamines and their metabolic products. Chem Res Toxicol 26(12):1782–1800

23. Novo L, Rizzo LY, Golombek SK, Dakwar GR, Lou B, Remaut K, Mastrobattista E, van Nostrum CF, Jahnen Dechent W, Kiessling F, Braeckmans K, Lammers T, Hennink WE (2014) Decationized polyplexes as stable and safe carrier systems for improved biodistribution in systemic gene therapy. J Control Release 195:162–175

24. Min SH, Park KC, Yeom YI (2014) Chitosan-mediated non-viral gene delivery with improved serum stability and reduced cytotoxicity. Biotechnol Bioproc E 19(6):1077–1082

25. Wytrwal M, Koczurkiewicz P, Wojcik K, Michalik M, Kozik B, Zylewski M, Nowakowska M, Kepczynski M (2014) Synthesis of strong polycations with improved biological properties. J Biomed Mater Res A 102(3):721–731

26. Bertrand E, Goncalves C, Billiet L, Gomez JP, Pichon C, Cheradame H, Midoux P, Guegan P (2011) Histidinylated linear PEI: a new efficient non-toxic polymer for gene transfer. Chem Commun 47(46):12547–12549

27. Billiet L, Gomez JP, Berchel M, Jaffres PA, Le Gall T, Montier T, Bertrand E, Cheradame H, Guegan P, Mevel M, Pitard B, Benvegnu T, Lehn P, Pichon C, Midoux P (2012) Gene transfer by chemical vectors, and endocytosis routes of polyplexes, lipoplexes and lipopolyplexes in a myoblast cell line. Biomaterials 33(10):2980–2990

28. Nuutila J, Lilius EM (2005) Flow cytometric quantitative determination of ingestion by phagocytes needs the distinguishing of overlapping populations of binding and ingesting cells. Cytometry A 65A(2):93–102

29. Monsigny M, Roche AC, Midoux P (1984) Uptake of Neoglycoproteins Via Membrane Lectin(S) of L1210 Cells Evidenced by Quantitative Flow Cytofluorometry and Drug Targeting. Biol Cell 51(2):187–196

30. Midoux P, Roche AC, Monsigny M (1987) Quantitation of the binding, uptake, and degradation of fluoresceinylated neoglycoproteins by flow-cytometry. Cytometry 8(3):327–334

31. Goncalves C, Mennesson E, Fuchs R, Gorvel JP, Midoux P, Pichon C (2004) Macropinocytosis of polyplexes and recycling of plasmid from clathrin-dependent pathway impair the transfection efficiency into human hepatocarcinoma cells. Mol Ther 10:373–385

32. Steinman RM, Mellman IS, Muller WA, Cohn ZA (1983) Endocytosis and the recycling of plasma-membrane. J Cell Biol 96(1):1–27

33. Erbacher P, Roche AC, Monsigny M, Midoux P (1996) Putative role of chloroquine in gene transfer into a human hepatoma cell line by DNA lactosylated polylysine complexes. Exp Cell Res 225(1):186–194

34. de Bruin K, Ruthardt N, von Gersdorff K, Bausinger R, Wagner E, Ogris M, Brauchle C (2007) Cellular dynamics of EGF receptor-targeted synthetic viruses. Mol Ther 15(7):1297–1305

35. Breuzard G, Tertil M, Goncalves C, Cheradame H, Geguan P, Pichon C, Midoux P (2008) Nuclear delivery of N kappa B-assisted DNA/polymer complexes: plasmid DNA quantitation by confocal laser scanning microscopy and evidence of nuclear polyplexes by FRET imaging. Nucleic Acids Res 36(12), e17

Chapter 11

Biodegradable Three-Layered Micelles and Injectable Hydrogels

Daniel G. Abebe, Rima Kandil, Teresa Kraus, Maha Elsayed, Tomoko Fujiwara, and Olivia M. Merkel

Abstract

Polymeric micelles have found a growing interest as gene vectors due to the serious safety concerns associated with viral vectors. In particular, the cationic polymer polyethylene imine (PEI) has shown relatively high condensation and transfection efficiencies. Additionally, polyethylene glycol (PEG) modification of polymeric gene vectors has dramatically improved their biological properties, including enhanced biocompatibility, prolonged circulation time, and increased bio-distribution. However, PEG grafting of PEI for subsequent condensation of nucleic acids (NAs) does not necessarily result in the formation of a PEI/NAs core with a PEG corona. But often times, the presence of PEG interferes with PEI's electrostatic interaction with NAs. We describe here a facile method to prepare multilayered biodegradable micelles which address some of the critical drawbacks associated with current PEI-based systems. The polyplex micelles have superb stability and stealth properties. Moreover, we describe a method to prepare fully biodegradable and biocompatible injectable hydrogels for use in localized gene therapy.

Key words DNA delivery, Micelles, Hydrogels, Biodegradable, Injectable, PEI, PEG, PLLA, Block copolymers

---

1 Introduction

Gene therapy has the potential to treat a wide array of inherited and acquired genetic disorders, including diabetes, cystic fibrosis, certain cancers, haemophilia, and cardiovascular and infectious diseases [1–4]. The development of gene delivery vectors has been a paramount feature in the overall maturation of gene therapy and has propelled it from a theoretical concept into a next generation treatment. Viral vectors were among the earliest investigated vectors and have continued to dominant clinical research due to the high transfection efficiency of viruses. However, there are inherent drawbacks associated with viral vectors, particularly the serious safety concerns of immunogenicity and oncogenicity [5]. Therefore, nonviral

Gabriele Candiani (ed.), *Non-Viral Gene Delivery Vectors: Methods and Protocols*, Methods in Molecular Biology, vol. 1445, DOI 10.1007/978-1-4939-3718-9_11, © Springer Science+Business Media New York 2016

vectors have found growing interest, of which cationic polymers are an attractive option. Polyethylene imine (PEI) is one of the most studied cationic polymers and has shown high condensation and superior transfection efficiencies [6]. The drawbacks with current PEI-based vectors are critical cytotoxicity due to the high molecular weight (MW) needed for high transfection and low in vivo stability of the PEI/DNA polyplexes [7–11]. Surface modification of PEI-based vectors with polyethylene glycol (PEG) has led to enhanced biocompatibility, prolonged circulation half-life, and improved bio-distribution [12–14]. The "stealth" properties achieved through PEG modification have allowed for the preparation of systemic gene delivery vectors which can be administered through conventional routes [15]. Stealth systemic delivery vectors with a distinct PEG layer have the ability to target a large array of disease states including penetration of the difficult blood-brain barrier [16]. Alternatively, localized gene delivery vectors, such as hydrogels, have found increasing popularity in the last decade. The emerging field of in situ forming (injectable) hydrogels possesses unique features, including minimal invasiveness, reduced surgery-related complications, and ability to mold to specific shapes/crevices [17, 18]. The encapsulation and delivery of nucleic acids (NAs) has been reported using both synthetic and natural polymer-based hydrogels. Both physical and chemical crosslinking methods have been investigated for hydrogel formation [19–22]. The main hurdle in the development of an efficient injectable hydrogel system is the fine balance needed between the gel's mechanical integrity and its biocompatibility and biodegradability.

We describe here a facile formulation method for the preparation of stealth three-layered polyplex micelles (3LM) for application as versatile gene delivery vectors [23]. A dual encapsulation procedure capable of condensing high MW DNA into a compact polyplex particle is outlined. Moreover, the procedure utilized relatively nontoxic low MW PEI to address the critical cytotoxicity associated with high MW PEI. The 3LM are prepared by a two-step procedure (Fig. 1). In the first step, DNA is encapsulated through electrostatic interaction and solvent-induced condensation in an organic solvent system. In the second step, the DNA-loaded organo-polyplex micelle is encapsulated with a PEG-based amphiphilic polymer system to yield aqueous-stabilized polyplex micelles. The different layers of the 3LM can be clearly observed using DNA labeling technique and transmission electron microscopy (TEM) (Fig. 2). The 3LM showed superb biological stability and stealth properties. Controlled and complete release of the encapsulated DNA was achieved at pH ~4.5 (late endosome environment), while negligible DNA release was observed at neutral pH. Furthermore, we describe here a method to prepare the injectable hydrogels from the DNA-loaded 3LM utilizing the stereocomplexation by enantiomeric L- and D-polylactides, PLLA and PDLA, respectively [24]. The resulting micelle solutions have controllable

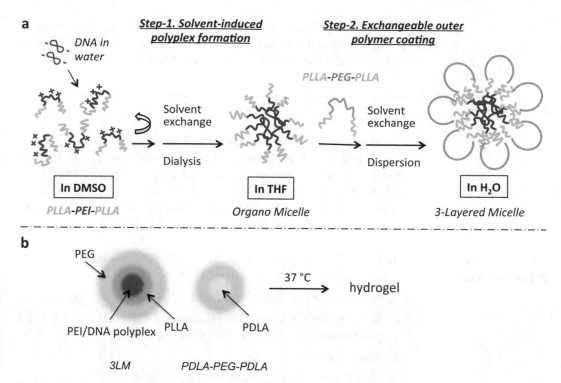

a   **Step-1. Solvent-induced polyplex formation**   **Step-2. Exchangeable outer polymer coating**

DNA in water

PLLA-*PEG*-PLLA

Solvent exchange

Dialysis

Solvent exchange

Dispersion

In DMSO   In THF   In H₂O

PLLA-*PEI*-PLLA   Organo Micelle   3-Layered Micelle

b

PEG

37 °C → hydrogel

PEI/DNA polyplex   PLLA   PDLA

3LM   PDLA-PEG-PDLA

Fig. 1 (**a**) 3LM and (**b**) hydrogel preparation. Reproduced with permission from Abebe et al. [23]. Copyright 2015 John Wiley and Sons

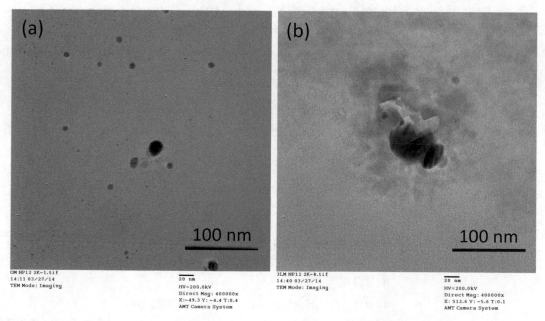

Fig. 2 TEM images of AgNO₃ pre-stained organo-micelles (**a**) and 3LM (**b**) at N/P 12

sol-to-gel phase transitions between 25 and 37 °C. The complete absence of relatively toxic chemical crosslinking reagents makes these hydrogels fully biodegradable and biocompatible.

2   Materials

For this particular formulation, PLLA-PEI-PLLA, PLLA-PEG-PLLA, and PDLA-PEG-PDLA block copolymers are needed. We describe here the use of PLLA-PEI-PLLA, PLLA-PEG-PLLA, PDLA-PEG-PDLA, and Folate-PEG-PLLA. These polymers can be freshly synthesized using high yielding and controllable synthetic protocols as described previously [23–25].

2.1   Formation of Organo-Micelles

1. PLLA-PEI-PLLA with MWs of 1700 and 2000 Da of the PLLA and PEI blocks, respectively.
2. Salmon sperm DNA (Sigma-Aldrich, St. Louis, MO).
3. Regenerated Cellulose (RC) dialysis tube with MWCO 3.5–5 k (Spectrum Labs, Rancho Dominguez, CA).
4. Tetrahydrofuran (THF).
5. 99.9 % pure dimethylsulfoxide (DMSO).
6. 20 mL glass scintillation vials (polypropylene cap, foamed PEI liner).
7. Magnetic stirrer.

2.2   3LM Formulation

1. Organo-micelles.
2. PLLA-PEG-PLLA with MWs of 800 and 2000 (Da) of the PLLA and PEG blocks, respectively.
3. Folate-PEG-PLLA with MWs of 800 and 3000 (Da) of the PLLA and PEG blocks, respectively.
4. THF.
5. Ultra-pure water (dH$_2$O) with resistivity close to 18 MΩ cm.
6. 20 mL glass scintillation vials (polypropylene cap, foamed PEI liner).
7. Fume hood.
8. Ice bath.

2.3   Hydrogels

1. 3LM.
2. PDLA-PEG-PDLA with MWs of 800 and 2000 Da of the PDLA and PEG blocks, respectively.
3. THF.
4. dH$_2$O with resistivity close to 18 MΩ cm.
5. 20 mL glass scintillation vials (polypropylene cap, foamed PEI liner).

6. Ice bath.

7. Water bath.

8. Sonicator.

2.4 Determination of DNA-Loading Efficiency

1. 3LM.

2. Trizol reagent (Invitrogen, Life Technologies, Carlsbad, CA).

3. Pure ethanol (EtOH).

4. 99.9 % pure chloroform ($CHCl_3$).

5. dH_2O with resistivity close to 18 $M\Omega$ cm.

6. 5 % (w/v) glucose in deionized water (dH_2O).

7. 100 mM sodium acetate (CH_3COONa) buffer, pH 4.5.

8. 8 mM sodium hydroxide (NaOH) in dH_2O.

9. 12.5 mg/mL of heparin in TE buffer (10 mM Tris–HCl, pH 7.5, and 1 mM ethylenediaminetetraacetic acid, EDTA).

10. Glass scintillation vials.

11. 2 mL polypropylene microcentrifuge tubes.

12. Tube centrifuge or rotor for 2 mL microcentrifuge tubes.

13. UV-Vis spectrophotometer.

2.5 Determination of 3LM Stability and Release Properties

1. 3LM.

2. 5–50 µg of dextran sulfate from Leuconostoc. spp (Sigma-Aldrich) dissolved in 10 µL of dH_2O.

3. Unmodified PEI, Lupasol G100, MW 5 k (BASF, Ludwigshafen, Germany).

4. 5 % (w/v) glucose in dH_2O.

5. 100 mM CH_3COONa buffer, pH 4.5.

6. 4× SYBR Gold solution (Life Technologies).

7. Opaque 96-well plates.

8. Fluorescence plate reader.

2.6 Silver Staining and TEM Imaging

1. 0.1 M silver nitrate ($AgNO_3$).

2. Copper-coated carbon grid (Ted Pella Inc. Redding, CA).

3. TEM equipped with a digital CCD camera.

3 Methods

3.1 Formation of DNA-Loaded Organo-Micelles

1. In a glass scintillation vial, weigh out 4.24 mg of PLLA-PEI-PLLA triblock copolymer (*see* **Note 1**).

2. Add 1 mL of DMSO to the vial and allow mixture to stir at room temperature (RT) to obtain a transparent faint orange solution.

3. Under vigorous stirring, add bulk 1 mg of DNA in 200 μL of dH$_2$O (*see* **Note 2**).

4. Allow the transparent faint orange mixture to stir for 60 min at 25 °C.

5. Under vigorous stirring, pipette in 5 mL of THF to the mixture.

6. Allow the transparent, clear solution to equilibrate at RT for 10 min.

7. Transfer the mixture to an RC dialysis tube and dialyze the solution against 1 L of THF for 4 h to obtain the organo-micelles (*see* **Note 3**).

3.2 Formation of Targeted PEG-Stabilized 3LM

1. In a glass scintillation vial, weigh out 4.24 mg of PLLA-PEG-PLLA triblock copolymer (*see* **Note 4**).

2. Combine the organo-micelle/THF solution (typically between 3 and 4 mL after dialysis) with the vial containing PLLA-PEG-PLLA copolymer.

3. Allow PLLA-PEG-PLLA to dissolve and equilibrate with the organo-micelles.

4. Add the THF solution drop-wise into 10 mL of dH$_2$O under vigorous stirring at 4 °C.

5. Remove THF by evaporation in a fume hood setup under a gentle stream of compressed air to obtain a transparent and clear aqueous solution of 3LM (*see* **Note 5**).

6. Concentrate the 3LM aqueous solution under a gentle stream of compressed air to the desired volume. For hydrogel formation, concentrate to the final volume of 50 μL to obtain a ~20% (w/v) solution (*see* **Note 6**).

3.3 Preparation of Injectable Hydrogels

1. In a glass scintillation vial, weigh out 100 mg of PDLA-PEG-PDLA triblock copolymer.

2. Add 300 μL of THF to dissolve the copolymer.

3. Add the THF solution drop-wise to 500 μL of dH$_2$O under vigorous stirring at 4 °C (*see* **Note 7**).

4. Allow THF to evaporate in a fume hood setup and obtain the PDLA-PEG-PDLA micelle solution at a final concentration of 20% (w/v) (*see* **Note 8**).

5. For hydrogel formation, first place the PDLA-PEG-PDLA micelle and 3LM solutions separately in an ice bath and equilibrate at 4 °C for 30 min.

6. In a test tube immersed in a sonication bath at 4 °C, add equal volumes of both micelle solutions. Allow the solution to mix and form a homogenous transparent aqueous dispersion.

7. Tightly seal the test tube and place it in a water bath at 37 °C to jellify.

3.4 Quantification of Encapsulated DNA

1. To isolate and quantify encapsulated DNA, pipette 100 μL of 3LM into a glass scintillation vial. Dilute the solution with 500 μL of TE buffer containing 12.5 mg/mL of heparin.

2. Add 200 μL of $CHCl_3$ and 500 μL of Trizol reagent to the vial.

3. Tightly seal the vial and stir vigorously at 37 °C for 60 min.

4. Transfer the mixture to a 2 mL polypropylene microcentrifuge tube.

5. Centrifuge the mixture at $12,000 \times g$ for 15 min at 4 °C to separate the phases.

6. Discard the aqueous top layer.

7. Add 300 μL of pure EtOH to the interphase and bottom organic layers; incubate for 10 min at 25 °C.

8. Centrifuge the solution at $2000 \times g$ for 5 min at 4 °C to pellet the DNA.

9. Discard the supernatant and wash DNA pellet with 75 % (v/v) EtOH by gentle inversion.

10. Centrifuge the mixture at $2000 \times g$ for 5 min at 4 °C to re-pellet the DNA. Repeat wash cycles three to four times to completely remove phenol.

11. Resuspend the DNA pellet by dissolving in 200 μL of 8 mM NaOH solution.

12. Centrifuge the solution at $12,000 \times g$ for 10 min at 4 °C to remove insoluble materials.

13. Measure UV absorbance to obtain concentration of DNA in ng/μL (*see* **Note 9**).

3.5 Determination of 3LM Stability and Release Properties

1. Dilute 3LM to obtain a final DNA concentration of 1 μg/90 μL in either 5 % glucose solution, pH 7.4, or 100 mM CH_3COONa buffer, pH 4.5.

2. Pipette 90 μL of the 3LM solution to an opaque 96-well plate (*see* **Note 10**).

3. To each well, add 30 μL of a 4× SYBR Gold solution and incubate the plate for 10 min at 25 °C.

4. Prepare dextran sulfate stock solution and dilute to achieve 10 μL aliquots at concentrations ranging from 0.5 to 5 μg/μL.

5. To each well containing 3LM, add 10 μL of dextran sulfate solution with increasing concentration.

6. Incubate the plate for 30 min, 1 h, 2 h, and 3 h at 25 °C.

7. Measure the fluorescence at each time interval with $\lambda_{ex} = 495$ nm and $\lambda_{em} = 537$ nm using a plate reader.

3.6 Silver Staining and TEM Imaging

1. Dissolve bulk 1 mg of DNA in 200 μL of dH$_2$O (*see* **Note 2**) and add 1 mL of 0.1 M AgNO$_3$ solution. Incubate for 2 h at RT to metallize the DNA. Purification is not necessary.

2. Proceed with the formation of organo-micelles (*see* Subheading 3.1), and with the formation of 3LM (*see* Subheading 3.2) (*see* **Note 11**).

3. Place one droplet of the organo-micelles or 3LM on a copper-coated carbon grid and allow drying at RT.

4. Take images of the grid with the TEM instrument operating from 80 kV to 120 kV at different magnifications.

4 Notes

1. To calculate the amount of PLLA-PEI-PLLA needed for a specific N/P, the following equation can be used. Here the calculation for N/P 12 for 1 mg of DNA is given.

$$m(PEI) = m(DNA)/330 \times (N/P) \times (43.1)$$
$$= (1 \text{ mg})/330 \times (12) \times (43.1)$$
$$= 1.57 \text{ mg}$$

Percentage PLLA/PEI block ratio in PLLA-PEI-PLLA (1700–2000–1700) triblock copolymer is (63:37).

$$m(PLLA\text{-}PEI\text{-}PLLA) = 1.57 \text{ mg}/PEI\% = 1.57 \text{ mg}/0.37 = 4.24 \text{ mg}$$

2. Prepare bulk DNA stock solution to achieve final concentration of 5 mg/mL. Use low volume pipette tips in order to minimize the size of the droplet, thus decreasing aggregation.

3. It is important to minimize contact of the organo-micelle/THF solution with the aqueous solution used for storage/preparation of dialysis tubes. The residual aqueous solution on the dialysis tube must be rinsed away with THF. Additionally, the rinsing step allows for straightforward loading of the organo-micelle/THF solution into the tube without spillage. To rinse the dialysis tube, simply pour in THF into the tubes, invert the tube several times, and discard solution. Repeat the rinse step until all residual H$_2$O is removed and the tube becomes rigid.

4. The amount of PLLA-PEG-PLLA can also be substituted by a predefined percentage of Folate-PEG-PLLA to prepare folate-targeted 3LM.

5. A special evaporation setup can be assembled to complete the evaporation steps in a timely manner. Attach a clean plastic hose to a plastic powder funnel, preferably large enough to completely cover the mouth rim of the evaporation beaker.

Attach the plastic hose to a compressed air line with a spigot. Place the powder funnel on top of the evaporation beaker; fasten to place using a clamp. Slowly turn the compressed air on until there is slight disruption of the solvent top layer. Allow the solution to stir on medium speed and gentle stream of compressed air to fasten the evaporation of the solvents.

6. The final stage of 3LM concentration to the final volume of 50 µL should be done in a 10 mL beaker or smaller container to prevent loss of material due to dryness. If the concentration step is difficult for handling, the whole procedures of organo-micelles and 3LM can be scaled up to obtain a ~20% (w/v) final 3LM aqueous solution. For in vitro characterization of 3LM, the final volume after evaporation was 500 µL.

7. The polymer/THF solution should be added in increments in order to obtain a transparent, slightly turbid micelle suspension. The increment addition should be ~50 µL, followed by 5 min stirring at 4 °C and 15 min at 25 °C. Place the beaker back in the ice bath before addition of the next increment; repeat the steps until all the polymer/THF solution is added.

8. Before addition of THF to the aqueous solution, the water level should be marked using a sharpie. Following the complete evaporation of THF, the aqueous solution is replaced to the marked level to maintain a final concentration of 20% (w/v).

9. Instead of measuring UV absorbance using a NanoDrop UV-Vis spectrophotometer, any other UV-Vis spectrophotometer can be used as well.

10. Include blank control wells of the same volume of glucose solution or CH_3COONa buffer only and positive control wells including free DNA in glucose solution or CH_3COONa buffer. To each control well containing free DNA, add 10 µL of glucose solution or CH_3COONa buffer, respectively.

11. If desired, the organo-micelles can be used for the TEM imaging as well.

Acknowledgments

OMM acknowledges the Wayne State University Start-Up grant. The Electron Microscopy Core Facility at Wayne State University is partially supported by NSF-MRI grant 0216084 and NSF-MRI grant 0922912. We are grateful to Dr. Zhi Mei for expert support with the TEM imaging of our samples.

References

1. Langer R, Tirrell DA (2004) Designing materials for biology and medicine. Nature 428(6982): 487–492

2. Vagner J, Qu HC, Hruby VJ (2008) Peptidomimetics, a synthetic tool of drug discovery. Curr Opin Chem Biol 12(3):292–296

3. Mavromoustakos T, Durdagi S, Koukoulitsa C, Simcic M, Papadopoulos MG, Hodoscek M, Grdadolnik SG (2011) Strategies in the rational drug design. Curr Med Chem 18(17): 2517–2530

4. Singh V (2014) Recent advancements in synthetic biology: current status and challenges. Gene 535(1):1–11

5. Hacein-Bey-Abina S, Von Kalle C, Schmidt M, McCcormack MP, Wulffraat N, Leboulch P, Lim A, Osborne CS, Pawliuk R, Morillon E, Sorensen R, Forster A, Fraser P, Cohen JI, de Saint BG, Alexander I, Wintergerst U, Frebourg T, Aurias A, Stoppa-Lyonnet D, Romana S, Radford-Weiss I, Gross F, Valensi F, Delabesse E, Macintyre E, Sigaux F, Soulier J, Leiva LE, Wissler M, Prinz C, Rabbitts TH, Le Deist F, Fischer A, Cavazzana-Calvo M (2003) LMO2-associated clonal T cell proliferation in two patients after gene therapy for SCID-X1. Science 302(5644):415–419

6. Wiseman JW, Goddard CA, McLelland D, Colledge WH (2003) A comparison of linear and branched polyethylenimine (PEI) with DCChol/DOPE liposomes for gene delivery to epithelial cells in vitro and in vivo. Gene Ther 10(19):1654–1662

7. Chollet P, Favrot MC, Hurbin A, Coll JL (2002) Side-effects of a systemic injection of linear polyethylenimine-DNA complexes. J Gene Med 4(1):84–91

8. Moghimi SM, Symonds P, Murray JC, Hunter AC, Debska G, Szewczyk A (2005) A two-stage poly(ethylenimine)-mediated cytotoxicity: Implications for gene transfer/therapy. Mol Ther 11(6):990–995

9. Breunig M, Lungwitz U, Liebl R, Goepferich A (2007) Breaking up the correlation between efficacy and toxicity for nonviral gene delivery. Proc Natl Acad Sci U S A 104(36):14454–14459

10. Merkel OM, Urbanics R, Bedocs P, Rozsnyay Z, Rosivall L, Toth M, Kissel T, Szebeni J (2011) In vitro and in vivo complement activation and related anaphylactic effects associated with polyethylenimine and polyethylenimine-graft-poly(ethylene glycol) block copolymers. Biomaterials 32(21):4936–4942

11. Moret I, Peris JE, Guillem VM, Benet M, Revert F, Dasi F, Crespo A, Alino SF (2001) Stability of PEI-DNA and DOTAP-DNA complexes: effect of alkaline pH, heparin and serum. J Control Release 76(1-2):169–181

12. Petersen H, Fechner PM, Fischer D, Kissel T (2002) Synthesis, characterization, and biocompatibility of polyethylenimine-graft-poly(ethylene glycol) block copolymers. Macromolecules 35(18):6867–6874

13. Kunath K, von Harpe A, Petersen H, Fischer D, Voigt K, Kissel T, Bickel U (2002) The structure of PEG-modified poly(ethylene imines) influences biodistribution and pharmacokinetics of their complexes with NF-kappa B decoy in mice. Pharm Res 19(6):810–817

14. Bauhuber S, Liebl R, Tomasetti L, Rachel R, Goepferich A, Breunig M (2012) A library of strictly linear poly(ethylene glycol)-poly(ethylene imine) diblock copolymers to perform structure-function relationship of non-viral gene carriers. J Control Release 162(2):446–455

15. Barratt G (2003) Colloidal drug carriers: achievements and perspectives. Cell Mol Life Sci 60(1):21–37

16. Mintzer MA, Simanek EE (2009) Nonviral vectors for gene delivery. Chem Rev 109(2): 259–302

17. Lee JI, Kim HS, Yoo HS (2009) DNA nanogels composed of chitosan and Pluronic with thermo-sensitive and photo-crosslinking properties. Int J Pharm 373(1-2):93–99

18. Giano MC, Ibrahim Z, Medina SH, Sarhane KA, Christensen JM, Yamada Y, Brandacher G, Schneider JP (2014) Injectable bioadhesive hydrogels with innate antibacterial properties. Nat Commun 5:9

19. Lei P, Padmashali RM, Andreadis ST (2009) Cell-controlled and spatially arrayed gene delivery from fibrin hydrogels. Biomaterials 30(22):3790–3799

20. Krebs MD, Salter E, Chen E, Sutter KA, Alsberg E (2010) Calcium alginate phosphate-DNA nanoparticle gene delivery from hydrogels induces in vivo osteogenesis. J Biomed Mater Res A 92A(3):1131–1138

21. Li ZH, Ning W, Wang JM, Choi A, Lee PY, Tyagi P, Huang L (2003) Controlled gene delivery system based on thermosensitive biodegradable hydrogel. Pharm Res 20(6):884–888

22. Kasper FK, Seidlits SK, Tang A, Crowther RS, Carney DH, Barry MA, Mikos AG (2005) In vitro release of plasmid DNA from oligo(poly(ethylene glycol) fumarate) hydrogels. J Control Release 104(3):521–539

23. Abebe DG, Kandil R, Kraus T, Elsayed M, Merkel OM, Fujiwara T (2015) Three-layered

biodegradable micelles prepared by two-step self-assembly of PLA-PEI-PLA and PLA-PEG-PLA triblock copolymers as efficient gene delivery system. Macromol Biosci 15(5):698–711

24. Abebe DG, Fujiwara T (2012) Controlled thermoresponsive hydrogels by stereocomplexed PLA-PEG-PLA prepared via hybrid

micelles of Pre-mixed copolymers with different PEG lengths. Biomacromolecules 13(6): 1828–1836

25. Patil YB, Toti US, Khdair A, Ma L, Panyam J (2009) Single-step surface functionalization of polymeric nanoparticles for targeted drug delivery. Biomaterials 30(5):859–866

Chapter 12

Cationic Lipid-Coated Polyplexes (Lipopolyplexes) for DNA and Small RNA Delivery

Alexander Ewe and Achim Aigner

Abstract

The delivery of nucleic acids (NA) like DNA for cell transfection or siRNAs for gene knockdown is of major interest for in vitro studies as well as for applications in vivo. The same is true for other small RNA molecules like miRNAs or miRNA inhibitors (antimiRs). Important nonviral gene delivery vectors include liposomes and cationic polymers. With regard to cationic polymers, polyethylenimines (PEIs) are well established for the delivery of NA, by acting as nanoscale delivery platforms (polyplexes). Their combination with liposomes comprising different phospholipids leads to the formation of lipopolyplexes and can further improve their efficacy and biocompatibility, by combining the favorable properties of lipid systems (high stability, efficient cellular uptake, low cytotoxicity) and PEI (NA condensation, facilitated endosomal release).

In this chapter, optimal lipopolyplex compositions containing different liposomes and certain branched or linear low-molecular weight PEIs are given. This also includes optimal parameters for lipopolyplex generation, based on various PEIs, N/P ratios, lipids, lipid/PEI ratios, and preparation conditions.

Importantly, certain lipopolyplexes retain their biological activity and physicochemical integrity upon prolonged storage at room temperature (RT), in the presence of serum and upon nebulization, thus extending their usefulness toward various applications in vivo.

Key words Lipopolyplexes, Liposomes, Polyethylenimine, PEI, RNAi, miRNA, siRNA, Gene knockdown, miRNA, AntimiR, Nanoparticles, Nebulization, Transfection

1 Introduction

Nucleic acids (NA) delivery is still a major bottleneck in many in vitro and in vivo applications. The development of nonviral carriers for the encapsulation and delivery of various NA has gained significant attention [1–3]. Beyond DNA, these include small RNA molecules like small interfering RNAs (siRNAs) for the induction of RNA interference (RNAi), aiming at targeted gene knockdown, as well as miRNAs or miRNA inhibitors (antimiRs) for the analysis of (patho-) physiological miRNA functions and potential therapeutic intervention.

In the context of NA and beyond, liposomal formulations, including those comprising different phospholipids, have been

Gabriele Candiani (ed.), *Non-Viral Gene Delivery Vectors: Methods and Protocols*, Methods in Molecular Biology, vol. 1445, DOI 10.1007/978-1-4939-3718-9_12, © Springer Science+Business Media New York 2016

explored. Phospholipids are the major component of cell membranes and are available in different structures with diverse aliphatic chain lengths and head groups. This offers a broad range of physicochemical characteristics and high biocompatibility. Precise formulations with synthetic lipids or semisynthetic (polyethylene glycol-lipids, PEG-lipids) allows for the generation of tailor-made carriers [4–6]. In fact, the delivery of NA with neutral or negatively charged liposomes represents an emerging field, and the encapsulation of NA in neutral or anionic charged liposomes has shown promising results in vitro and in vivo [7–9].

Likewise, polyethylenimines (PEIs) have been well established as NA delivery platform for in vitro and in vivo use [10–13]. PEIs are synthetic, water-soluble branched or linear polymers (bPEI and lPEI, respectively) available in a broad range of molecular weights (MW: 0.8–800 kDa). At physiological pH, they show a high cationic charge density [14–16] which allows for the formation of nanosized complexes (polyplexes) with negatively charged NA. These polymeric nanoparticles (NPs) are able to protect NA from nuclease digestion, mediate their endosomal/lysosomal release due to the so-called proton sponge effect [17, 18], and facilitate DNA entry into the nucleus [19, 20]. Transfection efficacy and cytotoxicity, however, strongly depend on the MW and structure, and optimal PEIs have been described [14, 21].

The combination of liposomes and PEIs (*see* Fig. 1) is a particularly intriguing concept with regard to combining favorable properties of both systems. Among others, this may lead to enhanced transfection efficiencies, lower cytotoxicities and increased colloidal stability, and concomitant protection from polyplex aggregation. Lipopolyplexes consisting of cationic liposomes and PEI indeed showed enhanced in vitro transfection efficiencies and improved serum stability [22–27]. Neutral, anionic, or PEG-modified (phospho-)lipids are still more promising candidates for lipopolyplex formation. This also allows prolonged storage [28].

Herein, lipopolyplexes comprising low-MW bPEI or lPEI and various phospholipids are described. These include the neutral

Complex preparation

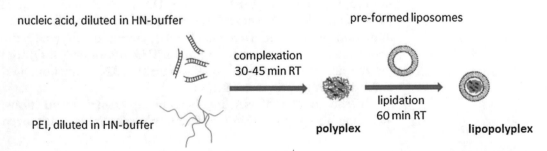

Fig. 1 Schematic overview of lipopolyplex formation. HN complexation buffer: 150 mM NaCl, 10 mM HEPES, pH 7.4

phospholipid 1,2-dipalmitoyl-*sn*-glycero-3-phosphocholine (DPPC) with or without the co-lipids 1,2-dipalmitoyl-*sn*-glycero-3-phospho-(1′-*rac*-glycerol) (DPPG) and 1,2-dipalmitoyl-*sn*-glycero-3-phosphoethanolamine (DPPE). These lipopolyplexes show high transfection efficacy and low toxicity. Additionally, they can be stored at room temperature (RT) [28] or can be nebulized [29], both without losing their physicochemical integrity and biological activity.

2 Materials

2.1 Preparation of PEI Complexes

1. Complexation Buffer: 150 mM NaCl, 10 mM HEPES, pH 7.4.

2. NA, i.e., siRNAs, miRNAs, antimiRs, or plasmid DNA (pDNA).

3. PEI F25-LMW (for preparation, *see* Subheading 3.1) or commercially available PEIs: 10 kDa bPEI and 25 kDa lPEIs or 2.5 kDa (linPEImax, Polysciences, Eppelheim, Germany) and 25 kDa bPEI (Sigma, St. Louis, MO, USA).

2.2 Preparation of Liposomes

1. DPPC.

2. DPPG.

3. DPPE.

4. Methanol (MeOH).

5. Chloroform ($CHCl_3$).

2.3 Tissue Culture

1. Dulbecco's phosphate-buffered saline (PBS) without Ca^{2+} and Mg^{2+}.

2. Trypsin-EDTA solution: 0.05 % (w/v) trypsin/0.02 % (w/v) ethylenediaminetetraacetic acid (EDTA).

3. Fetal calf serum (FCS).

4. Iscove's Modified Dulbecco's Modified Eagle Medium (IMDM) or any other cell culture medium, supplemented with 10 % (v/v) FCS.

2.4 Quantitative RT-PCR (RT-qPCR)

1. RNA extraction solution containing guanidinium thiocyanate, phenol, and $CHCl_3$ (TRI, e.g., peqGOLD TriFast™, PEQLAB, Erlangen, Germany).

2. Reverse Transcriptase (e.g., Revert Aid™ H Minus M-MuLV Reverse Transcriptase), 200 U/μL supplied with 5× reaction buffer.

3. 20× Random Hexamer Primer: 100 μM mixture of single-stranded random hexanucleotides with 5′- and 3′-hydroxyl ends.

4. 10 mM dNTP Mix. Store at –20 °C.

5. ABsolute QPCR Capillary Mix, 2× SYBR Green.

6. RT-qPCR primers specific for the gene of interest and for housekeeping gene(s), e.g., actin, GAPDH, RPLP0, dissolved in nuclease-free water.

7. Ethanol (EtOH).

8. DEPC-treated bidistilled water (ddH$_2$O).

2.5 Luciferase Assay

1. Luciferase Assay System (e.g., Promega, Madison, WI, USA).

2.6 Equipment and Supplies

1. Laminar flow bench and cell culture incubator.

2. Luminometer.

3. UV/Vis spectrophotometer.

4. PCR thermal cycle system.

5. Real-time PCR thermal cycle system.

6. Rotary evaporator.

7. Avanti Polar Lipids Mini-Extruder or similar.

8. Nebulizer (e.g., Aeroneb® Solo nebulizer, Aerogen, Galway, Ireland).

3 Methods

While the complexation of NA works with PEIs of various chain lengths and degrees of branching, the capability of the polyplexes to successfully deliver DNA or small RNA molecules into cells relies on several complex properties including size, surface charge, and stability of the complexes as well as complexation efficacy and biocompatibility/toxicity. Among others, these parameters are determined by the degree of PEI branching, its MW and chemical modifications, the buffer conditions employed during complexation, the ratio between PEI and NA (the so-called N/P referring to the nitrogen atoms of PEI and the NA phosphates), and, to a lesser extent, the MW of the NA (*see* e.g., 21, 28, 30).

The low-MW PEIs described for lipopolyplex formation (*see* Subheading 3.3) have been shown to be efficient on their own, i.e., without the addition of liposomes, as transfection reagents in vitro and in vivo. Yet, the subsequent generation of lipopolyplexes from these polyplexes leads to improved properties, as outlined in the Introduction. On the other hand, lipopolyplex formation from polyplexes based on inactive PEIs will not significantly enhance transfection efficacies. The generation of efficient lipopolyplexes thus relies on the use of optimal PEIs as well as well-suited liposomes. Finally, results will be influenced by the ratio between liposomes and PEI (lipid/PEI mass ratio). Albeit transfection efficacies do not appear to vary over a broader range, lipid/PEI mass ratios in the range 1–5 are recommended.

3.1 Preparation of PEI Complexes

Prepare complexation buffer with nuclease-free water (*see* **Note 1**) and adjust the pH with HCl. Store sterile filtered 50 mL aliquots at –20 °C or, once thawed, at 4 °C. Dissolve custom-made siR-NAs, miRNAs, or antimiRs according to the manufacturer's instructions in buffer or nuclease-free water. Likewise, purchase or isolate pDNA according to standard protocols (e.g., using commercially available kits for plasmid DNA preparation) and dissolve in nuclease-free water. Store aliquots of a 100 µM stock solution at –80 °C. Use a 20 µM dilution as working solution, which is stored at –20 °C to –80 °C. Prepare PEI F25-LMW from the commercially available 25 kD bPEI by gel filtration as described [21]. PEI F25-LMW is filter sterilized through a 0.2 µm filter and stored at 4 °C. Prepare all PEI stock solutions at a concentration of 1–5 mg/mL in dH$_2$O, without further adjusting the pH.

Optimal PEIs according to the criteria given above include the 2.5 kDa or 25 kDa lPEIs, the 10 kDa and 25 kDa bPEIs, and the bPEI F25-LMW (*see* **Note 2**). The N/P is critical for efficient formation and cellular uptake of the complexes, and depends on the PEI rather than on the NA. While recommendations regarding PEI/NA are given in this protocol, the reader is also referred to *see* **Note 3**.

N/Ps are calculated according to the following equitation:

$$\frac{N}{P} = \frac{m(\text{polymer})}{43 \text{ g}/\text{mol}} \times \frac{330 \text{ g}/\text{mol}}{m(\text{nucleic acid})}$$

The following PEI/NA mass ratios (*see* Table 1) are suggested for complex preparation (*see* **Note 3**):

3.1.1 Procedure and Amounts for the Transfection of a Single Well (24-Well Plate): (for Preparing Larger Amounts, See Notes 4 and 5)

1. Dilute 0.5 µg of NA in 25 µL of Complexation Buffer.

2. Mix and incubate for 5–10 min (Vial 1).

3. In parallel, prepare 25 µL of PEI solution: Add PEI solution to Complexation Buffer to yield appropriate PEI amounts (*see* Table 1) in 25 µL. Mix and incubate at RT for 10 min (Vial 2).

Table 1
Optimal PEI/NA ratios for different PEIs

PEI	PEI/NA mass ratio	N/P ratio	µg PEI/0.5 µg NA
2.5 kDa lPEI	5	38	2.5
25 kDa lPEI	2.5	19	1.25
10 kDa bPEI	7.5	57	3.5
25 kDa bPEI	3.5	27	1.75
PEI F25-LMW	5	38	2.5

4. For complex preparation, add the PEI solution (Vial 2) to the NA solution (Vial 1).

5. Mix by vortexing for 5 s.

6. Incubate the complexes for 30–60 min at RT and briefly vortex again prior to transfection.

3.2 Preparation of Liposomes

Prepare stock solutions of the phospholipids at a concentration of 1–5 mg/mL in 2:1 (v/v) $CHCl_3$/MeOH. Store the solutions in glass flasks under nitrogen atmosphere at −20 °C.

The different liposomes DPPC, 92:8 (molar ratio) DPPC/DPPG, and 85:15 (molar ratio) DPPC/DPPE are prepared by hydration of a dried lipid film, using a protocol as given here. For liposome storage, *see* **Note 6**.

1. Take 5 mg of the required lipids from stock solutions and dilute with 2:1 (v/v) $CHCl_3$/MeOH in a 5 mL round-bottom flask.

2. Evaporate the solvent at 55 °C using a rotary evaporator (when equipped with a programmable vacuum pump, use time/pressure steps 0 s/1000 mbar, 30 s/800 mbar, 5 min/500 mbar, 60 min/0 mbar).

3. Hydrate the lipid film with 1 mL of sterile dH_2O and incubate for 2 min above the phase transition temperature in an ultrasound bath sonicator.

4. Extrude 11 times through a 200 nm polycarbonate membrane in a Mini-Extruder and preheat to a temperature above phase transition (45°–50 °C).

3.3 Lipopolyplex Formation

For the preparation of lipopolyplexes, the PEI/NA complexes from Subheading 3.1 are mixed with the preformed liposomes from Subheading 3.2. To this end, appropriate amounts of liposomes based on the lipid/PEI mass ratio must be used, i.e., a lipid/PEI mass ratio 1–5.

1. Dilute the appropriate amount of liposomes in 50 μL of dH_2O (e.g., 2.5–12.5 μg of liposomes per polyplex containing 2.5 μg of PEI).

2. Add 50 μL of the polyplex suspension containing 2.5 μg of PEI/0.5 μg of NA.

3. Mix by vigorously pipetting up and down, vortex, and incubate for 60 min at RT.

4. The lipopolyplexes are now ready to use.

3.4 Use and Properties of Lipopolyplexes

3.4.1 Transfection

Lipopolyplexes prepared according to Subheading 3.3 are ready to use for transfection, by just adding them to the transfection media (*see* **Note 7**). Similarly, lipopolyplexes can also be used for NA delivery in vivo (*see* **Note 8**). A standard transfection protocol is as follows:

1. Seed cells into 24-well plates, 12-well plates, or 6-well plates at $\sim 3 \times 10^4$ cells/well, $\sim 6 \times 10^4$ cells/well, or $\sim 1.5 \times 10^5$ cells/well, respectively (equivalent to $\sim 1.5 \times 10^4$ cells/cm^2).

2. Transfect cells on the same day or 1 day later by adding lipo-polyplexes prepared as described above. Suggested amounts (*see* **Note 9**): 0.5 μg of NA per 24-well and 1 mL of medium; 1 μg of NA per 12-well and 1–2 mL of medium; 2 μg of NA per 6-well and 2 mL of medium (*see* **Note 10**).

3. Leave the transfection medium on the cells unless medium exchange after 24 h is required by the experiment.

4. Analyze the cells for knockdown or transfection at appropriate time points, usually after 48–96 h (*see* below for sample protocols and *see* **Note 11**).

3.4.2 Nebulization

For background information on the nebulization of lipopolyplexes, *see* **Note 12**.

1. Prepare the lipopolyplexes as described above (*see* Subheading 3.3). Typical sample sizes are lipopolyplexes containing 2.5 μg of NA in 500 μL of 75 mM NaCl, 5 mM HEPES buffer.

2. Apply the lipopolyplex-containing solution into the nebulizer reservoir as detailed in the manufacturer's instructions for use.

3. For analytical purposes, collect the aerosols in a sterile 15 mL tube. Upon briefly spinning down the condensate in a short centrifugation step, determine the biological efficacies in transfection experiments (*see* Subheading 3.5).

4. For in vivo application in mice, put the mouthpiece of Aeroneb® directly over the nose of the non-anaesthetized mouse which is firmly held for the duration of the exposure (~ 30 s).

3.4.3 Storage

Some lipopolyplexes can be stored at 4 °C (*see* **Note 13**).

3.5 Determination of Transfection Efficacies

*3.5.1 Determination of in Vitro Transfection Efficacies Using the Luciferase System (See **Note 14**)*

Using the luciferase quantitation kit, we employed the following, slightly modified protocol, which refers to experiments in the 24-well plate format. Luciferase assay system: store substrates in aliquots at −20 °C for up to 30 days or at −70 °C for up to 1 year. Protect from light.

1. Prepare the 1× lysis buffer by adding 4 volumes of dH$_2$O to 1 volume of 5× lysis buffer.

2. Remove the growth medium from adherent cells (or, in the case of cells in suspension, after spinning them down at $\sim 100 \times g$ and aspirating the medium).

3. Add 100 μL/well of lysis buffer to the cells and incubate on a rocking platform for 10 min at RT.

4. Check complete cell lysis under the microscope.

5. For the measurement of the luciferase activity in the luminometer, dispense 25 μL of the Luciferase Assay Reagent into a luminometer tube, add 10 μL of the cell lysate, mix both components by carefully tapping against the tube and measure immediately (*see* **Note 15**).

3.5.2 Determination of mRNA levels/mRNA Knockdown Efficacies

For background information on target gene knockdown, miRNA target molecule levels and alternative methods, *see* **Notes 16–18**.

Total RNA Isolation

Store phenol-containing RNA extraction solution at 4 °C, protect from the light. Work under a hood and avoid skin contact.

1. Grow cells in 6-well plate to achieve 60–70 % confluency.

2. Transfect the cells as described above and wait for 72–120 h after transfection.

3. Add 1 mL of TriFast™ reagent per well.

4. Incubate for 5 min at RT.

5. Mix cell lysate by pipetting up and down several times prior to its transfer into a 1.5 mL vial.

6. Add 0.2 mL of $CHCl_3$ to each mL of TriFast™ and shake vigorously for 15 s.

7. Incubate at RT for 3–10 min.

8. Centrifuge at $12,000 \times g$ for 10 min at 4 °C.

9. Transfer the aqueous upper phase containing the RNA into a new tube.

10. Add 0.5 mL of isopropanol per 1 mL of TriFast™ and incubate 5–15 min on ice for RNA precipitation.

11. Centrifuge at $12,000 \times g$ for 10 min at 4 °C.

12. Remove the supernatant and wash the RNA pellet with 75 % EtOH.

13. Centrifuge again at $7500 \times g$ for 5–10 min at 4 °C.

14. Air-dry the RNA pellet until all excess of EtOH is evaporated completely and then resuspend the RNA in 10–50 μL nuclease-free water. Freezing and incubating the solution for 5 min at 65 °C will aid the resolubilization of the RNA.

15. Determine quality/quantity of isolated RNA.

Target mRNA levels can now be determined by qRT-PCR. To this end, cDNA can be generated using the RevertAid™ H Minus M-MuLV Reverse Transcriptase in accordance with the following protocol.

Reverse Transcription

Store Reverse Transcriptase and Random Hexamer Primer 20× at −20 °C.

1. Dilute 1 µg of total RNA in 10 µL of DEPC-treated ddH$_2$O in a PCR tube and add 1 µL of Random Hexamer Primer.

2. Incubate for 5 min at 65 °C and chill on ice.

3. After spinning down the solution by short centrifugation, add 4 µL of 5× reaction buffer, 2 µL of 10 mM dNTP Mix, 2.5 µL of DEPC-treated ddH$_2$O, and 0.5 µL of RevertAid™ H Minus M-MuLV Reverse Transcriptase.

4. Mix all components, spin down the solution by brief centrifugation, and place the tubes into a thermal cycler.

5. The initial incubation is at 25 °C for 10 min, followed by the elongation step at 42 °C for 60 min and an enzyme inactivating step at 70 °C for 10 min.

6. The cDNA is cooled down to 4 °C and used directly for PCR, or stored at –20 °C.

Quantitative PCR

Store RT-qPCR primers as 100 µM stock solutions at –20 °C. Prepare 5 µM aliquots of a mix of forward and reverse primers and store at –20 °C.

1. Dilute 1:10 cDNA in DEPC-treated ddH$_2$O.

2. Combine 1 µL of primer mix, 5 µL of 2× SYBR Green Mix, and 4 µL of the cDNA dilution.

3. Mix the components thoroughly by pipetting the mixture up and down for at least ten times, and transfer 10 µL of the reaction mixture into a LightCycler capillary.

4. In the LightCycler, preincubate the reaction at 95 °C for 15 min to activate the HotStarTaq® DNA Polymerase.

5. Parameters for PCR are following: denaturation step 15 s/94 °C, annealing step 30 s/55 °C, extension step 30 s/72 °C for 55 cycles. Then cool down to 4 °C. The annealing temperature may vary dependent on the primers used and may require adjustment.

6. Run PCR reactions with target gene-specific and, for normalization, with housekeeping gene-specific primer sets (e.g., actin) in parallel for each sample, and determine expression levels of the gene of interest by the formula:

$$\text{Expression level} = \frac{2^{CP(\text{target gene})}}{2^{CP(\text{actin})}}$$

with CP = cycle number at the crossing point (0.3).

When performing experiments described here, the reader is also referred to *see* **Note 19**.

4 Notes

1. To avoid nuclease degradation, resuspension and dilution of NA should be performed with DNase- and RNase-free solutions. For the preparation of Complexation Buffer, DEPC-treated ddH_2O should be used.

2. 2.5 kDa or 25 kDa lPEI can be used for pDNA, while for small RNA molecules the 10 kDa and 25 kDa bPEIs may be better suited. The branched PEI F25-LMW has been found efficient for the delivery of both pDNA and small RNA molecules.

3. Optimal PEI/NA (N/P) ratios may vary dependent on the cell line and may thus benefit from some optimization in the range of ~ ×0.5 to ×2, if transfection efficacies are not satisfactory or cytotoxicity is observed. The given values, however, represent average values that usually work well.

4. For the preparation of larger amounts, the protocol can be upscaled accordingly. For complexation volumes > 1.5 mL, however, multiple complexation reactions should be run in parallel to avoid excessively large volumes. Upon completion of complex formation, combine the contents of the different vials and briefly vortex again. PEI F25-LMW-based complexes can be stored frozen (*see* **Note 5**).

5. Polyplexes with PEI F25-LMW and NA allow freezing. To this end, prepare appropriate ready-to-use aliquots and store at –20 °C or –80 °C until use. This procedure does not impair the biological activity of the complexes, including their subsequent use for lipopolyplex formation. Repeated freeze/thawing cycles should be avoided. Upon re-thawing, briefly vortex and incubate complexes for 30 min prior to use.

6. Depending on the lipid formulation, the liposomes can be stored at 4 °C for several weeks (30 days). In particular, liposomes comprising only neutral charged lipids (e.g., DPPC) tend to grow in size within a few days and should better be prepared freshly.

7. It is recommended to perform transfections in serum-containing medium. FCS in the transfection medium may impair transfection efficacy when using certain transfection reagents. For lipopolyplexes, however, no negative effects of FCS were observed and it is in fact even better to perform the transfection in serum-containing medium. Antibiotics can be added, but are not mandatory. If possible, the lipopolyplexes should be left on the cells without medium change.

8. Lipopolyplexes have also been found to be active in mouse models in vivo (Ewe et al., unpublished). Thus, transfection experiments in tissue culture may also serve as analytical tool for the determination of efficacies and biological effects prior to in vivo studies. For in vivo use, lipopolyplexes can be adminis-

tered for example by intraperitoneal or intravenous injection. Amounts equivalent to 10–20 μg of NA should be used per injection, with lipopolyplexes being prepared as described above. Injection volumes should not exceed 100–200 μL and injections can be performed repeatedly (e.g., three times/week).

9. Optimal NA amounts used for transfection may vary dependent on the cell line and on the type of NA (pDNA or small RNAs). They may thus benefit from some optimization; increase amounts if transfection efficacies are not satisfactory or decrease amounts when cytotoxicity is observed. The given values represent average values that usually work well.

10. In the case of small RNAs, e.g., for gene knockdown, the important control for nonspecific effects of the transfection reagent (here: the lipopolyplex) is relatively straightforward by including lipopolyplexes containing a nonspecific or scrambled siRNA/miRNA in parallel. Upon transfection, results from the cells treated with nonspecific NA will serve as a negative control in addition to non-transfected cells. Thus, this allows controlling for the absence of vector and/or NA-mediated off-target effects, stimulation of the innate immune system by the NA, and nonspecific cytotoxicity. In the case of DNA, the inclusion of an appropriate negative control is less straightforward, and the evaluation of cytotoxic or other adverse effects will have to rely for example on the visual assessment of the cells under the microscope or on cytotoxicity assays (e.g., LDH release assay).

11. Since transfection efficacies will depend on the cell line, the optimization of complexation conditions may be required. To this end, the knockdown of a reporter gene like luciferase can be performed, if the appropriate cells stably expressing the reporter are available. This approach is more facile in the case of DNA transfection by using an easy-to-quantitate reporter gene for transfection, e.g., luciferase or EGFP. It should be noted, however, that DNA transfection efficiency does not necessarily reflect siRNA/miRNA knockdown efficacies.

12. Lipopolyplexes prepared as detailed above (*see* Subheading 3.3) can be nebulized without loss of physical integrity or biological activity. In our studies, the Aeroneb® Pro-X control module with an Aeroneb® Solo nebulizer (Aerogen, Galway, Ireland) was used. The Aeroneb® Solo is a compact, single patient use nebulizer for aerosol therapy, featuring a vibrating mesh nebulization technology. As energy is applied to the vibrational element, each aperture within the mesh acts as a micropump, drawing liquid through the holes to form consistently sized droplets. The result is a fine particle, low velocity aerosol optimized for targeted drug delivery to the lungs. Other systems may work well, but have not been tested here.

13. Upon storage over 2 weeks, only minor losses of bioactivity were determined [28].

14. For the simple and accurate analysis of gene targeting efficacies, the determination of luciferase activity can be performed either in stably luciferase expressing cells (if available), e.g. SKOV-3-Luc [31], or in wild-type cells upon their prior transient transfection with a luciferase expression vector. Luciferase knockdown after siRNA transfection usually reaches maximum values at 48–96 h after siRNA transfection, but may depend on the target gene and the cell line, and thus require optimization. Likewise, successful transfection of a luciferase reporter pDNA can be measured in the same time range and using the same protocol. The activity of the luciferase enzyme is measured in a luminometer and expressed in relative light units (RLU).

15. To avoid background signals, no gloves should be worn when handling the luminometer tubes.

16. Knockdown efficacies can be determined on mRNA level by RT-PCR or, being more accurate, by quantitative RT-PCR. For the correct estimation of the RNAi knockdown efficacies of the selected target gene, control transfections with lipopolyplexes containing nonspecific siRNA need to be done in parallel. Knockdown efficacies are determined by the comparison of expression levels of the target gene in cells treated with the specific siRNA lipopolyplexes vs. control transfected cells, and are expressed in "% remaining expression over control" or in "% knockdown compared to control." The most reliable documentation of gene knockdown relies on the parallel determination of targeting efficacies on both mRNA and protein levels (*see* **Note 16**), and is often required by referees when submitting articles to peer-reviewed journals.

17. To determine the molecular effects of a given miRNA of interest, its inhibitory activity on potential (predicted in silico, as available in databases like www.mirdb.org) or already established target genes can be measured. Except for the conserved seed region, miRNAs, unlike siRNAs, show incomplete sequence complementarity with their target mRNA and thus exert their effects of preventing protein biosynthesis often by the inhibition of protein translation rather than mRNA cleavage. Consequently, effects of the miRNA or of its inhibition upon antimiR transfection may not be seen on mRNA level, and it is necessary to determine the protein expression of the target molecule. The method of choice for the quantitation of protein levels will strongly depend on the protein of interest and the assays or reagents available (antibodies, substrates, distinct signal transduction pathways). This includes Western blotting, ELISA, FACS, and assays for enzyme activity, substrate binding or downstream effects of the target protein.

18. To confirm the enrichment of the transfected miRNA in the cells, a quantification of this miRNA may be performed by PCR using stem-loop primers [32]. The cell or tissue lysate is subjected to RNA extraction with enriching small RNAs. For reverse transcription, stem-loop primers are employed due to the shortness of the miRNA sequence. These primers are ~50 nt in length and have an overhang on one side of the stem that is complementary to the miRNA sequence, thus forming a cDNA hybrid of miRNA and primer. For the quantitative PCR reaction, one primer specific for the miRNA and one recognizing the loop sequence are used.

Likewise, alterations in miRNA target genes as known from the literature or identified in databases (e.g., mirBase) can be determined upon transfection of the respective miRNA or antimiR and comparison of the results with a nonspecific negative control.

19. Experiments described here may include the work with potentially hazardous or genetically modified material. Please consult the safety guidelines in your lab for proper handling.

Acknowledgments

This work was supported by grants from the Saxonian Ministry for Science and Art (Sächsisches Ministerium für Wissenschaft und Kunst, SMWK), the Deutsche Forschungsgemeinschaft (DFG), and the German Cancer Aid (Deutsche Krebshilfe).

References

1. Piskin E, Dincer S, Turk M (2004) Gene delivery: intelligent but just at the beginning. J Biomater Sci 15(9):1181–1202

2. Basarkar A, Singh J (2007) Nanoparticulate systems for polynucleotide delivery. Int J Nanomedicine 2(3):353–360

3. Aigner A (2008) Cellular delivery *in vivo* of siRNA-based therapeutics. Curr Pharm Des 14(34):3603–3619

4. Hadinoto K, Sundaresan A, Cheow WS (2013) Lipid-polymer hybrid nanoparticles as a new generation therapeutic delivery platform: a review. Eur J Pharm Biopharm 85 (3 Pt A):427-443.

5. Torchilin VP (2005) Recent advances with liposomes as pharmaceutical carriers. Nat Rev 4(2):145–160

6. Maurer N, Fenske DB, Cullis PR (2001) Developments in liposomal drug delivery systems. Expert Opin Biol Ther 1(6):923–947

7. Landen CN Jr, Chavez-Reyes A, Bucana C, Schmandt R, Deavers MT, Lopez-Berestein G, Sood AK (2005) Therapeutic EphA2 gene targeting *in vivo* using neutral liposomal small interfering RNA delivery. Cancer Res 65(15): 6910–6918

8. Srinivasan C, Burgess DJ (2009) Optimization and characterization of anionic lipoplexes for gene delivery. J Control Release 136(1):62–70

9. Chao M, Jiawei X, Zhongxin J, Kuang A (2010) Anionic long-circulating liposomes for delivery of radioiodinated antisense oligonucleotides. Eur J Lipid Sci Technol 112:545–551

10. Boussif O, Lezoualc'h F, Zanta MA, Mergny MD, Scherman D, Demeneix B, Behr JP (1995) A versatile vector for gene and oligonucleotide transfer into cells in culture and *in vivo*: polyethylenimine. Proc Natl Acad Sci U S A 92(16):7297–7301

11. Neu M, Fischer D, Kissel T (2005) Recent advances in rational gene transfer vector design

based on poly(ethylene imine) and its derivatives. J Gene Med 7(8):992–1009

12. Lai WF (2011) *In vivo* nucleic acid delivery with PEI and its derivatives: current status and perspectives. Expert Rev Med Devices 8(2):173–185

13. Hobel S, Aigner A (2013) Polyethylenimines for siRNA and miRNA delivery in vivo. Wiley Interdiscip Rev Nanomed Nanobiotechnol 5(5):484–501

14. Godbey WT, Wu KK, Mikos AG (1999) Size matters: molecular weight affects the efficiency of poly(ethylenimine) as a gene delivery vehicle. J Biomed Mater Res 45(3):268–275

15. Tang MX, Szoka FC (1997) The influence of polymer structure on the interactions of cationic polymers with DNA and morphology of the resulting complexes. Gene Ther 4(8):823–832

16. Lungwitz U, Breunig M, Blunk T, Gopferich A (2005) Polyethylenimine-based non-viral gene delivery systems. Eur J Pharm Biopharm 60(2):247–266

17. Zuber G, Dauty E, Nothisen M, Belguise P, Behr JP (2001) Towards synthetic viruses. Adv Drug Deliv Rev 52(3):245–253

18. Behr JP (1997) The proton sponge: a trick to enter cells the viruses did not exploit. Chimia 51:34–36

19. Godbey WT, Wu KK, Mikos AG (1999) Tracking the intracellular path of poly(ethylenimine)/DNA complexes for gene delivery. Proc Natl Acad Sci U S A 96(9):5177–5181

20. Pollard H, Remy JS, Loussouarn G, Demolombe S, Behr JP, Escande D (1998) Polyethylenimine but not cationic lipids promotes transgene delivery to the nucleus in mammalian cells. J Biol Chem 273(13):7507–7511

21. Werth S, Urban-Klein B, Dai L, Hobel S, Grzelinski M, Bakowsky U, Czubayko F, Aigner A (2006) A low molecular weight fraction of polyethylenimine (PEI) displays increased transfection efficiency of DNA and siRNA in fresh or lyophilized complexes. J Control Release 112(2):257–270

22. Garcia L, Bunuales M, Duzgunes N, Tros de Ilarduya C (2007) Serum-resistant lipopolyplexes for gene delivery to liver tumour cells. Eur J Pharm Biopharm 67(1):58–66

23. Lee CH, Ni YH, Chen CC, Chou C, Chang FH (2003) Synergistic effect of polyethylenimine and cationic liposomes in nucleic acid delivery to human cancer cells. Biochim Biophys Acta 1611(1-2):55–62

24. Pelisek J, Gaedtke L, DeRouchey J, Walker GF, Nikol S, Wagner E (2006) Optimized lipopolyplex formulations for gene transfer to human colon carcinoma cells under *in vitro* conditions. J Gene Med 8(2):186–197

25. Gaedtke L, Pelisek J, Lipinski KS, Wrighton CJ, Wagner E (2007) Transcriptionally targeted nonviral gene transfer using a beta-catenin/TCF-dependent promoter in a series of different human low passage colon cancer cells. Mol Pharm 4(1):129–139

26. Hanzlikova M, Soininen P, Lampela P, Mannisto PT, Raasmaja A (2009) The role of PEI structure and size in the PEI/liposome-mediated synergism of gene transfection. Plasmid 61(1):15–21

27. Schafer J, Hobel S, Bakowsky U, Aigner A (2010) Liposome-polyethylenimine complexes for enhanced DNA and siRNA delivery. Biomaterials 31(26):6892–6900

28. Ewe A, Schaper A, Barnert S, Schubert R, Temme A, Bakowsky U, Aigner A (2014) Storage stability of optimal liposome-polyethylenimine complexes (lipopolyplexes) for DNA or siRNA delivery. Acta Biomater 10:2663–2673

29. Ewe A, Aigner A (2014) Nebulization of liposome–polyethylenimine complexes (lipopolyplexes) for DNA or siRNA delivery: Physicochemical properties and biological activity. Eur J Lipid Sci Technol 116(9):1195–1204

30. Malek A, Czubayko F, Aigner A (2008) PEG grafting of polyethylenimine (PEI) exerts different effects on DNA transfection and siRNA-induced gene targeting efficacy. J Drug Target 16(2):124–139

31. Urban-Klein B, Werth S, Abuharbeid S, Czubayko F, Aigner A (2005) RNAi-mediated gene-targeting through systemic application of polyethylenimine (PEI)-complexed siRNA *in vivo*. Gene Ther 12(5):461–466

32. Chen C, Ridzon DA, Broomer AJ, Zhou Z, Lee DH, Nguyen JT, Barbisin M, Xu NL, Mahuvakar VR, Andersen MR, Lao KQ, Livak KJ, Guegler KJ (2005) Real-time quantification of microRNAs by stem-loop RT-PCR. Nucleic Acids Res 33(20), e179

Chapter 13

Preparation of Targeted Anionic Lipid-Coated Polyplexes for MicroRNA Delivery

Xiaomeng Huang, Mengzi Zhang, Xinmei Wang, L. James Lee, and Robert J. Lee

Abstract

As nonviral nucleic acid delivery vehicles, lipid nanoparticles (LNPs) have been widely used. Here we describe the synthesis and evaluation of LNPs based on targeted anionic lipid-coated polyplexs for therapeutic delivery of microRNA (miRNA) mimics. These LNPs are particularly suited for therapeutic delivery of oligonucleotide agents to leukemia cells.

Key words Anionic lipid, Targeted delivery, Lipid nanoparticles, microRNA delivery

1 Introduction

Many nonviral delivery methods have been developed for synthetic short interfering RNAs (siRNAs) or microRNA (miRNA) mimics. Among them are notably the incorporation into lipid-based or polymer-based nanocarriers and chemical conjugation to cholesterol. Cholesterol-conjugated siRNA can be efficiently delivered to liver cells that express low-density lipoprotein (LDL) [1, 2]. Polymers such as poly-L-lysine (PLL), polyethylenimine (PEI) [3], chitosan [4–8], cationic polymeric cyclodextrin [9, 10], and polyamidoamine (PAMAM) dendrimer [11–14] are biodegradable, biocompatible, and non-toxic, which are desirable properties for *in vivo* delivery system [3]. Cationic lipids such as dioleoyl trimethylammonium propane (DOTAP), $3\beta[N\text{-}(N',N'\text{-dimethylaminoethane})\text{-carbamoyl}]$ cholesterol (DC-Chol), and $N\text{-}[1\text{-}(2,3\text{-dioleoyloxy})$ propyl]-N,N,N-trimethylammonium chloride (DOTMA) have been used in lipid-based carriers because they can form complexes with nucleic acids and enhance their cellular uptake, taking advantage of electrostatic interactions [15–18]. However the high positive surface charge of cationic carriers can cause toxicity and unwanted immunoreaction. The alternative is to use anionic lipids.

Gabriele Candiani (ed.), *Non-Viral Gene Delivery Vectors: Methods and Protocols*, Methods in Molecular Biology, vol. 1445, DOI 10.1007/978-1-4939-3718-9_13, © Springer Science+Business Media New York 2016

For example, the LPDII vector developed for plasmid delivery is based on anionic lipids coating of a cationic polymer condensed DNA core [19]. Commonly used anionic lipids including cholesteryl hemisuccinate (CHEMS), oleic acid, dicetyl-phosphate (DCP) [20], linoleic acid [21], and linolenic acid [22].

We have designed a novel LNP formulation based on anionic lipid-coated polyplex composed of fusogenic neutral lipid, dioleoylphosphatidylethanolamine (DOPE), an anionic lipid linoleic acid, a polyethylene glycol (PEG) derivative 1,2-dimyristoyl-sn-glycerol-methoxypolyethylene glycol (DMG-PEG) [21, 23, 24]. Low-molecular weight (MW) PEI was selected as a cationic agent to condense miRNA molecules. In addition, the interaction between linoleic acid and PEI may enhance the dissociation of miRNAs from the lipopolyplex after endocytosis and facilitate target gene down-regulation [22]. Furthermore, LNPs are protected from reticuloendothelial system clearance by the inclusion of 2 % molar DMG-PEG to achieve long circulation times [25] and, thus, more efficient delivery in hematopoietic tissues, including bone marrow. This anionic lipid-based formulation of LNPs was designed to avoid the nonspecific immune response caused by cationic lipids, which is triggered by activation of TLR4 and NF-κB pathways, leading to pro-inflammatory cytokine production [26, 27]. Moreover, the overall neutral surface charge of the particles results in reduced plasma protein binding and nonspecific cellular uptake [28].

To increase specific delivery to tumor cells, LNPs may be conjugated with targeting molecules. Delivering miRNA with targeted LNP carriers provides opportunities for targeting a specific tissue or cell type, as well as enhancing circulation time and desired cellular uptake and decreasing systemic toxicity. Commonly used targeting molecules include peptides, antibodies, and small molecule ligands. Transferrin (Tf) was used as a targeting molecule in our formulation since many acute myeloid leukemia cells have high expression of Tf receptor [21, 23, 24, 29, 33, 34].

2 Materials

All solutions were prepared with sterilized DNA/RNase free ultra-pure water (dH$_2$O) or 200 proof ethanol (EtOH).

2.1 Stock Solutions of Lipid Components in Ethanol

1. 25 mg/mL of DOPE (Avanti Polar Lipids, Alabaster, AL) dissolved in EtOH (*see* **Note 1**). Store at −20 °C.

2. 20 mg/mL of DMG-PEG (NOF America Corporation, White Plains, NY) dissolved in EtOH. Store at −20 °C.

3. 100 mg/mL of linoleic acid dissolved in EtOH. Store at −20 °C.

2.2 Aqueous Solutions

1. 20 mM 4-(2-hydroxyethyl)-1-piperazineethanesulfonic acid (HEPES) buffer, pH 7.4.

2. 1× phosphate buffered saline (PBS), pH 6.5, pH 7.4, and PBS adjusted to pH 8.0.

3. Sterile nuclease-free dH_2O.

4. Traut's reagent (2-iminothiolane): 1 mg/mL Traut's reagent (Thermo Fisher Scientific, Grand Island, NY) in PBS, pH 8.0 (*see* **Note 2**).

5. Holo-transferrin (Tf) (Sigma Aldrich, St. Louis, MO) solution: 5 mg/mL of Holo-Tf in PBS, pH 8.0 (*see* **Note 3**).

6. Maleimide-PEG-DSPE (Mal-PEG-DSPE) solution: 10 mg/mL of Mal-PEG-DSPE (Avanti Polar Lipids) dissolved in PBS, pH 6.5 (*see* **Note 4**).

7. Antibody solution: 0.5 mg/mL purified anti-mouse CD45.2 antibody (without BSA and other proteins) (*see* **Note 5**).

8. 0.5 % (w/v) sodium dodecyl sulfate (SDS) in dH_2O.

9. PEI solution: 10 mg/mL of polyethylenimine (PEI) (Sigma Aldrich; 50 wt. % solution in dH_2O; MW ~2000; density ~1.08 g/mL at 25 °C) stock solution in 20 mM HEPES buffer, pH 7.4. Then further dilute to 1 mg/mL with 20 mM HEPES buffer, pH 7.4, as the working solution.

10. Oligonucleotides solution. 100 µM of synthetic miRNA mimic (Ambion®, Thermo Fisher Scientific; MW ~14,000) is dissolved in sterile nuclease-free dH_2O. For in vivo study, 7 µg/µL of miRNA duplex mimic (Ambion®; MW ~14,000) is dissolved in sterile nuclease-free dH_2O. Alternatively, 5 µg/µL of single strand miRNA oligodeoxynucleotide (ODN; MW ~7000; Sigma Aldrich) is dissolved in sterile nuclease-free dH_2O.

11. Urea-polyacrylamide gel (Invitrogen, Thermo Fisher Scientific).

2.3 Equipments

1. Water bath sonicator.

2. UV spectrometer (Nanodrop, Thermo Fisher Scientific).

3. Particle size analyzer (NICOMP Particle Sizer Model 370, Particle Sizing Systems, Santa Barbara, CA).

4. ZetaPALS, Zeta Potential Analyzer (Brookhaven Instruments Corp., Worcestershire, NY).

2.4 Supplies

1. PD10 column (GE Healthcare, Piscataway, NJ).

2. 1.5 mL polypropylene microcentrifuge tubes.

3. 5 mL polypropylene Round-Bottom flow tubes (BD Falcon, Franklin Lakes, NJ).

4. U100 insulin syringes with $29_G\frac{1}{2}''$ gage (BD).

5. 0.22 µm sterile filters (Thermo Fisher Scientific).

6. Centrifugal Filter Unit (Microcon®-10; EMD Millipore, Darmstadt, Germany).

7. Centrifugal Filter Tubes (Amicon Ultra-15; EMD Millipore).

2.5 Protein Assay Dye Reagent

Protein assay dye reagent (Bio-Rad, Hercules, CA) diluted 1:4 with dH₂O.

2.6 Cells and Medium

1. Kasumi-1, acute myeloid leukemia cell line (ATCC, Manassas, VA).

2. Complete cell-culture medium: RPMI-1640 medium supplement with 20% (v/v) fetal bovine serum (FBS) (*see* **Note 6**).

3 Methods

3.1 Empty LNP Preparation

1. Mix 1069.3 µL of DOPE, 96.7 µL of linoleic acid, 179.7 µL of DMG-PEG, and 654.3 µL of EtOH (50:48:2 molar ratio) (DOPE:linoleic acid:DMG-PEG), to obtain a total volume of 2 mL at a final 20 mg/mL lipids mixture concentration.

2. Transfer 300 µL of lipid mixture into a 1.5 mL polypropylene microcentrifuge tube.

3. Transfer 2.7 mL of 20 mM HEPES buffer, pH 7.4, into 5 mL polypropylene Round-Bottom flow tube.

4. Draw 300 µL of lipids mixture into U100 Insulin syringe with 29ᴳ½″ gage.

5. Put needle tip under the HEPES buffer surface and inject lipids solution as quickly as possible to form empty LNPs.

6. Vortex for 10 s.

7. Sonicate empty LNP solution in a bath sonicator (120 Volts 2 Amps 50/60 Hz) for 3–5 min (*see* **Note 7**) to give a final concentration of 2 mg/mL empty LNPs.

8. Store empty LNPs at 4 °C until use (*see* **Note 8**).

3.2 Tf-PEG-DSPE Synthesis

1. Mix 5 mg of Tf solution with 86 µL (0.086 mg) of Traut's reagent at 1:10 molar ratio for 2 h at room temperature (RT) to yield Tf-SH (*see* **Note 9**).

2. Remove extra Traut's reagent by PD10 column (following **steps 3-8** below).

3. Wash the column with 3 column-volumes of PBS, pH 6.5.

4. Load Tf and Traut's mixture solution onto the column.

5. Add 500 µL of PBS, pH 6.5, twice.

6. Start to collect 8 tubes of elution solution.

7. Transfer 10 μL from each collected tube into 1.5 mL polypropylene microcentrifuge tube, then add 300 μL of diluted protein assay dye reagent and mix thoroughly.

8. Pool all Tf-SH fractions in which the corresponding dye reagent test turns blue.

9. Mix pooled Tf-SH from last step with 1.83 mg of Mal-PEG-DSPE at 1:10 (mol/mol) overnight at RT to yield micelles of Tf-PEG-DSPE (*see* **Notes 10** and **11**).

10. Filter Tf-PEG-DSPE through a 0.22 μm filter.

11. Measure the Tf concentration by means of a spectrophotometer at λ = 280 nm.

12. Store Tf-PEG-ESPE at 4 °C until use (*see* **Note 12**).

3.3 Antibody-PEG-DSPE Synthesis (See Note 13)

1. Load anti-mouse CD45.2 antibody solution in a Centrifugal Filter Unit. Concentrate antibody by centrifugation at 16,800 × *g* for 20 min. Wash twice with PBS, pH 8.0. Dilute antibody with PBS, pH 8.0, to a total volume of 500 μL.

2. Mix 500 μL of antibody solution in PBS, pH 8.0 from above step with 4.6 μL (4.6 μg) of Traut's reagent at 1:10 (molar ratio) for 2 h at RT.

3. Remove extra Traut's by loading the mixture solution into Centrifugal Filter Unit and centrifuging at 16,800 × *g* for 25 min.

4. Wash with 400 μL of PBS, pH 6.5.

5. Refill filter cartridge with 400 μL of PBS, pH 6.5.

6. Mix antibody-SH from above step (total volume ~500 μL) with 98 μL (98 μg) of Mal-PEG-DSPE in PBS, pH 6.5, at 1:10 (mol/mol) for 2 h at RT.

7. Measure antibody concentration by means of a spectrophotometer at λ = 280 nm (*see* **Note 14**).

8. Store antibody-PEG-DSPE at 4 °C until use (*see* **Note 15**).

3.4 Targeted Lipopolyplex LNP Preparation for In Vitro Study

1. Calculate the amount of miRNA based on the required final miRNA concentration and calculate the amount of PEI and empty LNP needed (*see* **Note 16**).

2. Dilute 4 μL of 100 μM miRNA stock solution in 18 μL of 20 mM HEPES buffer (*see* **Note 17**).

3. Dilute 7 μL of PEI in 15 μL of 20 mM HEPES buffer (*see* **Note 17**).

4. Add miRNA solution to PEI solution and mix by vortex.

5. Incubate mixture for 3–5 min at RT.

6. Dilute empty LNP with 20 mM HEPES buffer to a final concentration of 1 mg/mL.

7. Add 56 μL of empty LNPs to the PEI/miRNA mixture.

8. Vortex and then sonicate in water bath sonicator (120 V, 2 A, 50/60 Hz) for 3–5 min.

9. Incubate for 10 min at RT.

10. Add 3.2 μg of Tf-PEG-DSPE to 100 μL miRNA-loaded LNPs from above step and mix by vortex. Tf/lipid molar ratio is 1:2000. Otherwise add antibody-PEG-DSPE to miRNA-loaded LNPs and mix by vortex. The optimal antibody/lipid molar ratio can be determined by cellular uptake assay (*see* **Note 18**). The amount of antibody-PEG-DSPE needed can be calculated based on the optimal antibody/lipid molar ratio.

11. Incubate the mixture for ~1 h at 37 °C.

12. Store at 4 °C until use (*see* **Note 19**) (Fig. 1).

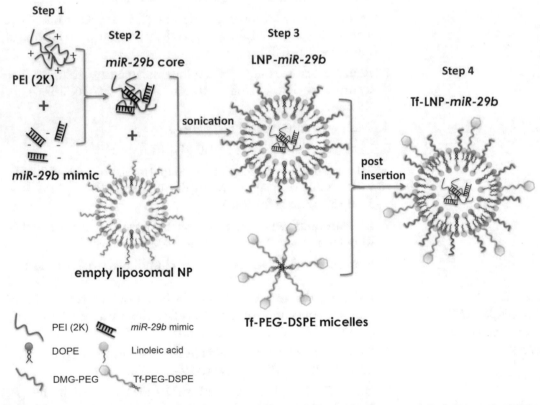

Fig. 1 Preparation of miRNA-loaded Tf-conjugated-LNPs (Tf-LNP-miRNA). The preparation of Tf-LNP-miRNA is schematically illustrated. *Step 1*: negatively charged miRNA molecules are mixed with positively charged PEI to form a miRNA-PEI core structure. *Step 2*: empty LNP are formed by injection of a lipid EtOH solvent into 20 mM HEPES buffer. *Step 3*: the miRNA-PEI are mixed with the empty LNP and sonicated to load the miRNA PEI core into the LNP. *Step 4*: LNP-miRNA are modified to incorporate Tf-PEG-DSPE micelles to form the Tf-LNP-miRNAs

Table 1
Particle size distribution and ζ-potential of LNPs

	Particle size (nm)	ζ-potential (mV)
Empty LNP	129.6 ± 1.0	−9.8 ± 1.5
LNP-miRNA	137.6 ± 1.0	+22.5 ± 1.4
Tf-LNP-miRNA	147.3 ± 4.8	+5.8 ± 1.9

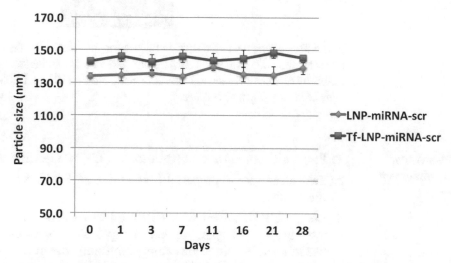

Fig. 2 Colloidal stability of the miRNA-scramble (miRNA-scr) loaded LNP. Tf-LNP-miRNA-scr (*quadrangle*) and LNP-miRNA-scr (*circle*) during storage at 4 °C. The values in the plot were by means of three separate experiments

3.5 Measurement of the Size and ζ-Potential of LNPs

1. Prepare miRNA-loaded and Tf-conjugated LNPs as described above.

2. Load empty LNP, miRNA-loaded and Tf-conjugated LNPs solutions to cartridge of Particle Sizer individually. Measure the particle size thrice for each sample (*see* Table 1).

3. Load empty LNP, miRNA-loaded and Tf-conjugated LNPs solutions to cartridge of ζ-potential Analyzer individually. Measure thrice the ζ-potential for each sample (*see* Table 1).

3.6 Measurement of the Stability of LNPs

1. Prepare miRNA-loaded and Tf-conjugated LNPs as described above. Store at 4 °C.

2. At days 1, 3, 7, 11, 16, 21, and 28, take prepared miRNA-loaded and Tf-conjugated LNPs and load the LNP solution to cartridge of Particle Sizer. Measure the particle size thrice each day [23] (Fig. 2).

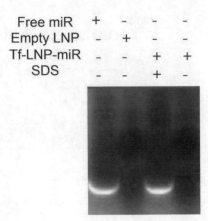

Fig. 3 miRNA entrapment efficiency. To release the miRNA, 0.5 % SDS was used to dissolve the LNPs. The samples were compared before and after dissolution by SDS by agarose gel electrophoresis of RNA. Free miRNA and SDS treated empty LNPs are shown as controls

3.7 Measurement of miRNA Entrapment Efficiency

1. Prepare Tf-conjugated miRNA-loaded LNPs as described above.

2. Take an aliquot of prepared LNP and use 0.5 % SDS to dissolve the LNPs.

3. Load LNP dissolved with SDS and not dissolved with SDS into urea-polyacrylamide gel for gel electrophoresis. Load naked miRNA mimic and empty LNP into the gel at the same time as controls (Fig. 3).

3.8 Cell Treatment

This design of LNP is tailored for suspended cell transfection to give low cytotoxicity and high transfection efficiency.

1. Spin down Kasumi-1 cells and change media 24 h before the treatment.

2. Count the cells and spin down the desired amount of cells and resuspend with warm complete cell-culture medium. The cell concentration should be $3–5 \times 10^5$/mL for cell line and 1×10^6/mL for patient leukemoblasts.

3. Slowly add the prepared LNPs into media with cells. Shake the plate or flask while adding the LNPs, if possible. Make sure that LNPs are distributed evenly in the media.

4. Incubate cells at 37 °C.

3.9 LNP Preparation for In Vivo Study

1. Calculate how much miRNA will be used based on the weight of the animal (*see* **Note 20**).

2. Calculate how much PEI and empty LNP will be needed (*see* **Note 21**).

3. Prepare ~400 µL of LNP solution by mixing miRNA, PEI, empty LNPs, and Tf-PEG-DSPE as described in Subheading 3.4. Use empty LNPs at a concentration of 2 mg/mL (*see* **Note 22**).

4. (Optional) Load prepared LNPs up to 15 mL in Centrifual Filter Tube and centrifuge at $2106 \times g$ for 30 min (*see* **Note 23**).

4   Notes

1. Usually DOPE is difficult to dissolve at RT. Raising the solution temperature in a 37 °C water bath is recommended.

2. Traut's reagent solution should be made fresh. Dissolved Traut's reagent should be used in the same day and unused portion disposed off.

3. Make 5 mg/mL of Holo-Tf stock solution right before use. Otherwise store as powder at 4 °C.

4. Weigh the amount of Mal-PEG-DSPE needed and make 10 mg/mL solution right before use. Otherwise store as powder at –20 °C.

5. This protocol can be applied to other types of oligonucleotides, such as siRNA, antisense oligo, and anti-miR oligo, and other antibodies as targeting entities.

6. This protocol can be applied to other suspended cells.

7. Sonication can be used to make smaller particle size [30, 31].

8. Empty LNPs can be stored at 4 °C up to 120 days.

9. The MW of Traut's reagent is 137.63 g/mol while that of Tf is 80,000 g/mol. The amount of Traut's reagent (in mg) needed to react with 5 mg of Tf is:

$$\frac{5\,mg}{80,000\,\dfrac{g}{mol}} \times \frac{10}{1} \times 137.63\,\frac{g}{mol}$$

10. The MW of Mal-PEG-DSPE is 2941 g/mol. The amount of Mal-PEG-DSPE needed (in mg) to react with Tf-SH is:

$$\frac{5\,mg}{80,000\,\dfrac{g}{mol}} \times \frac{10}{1} \times 2941\,\frac{g}{mol}$$

11. Gently shake or rotate the tube while mixing Tf-SH and Mal-PEG-DSPE.

12. Tf-PEG-DSPE is stable at 4 °C for 2 months.

13. Since there is no sterile filtration performed at the end, try to keep every step as sterile as possible.

14. Final antibody recovery rate is ~60–70%.

15. Antibody-PEG-DSPE should be used within a month.

16. The weight ratios of miRNA:PEI and miRNA:lipid are 1:1.25 and 1:10, respectively. For example, to treat 4 mL of suspended cells with 100 nM of miRNA, 5.6 µg of miRNA would be needed, which is 4 µL of 100 µM miRNA stock. Meanwhile, 7 µg of PEI and 56 µg empty LNPs are needed.

17. Before mixing PEI and miRNA, it is better to use 20 mM HEPES buffer, pH 7.4, to dilute both reagents to the same volume.

18. When using antibodies as targeting molecules, it may be necessary to optimize the lipid/antibody ratio. A given ratio is selected depending on the size of the antibody and the expression of antigen on the surface of targeted cells. We usually prepare LNPs encapsulating fluorescence-labeled short RNAs. Next, the antibody-PEG-DSPE is post-inserted to LNPs at various lipid/antibody molar ratios, ranging from 200:1 to 50,000:1. Then cells are treated with antibody-conjugated LNP for at least 4 h and flow cytometry (FACS) is used to count fluorescence positive cells. The ratio that gives the highest cellular uptake is then chosen. For example, we prepared anti-CD45.2-LNP-Cy3-Oligonucleotide at various lipid/antibody molar ratios from 200:1 to 2000:1 in the first trial and from 2000:1 to 50,000:1 in the second one to treat CD45.2(+) leukemic cells for 24 h. The percentages of Cy3 positive cells are given in Fig. 4 [32]. The cellular uptake was the highest when the 10,000:1 lipid/antibody ratio was used.

19. The final product should preferably be used within 24 h. If necessary, store at 4 °C. During the storage time, if the aggregation of LNPs occurs, re-disperse by vortexing.

20. We used up to 2.4 mg of oligonucleotides per 1 kg/mouse. The same protocol can be applied to doses lower than 2.4 mg/kg. If the dose is higher than 2.4 mg/kg, a step for concentrating LNPs is needed.

21. For example, if the dose is 2.4 mg/kg of miRNA and a mouse weighs 25 g, 60 ng of miRNA, 75 ng of PEI, 600 ng of empty LNPs, and 34 ng of Tf-PEG-DSPE are needed.

22. The total volume should be less than 400 µL for tail vein injection in mice.

23. The volume of LNPs can be reduced to half.

Anti-CD45.2 antibody conjugated LNP cellular uptake

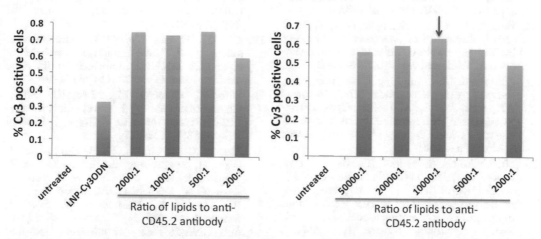

Fig. 4 Optimization of lipid-to-antibody ratio. Anti-CD45.2-LNP-Cy3-ODN were prepared at various molar ratios of lipid to antibody from 200:1 to 2000:1 in the first trial (**a**) and from 2000:1 to 50,000:1 in the second trial (**b**) to treat CD45.2(+) leukemic cells for 24 h. Then Cy3-positive cells were recognized by FACS

Acknowledgement

This work was supported in part by National Science Foundation under grant EEC-0914790.

References

1. Soutschek J, Akinc A, Bramlage B, Charisse K, Constien R, Donoghue M, Elbashir S, Geick A, Hadwiger P, Harborth J, John M, Kesavan V, Lavine G, Pandey RK, Racie T, Rajeev KG, Rohl I, Toudjarska I, Wang G, Wuschko S, Bumcrot D, Koteliansky V, Limmer S, Manoharan M, Vornlocher HP (2004) Therapeutic silencing of an endogenous gene by systemic administration of modified siRNAs. Nature 432(7014):173–178

2. Wolfrum C, Shi S, Jayaprakash KN, Jayaraman M, Wang G, Pandey RK, Rajeev KG, Nakayama T, Charrise K, Ndungo EM, Zimmermann T, Koteliansky V, Manoharan M, Stoffel M (2007) Mechanisms and optimization of in vivo delivery of lipophilic siRNAs. Nat Biotechnol 25(10):1149–1157

3. Guo P, Coban O, Snead NM, Trebley J, Hoeprich S, Guo S, Shu Y (2010) Engineering RNA for targeted siRNA delivery and medical application. Adv Drug Deliv Rev 62(6): 650–666

4. Salva E, Turan SO, Kabasakal L, Alan S, Ozkan N, Eren F, Akbuga J (2014) Investigation of the therapeutic efficacy of codelivery of psiRNA-vascular endothelial growth factor and pIL-4 into chitosan nanoparticles in the breast tumor model. J Pharm Sci 103(3):785–795

5. Matokanovic M, Barisic K, Filipovic-Grcic J, Maysinger D (2013) Hsp70 silencing with siRNA in nanocarriers enhances cancer cell death induced by the inhibitor of Hsp90. Eur J Pharm Sci 50(1):149–158

6. Xia H, Jun J, Wen-Ping L, Yi-Feng P, Xiao-Ling C (2013) Chitosan nanoparticle carrying small interfering RNA to platelet-derived growth factor B mRNA inhibits proliferation of smooth muscle cells in rabbit injured arteries. Vascular 21:301–306

7. Malmo J, Sandvig A, Varum KM, Strand SP (2013) Nanoparticle mediated P-glycoprotein silencing for improved drug delivery across the blood-brain barrier: a siRNA-chitosan approach. PLoS One 8(1), e54182

8. Yang J, Li S, Guo F, Zhang W, Wang Y, Pan Y (2013) Induction of apoptosis by chitosan/HPV16 E7 siRNA complexes in cervical cancer cells. Mol Med Rep 7(3):998–1002

9. Chaturvedi K, Ganguly K, Kulkarni AR, Kulkarni VH, Nadagouda MN, Rudzinski WE, Aminabhavi TM (2011) Cyclodextrin-based siRNA delivery nanocarriers: a state-of-the-art review. Expert Opin Drug Deliv 8(11):1455–1468

10. Hu-Lieskovan S, Heidel JD, Bartlett DW, Davis ME, Triche TJ (2005) Sequence-specific knockdown of EWS-FLI1 by targeted, nonviral delivery of small interfering RNA inhibits tumor growth in a murine model of metastatic Ewing's sarcoma. Cancer Res 65(19): 8984–8992

11. Liu J, Gu C, Cabigas EB, Pendergrass KD, Brown ME, Luo Y, Davis ME (2013) Functionalized dendrimer-based delivery of angiotensin type 1 receptor siRNA for preserving cardiac function following infarction. Biomaterials 34(14):3729–3736

12. Liu X, Li G, Su Z, Jiang Z, Chen L, Wang J, Yu S, Liu Z (2013) Poly(amido amine) is an ideal carrier of miR-7 for enhancing gene silencing effects on the EGFR pathway in U251 glioma cells. Oncol Rep 29(4): 1387–1394

13. Arima H, Yoshimatsu A, Ikeda H, Ohyama A, Motoyama K, Higashi T, Tsuchiya A, Niidome T, Katayama Y, Hattori K, Takeuchi T (2012) Folate-PEG-appended dendrimer conjugate with alpha-cyclodextrin as a novel cancer cell-selective siRNA delivery carrier. Mol Pharm 9(9):2591–2604

14. Liu XX, Rocchi P, Qu FQ, Zheng SQ, Liang ZC, Gleave M, Iovanna J, Peng L (2009) PAMAM dendrimers mediate siRNA delivery to target Hsp27 and produce potent antiproliferative effects on prostate cancer cells. ChemMedChem 4(8):1302–1310

15. Behlke MA (2006) Progress towards in vivo use of siRNAs. Mol Ther 13(4):644–670

16. Deng Y, Wang CC, Choy KW, Du Q, Chen J, Wang Q, Li L, Chung TK, Tang T (2014) Therapeutic potentials of gene silencing by RNA interference: principles, challenges, and new strategies. Gene 538(2):217–227

17. Kim SS, Garg H, Joshi A, Manjunath N (2009) Strategies for targeted nonviral delivery of siR-NAs in vivo. Trends Mol Med 15(11): 491–500

18. Grijalvo S, Avino A, Eritja R (2014) Oligonucleotide delivery: a patent review (2010–2013). Expert Opin Ther Pat 24(7):801–819

19. Lee RJ, Huang L (1996) Folate-targeted, anionic liposome-entrapped polylysine-condensed DNA for tumor cell-specific gene transfer. J Biol Chem 271(14):8481–8487

20. Guo W, Gosselin MA, Lee RJ (2002) Characterization of a novel diolein-based LPDII vector for gene delivery. J Control Release 83(1):121–132

21. Huang X, Schwind S, Yu B, Santhanam R, Wang H, Hoellerbauer P, Mims A, Klisovic R, Walker AR, Chan KK, Blum W, Perrotti D, Byrd JC, Bloomfield CD, Caligiuri MA, Lee RJ, Garzon R, Muthusamy N, Lee LJ, Marcucci G (2013) Targeted delivery of microRNA-29b by transferrin-conjugated anionic lipopolyplex nanoparticles: a novel therapeutic strategy in acute myeloid leukemia. Clin Cancer Res 19(9):2355–2367

22. Yu B, Hsu SH, Zhou C, Wang X, Terp MC, Wu Y, Teng L, Mao Y, Wang F, Xue W, Jacob ST, Ghoshal K, Lee RJ, Lee LJ (2012) Lipid nanoparticles for hepatic delivery of small interfering RNA. Biomaterials 33(25):5924–5934

23. Wang X, Huang X, Yang Z, Gallego-Perez D, Ma J, Zhao X, Xie J, Nakano I, Lee LJ (2014) Targeted delivery of tumor suppressor microRNA-1 by transferrin-conjugated lipopolyplex nanoparticles to patient-derived glioblastoma stem cells. Curr Pharm Biotechnol 15(9):839–846

24. Havelange V, Ranganathan P, Geyer S, Nicolet D, Huang X, Yu X, Volinia S, Kornblau SM, Andreeff M, Croce CM, Marcucci G, Bloomfield CD, Garzon R (2014) Implications of the miR-10 family in chemotherapy response of NPM1-mutated AML. Blood 123(15):2412–2415

25. Litzinger DC, Buiting AM, van Rooijen N, Huang L (1994) Effect of liposome size on the circulation time and intraorgan distribution of amphipathic poly(ethylene glycol)-containing liposomes. Biochim Biophys Acta 1190(1): 99–107

26. Tanaka T, Legat A, Adam E, Steuve J, Gatot JS, Vandenbranden M, Ulianov L, Lonez C, Ruysschaert JM, Muraille E, Tuynder M, Goldman M, Jacquet A (2008) DiC14-amidine cationic liposomes stimulate myeloid dendritic cells through Toll-like receptor 4. Eur J Immunol 38(5):1351–1357

27. Lonez C, Vandenbranden M, Ruysschaert JM (2008) Cationic liposomal lipids: from gene carriers to cell signaling. Prog Lipid Res 47(5): 340–347

28. Alexis F, Pridgen E, Molnar LK, Farokhzad OC (2008) Factors affecting the clearance and biodistribution of polymeric nanoparticles. Mol Pharm 5(4):505–515

29. Yang Z, Yu B, Zhu J, Huang X, Xie J, Xu S, Yang X, Wang X, Yung BC, Lee LJ, Lee RJ, Teng L (2014) A microfluidic method to synthesize transferrin-lipid nanoparticles loaded with siRNA LOR-1284 for therapy of acute myeloid leukemia. Nanoscale 6(16):9742–9751

30. Huang X, Caddell R, Yu B, Xu S, Theobald B, Lee LJ, Lee RJ (2010) Ultrasound-enhanced microfluidic synthesis of liposomes. Anticancer Res 30(2):463–466

31. Yu B, Zhu J, Xue W, Wu Y, Huang X, Lee LJ, Lee RJ (2011) Microfluidic assembly of lipid-based oligonucleotide nanoparticles. Anticancer Res 31(3):771–776

32. Huang X (2014) Targeted Delivery of MicroRNAs by Nanoparticles: A Novel Therapeutic Strategy in Acute Myeloid Leukemia. Dissertation, Ohio State University

33. Dorrance AM, Neviani P, Ferenchak G, Huang X, Nicolet D, Maharry K, Ozer HG, Hoellerbauer P, Khalife J, Hill E, Yadav M, Bolon B, Lee RJ, Lee LJ, Croce CM, Garzon R, Caligiuri MA, Bloomfield C, Marcucci G (2015) Targeting Leukemia Stem Cells in vivo with AntagomiR-126 Nanoparticles in Acute Myeloid Leukemia. Leukemia 29(11):2143–2153. doi:10.1038/leu.2015.139

34. Khalife J, Radomska H, Santhanam R, Huang X, Neviani P, Saultz J, Wang H, Wu YZ, Alachkar H, Anghelina M, Dorrance A, Curfman J, Bloomfield C, Medeiros B, Perrotti D, Lee LJ, Lee RJ, Caligiuri M, Pichiorri F, Croce C, Garzon R, Guzman M, Mendler J, Marcucci G (2015) Pharmacological Targeting of miR-155 via the NEDD8-Activating Enzyme Inhibitor MLN4924 (Pevonedistat) in Acute Myeloid Leukemia. Leukemia 29:1981–1992

Part II

Stimuli-Responsive Bolus Gene Delivery Vectors

Chapter 14

Characterization and Investigation of Redox-Sensitive Liposomes for Gene Delivery

Daniele Pezzoli, Elena Tallarita, Elena Rosini, and Gabriele Candiani

Abstract

A number of smart nonviral gene delivery vectors relying on bioresponsiveness have been introduced in the past few years to overcome the limits of the first generation of gene carriers. Among them, redox-sensitive lipidic and polymeric vectors exploit the presence of disulfide bonds in their structure to take advantage of the highly reductive intracellular milieu and to promote complex unpacking and nucleic acids release after cellular uptake (disulfide linker strategy). Glutathione (GSH) has been often identified as the leading actor in the intracellular reduction of bioreducible vectors but their actual mechanisms of action have been rarely investigated in depth and doubts about the real effectiveness of the disulfide linker strategy have been raised. Herein, we outline a simple protocol for the preparation and investigation of nanosized reducible cationic liposomes, focusing on their thorough characterization and optimization as gene delivery vectors. In addition, we carefully describe the techniques and procedures necessary for the assessment of the bioreducibility of the vectors and to demonstrate that the GSH-mediated intracellular cleavage of disulfide bonds is a pivotal step in their transfection process. Liposomes composed of 1,2-dioleoyl-sn-glycero-3-phosphocholine (DOPC), 1,2-dioleoyl-sn-glycero-3-phosphatidylethanolamine (DOPE), and of the reducible cationic lipid SS14 are reported as a practical example but the proposed protocol can be easily shifted to other formulations of reducible lipids/liposomes and to reducible polymers.

Key words Gene delivery, Nonviral vector, Liposome, Redox-sensitive vector, Glutathione, GSH depletion/repletion, Transfection efficiency, Cytotoxicity

1 Introduction

Gene delivery can be defined as the introduction of exogenous genetic material (i.e., DNA and RNA) into cells to control their protein expression [1]. The range of its therapeutic applications (gene therapy) has thoroughly expanded since the recent accomplishment of the Human Genome Project (HGP), leading to increased efforts in the investigation of gene delivery techniques. Aiming to obtain adequate delivery rates of nucleic acids to cells, two major classes of gene delivery agents have been developed so far, viral and nonviral vectors. Since their introduction in the late 1980s, nonviral synthetic gene vectors (transfectants) have been

Gabriele Candiani (ed.), *Non-Viral Gene Delivery Vectors: Methods and Protocols*, Methods in Molecular Biology, vol. 1445, DOI 10.1007/978-1-4939-3718-9_14, © Springer Science+Business Media New York 2016

thoroughly developed and investigated as promising alternatives to viruses mainly because they are easy-to-use, cheap, and have a safer profile, thus often making them the vectors of choice for in vitro laboratory research [2]. Nonviral vectors for gene delivery can be divided into two major families, cationic lipids and cationic polymers. Both lipids and polymers can self-assemble with anionic nucleic acids forming nano-/micro-scaled particles respectively named lipoplexes and polyplexes, which can interact with the plasma membrane and mediate cellular uptake. However, to date, the lower efficiency in delivering the genetic material to the target cells as compared to viruses has limited the use of nonviral gene delivery vectors in clinics. In order to overcome the major bottlenecks hindering effective nonviral gene delivery, recently a new generation of polymeric and lipidic vectors relying on bioresponsiveness has been developed [2].

Among these new gene carriers, redox-sensitive vectors have received increasing attention, owing to their peculiar ability to exploit the reductive intracellular milieu to increase the release of nucleic acids from the complexes after cellular uptake, considered as one of the main open issues in nonviral gene delivery. In fact, by introducing disulfide bonds within the chemical structure of vectors, an approach known as the "disulfide linker strategy", their stability can be spatially controlled thanks to the gradient in redox potential existing between the extracellular and the intracellular environment. More precisely, disulfides are highly stable in the oxidizing extracellular environment but they are quickly reduced to sulfhydryls by the high levels of cytoplasmic glutathione (GSH, 1–11 mM), eventually causing the intracellular disassembly of reducible lipoplexes and polyplexes [3, 4]. A number of redox-sensitive lipidic and polymeric transfectants have been synthesized and studied so far but often the investigation of the actual mechanism of transfection has been overlooked and some authors raised doubts about the real effectiveness of the disulfide linker strategy in gene delivery, suggesting that other factors, such as changes in the ability to promote endosomal escape, may influence to a greater extent the overall efficiency of reducible vectors [5]. In this context, our group has recently developed several techniques and methodologies aimed at developing and optimizing redox-sensitive lipid-based systems for gene delivery and at adequately demonstrating the key role of bioreducibility in their transfection process [3, 4, 6, 7].

The overall goal of this book chapter is to outline a simple protocol for the characterization, optimization, and investigation of redox-sensitive liposomes as gene delivery vectors describing, as a practical example, the development of reducible liposomes composed by 1,2-dioleoyl-sn-glycero-3-phosphocholine (DOPC), 1,2-dioleoyl-sn-glycero-3-phosphatidylethanolamine (DOPE), and SS14, a reducible *gemini* lipid previously synthesized and investigated by our group [3, 4, 6, 7]. After first outlining a quick method to formulate and extrude nanometer-sized three-component unilamellar liposomes (16.7:33.3:50 molar ratio) DOPC/DOPE/SS14 in water), the first part of the protocol is focused on their overall physicochemical and biological characterization: (1) determination of the mean diameter and overall surface charge (ζ-potential) of liposomes and lipoplexes by Dynamic Light Scattering (DLS) and Laser Doppler Microelectrophoresis (LDM) techniques; (2) investigation of the ability to complex and condense DNA by fluorophore (SYBR® Green I)-exclusion assay; (3) evaluation of transfection efficiency and cytotoxicity using the Enhanced Green Fluorescent Protein (EGFP) as reporter gene (pEGFP-N1 plasmid) and AlamarBlue® as cell viability assay; and (4) identification of the best transfection conditions. The second part of the protocol highlights the key experiments necessary to assess if the presence of disulfides in the lipid structure really impart bioresponsiveness to the resulting lipoplexes: (1) evaluation of DNA release from lipoplexes in the presence of reducing agents; (2) transfection experiments in GSH-depleted cells.

The protocol described herein reports specific transfection conditions for the DOPC/DOPE/SS14 (16.7:33.3:50) liposomes and for MG63 cells as model cell line, anyway, it could be easily shifted to other formulations and types of reducible transfectants (e.g., polymers) and to other types of cells following the suggestions reported in the Subheading 4.

2 Materials

2.1 Cationic Liposome and Lipoplex Preparation and Characterization

1. DOPC (Avanti Polar Lipids, Alabaster, AL). Store at −20 °C.

2. DOPE (Avanti Polar Lipids). Store at −20 °C.

3. SS14 reducible cationic lipid [6].

4. Chloroform ($CHCl_3$).

5. Ultrapure water (dH_2O) with resistivity values greater than 5 MΩ-cm at 25 °C.

6. Plasmid DNA (pDNA) encoding for Enhanced Green Fluorescent Protein, pEGFP-N1 Control Vector (Clontech Laboratories, Mountain View, CA).

7. pDNA encoding for Gaussia Luciferase, pCMV-GLuc Control pDNA (New England Biolabs, Ipswich, MA).

8. SYBR® Green I (Sigma-Aldrich, St. Louis, MO).

9. LiposoFast™ apparatus equipped with two 1.0 mL gas-tight syringes, glass syringe, and polycarbonate membranes with pore size of 100 nm (Avestin, Ottawa, Canada; see **Note 1**).

10. DLS and LDM apparatus: Malvern Zetasizer Nano ZS apparatus (Malvern Instruments Ltd, Worcestershire, UK).

11. Disposable capillary cells for ζ-potential measurements (Malvern Instruments Ltd).

12. 1.5 mL and 15 mL polypropylene microcentrifuge tubes.

13. Polystyrene multiwell plates.

14. Absorbance and fluorescence microplate reader.

15. Rotary evaporator.

16. Vortex mixer.

2.2 Cell Culture

1. MG63, human osteosarcoma cell line (European Collection of Cell Cultures, ECACC, Salisbury, UK).

2. 4.5 g/L high-glucose Dulbecco's Modified Eagle Medium (DMEM), stored at 4 °C.

3. Fetal bovine serum (FBS), aliquoted under sterile conditions and stored at –20 °C.

4. 100× penicillin–streptomycin sterile solution: 10,000 U/mL penicillin and 10 mg/mL streptomycin, aliquoted under sterile conditions and stored at –20 °C.

5. 200 mM sterile L-glutamine, aliquoted under sterile conditions and stored at –20 °C.

6. 1 M sterile HEPES buffer, pH 7.0–7.6, stored at 4 °C.

7. 100 mM sterile sodium pyruvate in dH$_2$O, stored at 4 °C.

8. Complete cell-culture medium: high-glucose DMEM supplemented with 10 % (v/v) FBS, 2 mM L-glutamine, 100 U/mL penicillin, 100 µg/mL streptomycin, 1 mM sodium pyruvate, and 10 mM HEPES buffer. Prepare complete cell-culture medium under sterile conditions and store at 4 °C. Prewarm it to 37 °C prior to use.

9. Dulbecco's Phosphate Buffered Saline (PBS), sterile solution. Store at 4 °C and prewarm it to 37 °C prior to use.

10. Trypsin-ethylenediamminetetracetic acid (EDTA) sterile solution: 0.5 mg/mL of porcine trypsin, 0.2 g/L of EDTA, aliquoted under sterile conditions and stored at –20 °C.

11. 1.5 mL and 15 mL polypropylene microcentrifuge tubes.

12. Polystyrene multiwell plates.

13. Benchtop centrifuge and microcentrifuge.

14. Cell-culture incubator.

2.3 Transfection Experiments and Post-Transfection Assays

1. Transfection medium: high-glucose DMEM supplemented with 10 % FBS, 2 mM of L-glutamine, 10 mM HEPES, and 1 mM of sodium pyruvate (*see* **Note 2**). Prepare transfection medium under sterile conditions and store at 4 °C. Prewarm it to 37 °C prior to use.

2. 10× AlamarBlue® solution (Thermo Fisher Scientific, Waltham, MA).

3. Fixation buffer: 4% (w/v) paraformaldehyde (PFA) in PBS. Store at −20 °C.

4. 1.5 mL polypropylene microcentrifuge tubes.

5. Polystyrene multiwell plates.

6. Flow cytometer (FCM).

2.4 Glutathione Depletion/Repletion Studies

2.4.1 GSH Quantification

1. 2′,7′-dichloro-dihydrofluorescein-diacetate (DCFH-DA, Thermo Fisher Scientific).

2. Glutathione Assay Kit (Sigma-Aldrich).

3. 5% (w/v) 5-sulfosalicylic acid in dH_2O (SSA, Sigma-Aldrich).

4. Working mixture (without GSH Reductase): 40 μg/mL of 5,5′-dithiobis(2-nitrobenzoic acid) (DTNB) in 1× Assay Buffer (Glutathione Assay Kit, 100 mM potassium phosphate buffer, pH 7.0, with 1 mM EDTA).

5. GSH Reductase-NADPH solution: 0.5 U/mL of GSH Reductase, 0.16 mg/mL of β-nicotinamide adenine dinucleotide 2′-phosphate (NADPH) in 1× Assay Buffer.

6. BCA Protein Assay Kit (Thermo Fisher Scientific).

7. 1.5 mL and 15 mL polypropylene microcentrifuge tubes.

8. Polystyrene multiwell plates.

9. Absorbance and fluorescence microplate reader.

3 Methods

3.1 Preparation of Tri-Component Cationic Liposomes

1. Prepare stock solutions of cationic lipids by dissolving in $CHCl_3$ DOPC, DOPE, and SS14 in three separate glass vials to a final concentration of 20 mM (*see* **Note 3**).

2. Prepare the lipid ternary mixture at a DOPC/DOPE/SS14 molar ratio of 16.7:33.3:50 by adding the correct amounts of lipid solutions in a round-bottomed flask using a glass syringe (*see* **Note 4**) and mix well. For example, for 1 mL, add 167 μL of 20 mM DOPC, 333 μL of DOPE and 500 μL of SS14.

3. Use a rotary evaporator at 40 °C to remove $CHCl_3$ up to the formation of a dry lipid film on inner surface of the flask.

4. Dry under vacuum overnight to completely remove the organic solvent.

5. Add dH_2O to a final total lipid concentration of 20 mM (*see* **Note 5**).

6. Hydrate the lipid film by vortexing thoroughly until a clear solution, containing large multilamellar vesicles, is obtained (*see* **Note 6**).

222 Daniele Pezzoli et al.

7. Freeze/thaw eight times (or at least five times) and bring to room temperature (RT).

8. Transfer the lipid dispersion (maximum 1 mL) in one of the gas-tight syringes (loading syringe).

9. Mount two 100 nm-pore polycarbonate membranes (*see* **Note 7**) and both the loading syringe and the empty receiving syringe onto the LiposoFast™ apparatus.

10. Extrude 27 times (*see* **Note 8**) the lipid dispersion.

11. Harvest the obtained liposome dispersion in a sterile plastic vial and store at 4 °C (*see* **Note 9**).

3.2 Characterization of Liposomes

3.2.1 Dynamic Light Scattering (DLS)

1. Dilute 50 μL of liposome suspension 1:20 in dH$_2$O (*see* **Note 10**) inside a disposable 12 mm square polystyrene cuvette.

2. Measure particle size using a DLS apparatus checking that the polydispersity index (PDI) of the Cumulant analysis is below 0.2 (*see* **Note 11**).

3.2.2 Laser Doppler Microelectrophoresis (LDM)

1. Transfer 750 μL of diluted liposome suspension, the same used for DLS measurement, into a disposable capillary cell for ζ-potential measurements.

2. Measure ζ-potential using a LDM apparatus and verify that the obtained value is positive (*see* **Note 12**).

3.3 Preparation and Characterization of Lipoplexes

3.3.1 Lipoplex Preparation

1. Dilute pDNA (pEGFP-N1) in dH$_2$O (*see* **Note 10**) to a final concentration of 0.04 μg/μL, corresponding to a phosphate (PO$_4$) concentration of 121.2 μM (DNA solution) (*see* **Note 13**).

2. Dilute liposome suspension in dH$_2$O so that the final concentration of net positive charges is X times higher than PO$_4$ concentration in the DNA solution (*see* **Note 14**), where X is the desired charge ratio (CR, +/−).

3. Mix equal volumes of DNA solution with liposome suspension and incubate at RT for 30 min (lipoplex suspension, *see* **Note 15**).

3.3.2 Evaluation of DNA Condensation

1. Prepare 20 μL of lipoplex suspension at different CRs (1–10) as described in Subheading 3.3.1 and 20 μL of pDNA at 0.02 μg/μL in dH$_2$O (CR 0).

2. Add 100 μL of dH$_2$O (*see* **Note 10**), containing 2× SYBR® Green I and incubate for 10 min at RT (*see* **Note 16**).

3. Add 100 μL of dH$_2$O containing 2× SYBR® Green I to 20 μL of dH$_2$O to prepare a blank sample.

4. Place 35 μL aliquots of the resulting solutions in triplicate in the wells of a black polystyrene 384 well plate (*see* **Note 17**).

5. Read fluorescence by using a fluorescence microplate reader with an excitation wavelength $\lambda_{ex} = 497$ nm and an emission wavelength $\lambda_{em} = 520$ nm.

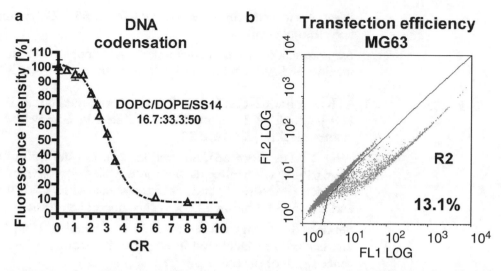

Fig. 1 (**a**) Evaluation of DNA condensation by 16.7:33.3:50 (molar ratio) DOPC/DOPE/SS14 liposomes as a function of CR by fluorophore (SYBR® Green I)-exclusion assay. Results are presented as fluorescence % with respect to uncomplexed DNA; adapted from [3]. (**b**) Example of cytofluorimetric analysis; a FL1 (*green fluorescence*) vs. FL2 (*orange fluorescence*) dot plot of MG63 transfected cells is reported. EGFP-expressing cells appear as a population delineated by region 2 (R2) (where FL1 > FL2) identified by the analysis of mock-transfected (pCMV-GLuc) cells

6. Identify the minimal fluorescence plateau, corresponding to maximum pDNA condensation, by plotting samples average fluorescence signal (subtracted of blank average signal) as a function of CR (*see* **Note 18**). An example of a typical condensation curve is reported in Fig. 1a for DOPC/DOPE/SS14 (16.7:33.3:50) liposomes.

3.3.3 Lipoplex Characterization

1. Prepare 100 μL of lipoplex suspension at the desired CR as described in Subheading 3.3.1 and dilute them 1:10 in dH$_2$O.

2. Measure particle size and ζ-potential of the obtained diluted lipoplex suspensions as described in Subheadings 3.2.1 and 3.2.2 (*see* **Note 19**).

3.4 Transfection Experiments

3.4.1 Cell Transfection

1. Seed MG63 cells at a density of 1.0×10^4 cells/cm^2 (*see* **Note 20**) in a 12-well cell-culture plate containing 800 μL/well of complete cell-culture medium (*see* **Note 21**).

2. 24 h after seeding, remove old medium, rinse cells with 800 μL of PBS (*see* **Note 22**) and add 800 μL/well of transfection medium.

3. Prepare 72 μL of lipoplex suspension at different CRs as described above, using both pEGFP-N1 and pCMV-GLuc.

4. Add 16 μL/well of lipoplex suspension at different CRs (pDNA dose: 0.32 μg/well). It is recommended to prepare at least 4 replicates per CR.

5. Place cells in a cell-culture incubator (37 °C, 5 % CO_2, humidified atmosphere).

6. Facultative: after 4 h of incubation, remove lipoplex-containing medium and add complete cell-culture medium (*see* **Note 23**).

3.4.2 *Cytotoxicity Assay*

1. 48 h after transfection (*see* **Note 24**), remove medium and add 800 μL/well of 1× AlamarBlue® (diluted in complete cell-culture medium, *see* **Note 25**).

2. After 2 h (*see* **Note 26**), for each sample, transfer 100 μL of AlamarBlue®-containing medium into a black polystyrene 96 well plate (*see* **Note 17**) and read fluorescence with $\lambda_{ex} = 540$ nm and $\lambda_{em} = 585$ nm using a fluorescence microplate reader.

3. Subtract the average fluorescence of blank samples (100 μL of 1× AlamarBlue® incubated in empty wells) from the fluorescence signal of the samples.

Average the net fluorescence signal of each quadruplicate and calculate cell viability as:

$$\text{Viability} \left[\%\right] = \frac{\text{Sample fluorescence}}{\text{CTRL fluorescence}} \times 100$$

and cytotoxicity as:

$$\text{Cytotoxicity} \left[\%\right] = 100\% - \text{Viability} \left[\%\right]$$

where CTRL fluorescence is the net fluorescence signal of positive controls (non-transfected cells).

3.4.3 *Preparation of Samples for Cytofluorimetric Analysis*

1. After AlamarBlue® assay (*see* Subheading 3.4.2), rinse cells with 500 μL of PBS.

2. Add 100 μL/well of trypsin-EDTA solution.

3. Incubate at 37 °C for 3 min (*see* **Note 27**).

4. Once cells are detached, add 250 μL of complete cell-culture medium to block trypsin activity.

5. Mix by pipetting and then transfer 350 μL of cell suspension into a clean 1.5 mL polypropylene microcentrifuge tube.

6. Rinse the well with 350 μL of complete cell-culture medium and transfer them in the same tube of **step 5** to collect the remaining cells.

7. Centrifuge the tube containing cell suspension at $1000 \times g$ at 4 °C for 5 min.

8. Remove 650 μL of supernatant and add 450 μL of PBS.

9. Centrifuge the tube at $1000 \times g$ at 4 °C for 5 min.

10. Discard the supernatant.

11. Resuspend cell pellet in 300 μL of fixation buffer.

12. Store at 4 °C until cytofluorimetric analyses are performed.

3.4.4   Evaluation of Transfection Efficiency by Cytofluorimetry

1. Transfer cells from Subheading 3.4.3, **step 12** in a round bottom 12×75 mm tube (compatible with the available FCM instrument).

2. Load the sample on the FCM.

3. Analyze at least 1.0×10^4 events exciting cells at $\lambda_{ex} = 488$ nm and measure fluorescence at $\lambda_{em} = 520$ nm (green fluorescence) and $\lambda_{em} = 575$ nm (orange fluorescence) to enable correction for autofluorescence by diagonal gating as described below and as shown in Fig. 1b.

4. Using a cytometry software, create a dot plot and graph green fluorescence (FL1) on the X axis and orange fluorescence (FL2) on the Y axis. Using mock-transfected cells (cells transfected with an empty plasmid or a plasmid encoding a nonfluorescent protein such as Luciferase, herein pCMV-GLuc, *see* **Note 28**), identify and define the region of positive (green fluorescent) cells, on the right of the population of mock-treated cells which should lie nearby the diagonal of the quadrant (the percentage of cells present in the defined positive region should be lower than 1 % in all mock-treated samples).

5. Use the identified region to calculate the percentage of positive (green fluorescent) cells of all the samples.

3.4.5   Choice of the Best Transfection Conditions

1. Identify the best CR for transfection experiments taking into account both cytotoxicity and transfection efficiency results.

2. Among low cytotoxic conditions, a good compromise between high transfection efficiency and low cytotoxicity should be chosen. For 16.7:33.3:50 (molar ratio) DOPC/DOPE/SS14 liposomes, CR 5 was chosen.

3.5   Lipoplex Disassembly in a Reducing Environment

1. Prepare 16 μL of lipoplexes at the identified working CR as described in Subheading 3.3.1 and incubate at RT for 30 min.

2. Add 304 μL (1:19 dilution) of aqueous solution of 10 mM GSH or 10 mM GSSG containing 2× SYBR® Green I.

3. Place 3×100 μL aliquots (*see* **Note 17**) of the resulting solutions in a black polystyrene 384 well plate and monitor the fluorescence ($\lambda_{ex} = 495$ nm; $\lambda_{em} = 520$ nm) using a fluorescence microplate reader every 30 s for at least 2 h.

4. Plot the samples average fluorescence signal (subtracted of blank average signal) as a function of time. An increase in fluorescence signal of samples containing GSH, compared to GSSG, indicates that the reduction of lipoplexes components (i.e., SS14) by the reducing agent led to the release of nucleic acids (Fig. 2a, *see* **Note 29**).

3.6 Glutathione Depletion/Repletion Studies

GSH depletion/repletion studies are aimed at proving that the transfection process of redox-sensitive liposomes is strictly dependent on the intracellular reduction by the reducing environment, specifically by the high levels of reduced GSH. Results of GSH depletion/repletion studies for DOPC/DOPE/SS14 (16.7:33.3:50 molar ratio) lipoplexes prepared at CR 5 are reported in Fig. 2.

3.6.1 Transfection Experiments After Glutathione Depletion/Repletion

The complete experimental procedure for GSH depletion/repletion experiments is outlined in Fig. 2b.

1. Seed MG63 cells in T25 flasks (*see* **Note 30**) at a density of 1.0×10^4 cells/cm^2 in 5 mL of complete cell-culture medium (*see* **Note 31**).

2. Seed MG63 cells in 24-well plates at a density of 1.0×10^4 cells/cm^2 in 400 μL of complete cell-culture medium (*see* **Notes 30** and **31**).

3. After 8 h, supplement medium with BSO to a final concentration of 0.05 mM (*see* **Note 32**).

4. After 20 h, wash cells with PBS and add fresh complete cell-culture medium supplemented with either 0.05 mM BSO, 1 mM NAC, or 0.2 mM Vit-C (*see* **Note 32**) and incubate in a cell-culture incubator.

5. After further 20 h (this time point is defined as t_0 in Fig. 2), wash cells with PBS, add fresh transfection medium and transfect cells by adding 16.7:33.3:50 (molar ratio) DOPC/DOPE/SS14 reducible lipoplexes prepared at CR 5 (100 μL/flask for T25 flasks and 8 μL/well for 24-well plates, *see* Subheading 3.4.1) and incubate in a cell-culture incubator for 48 h (t_{final}).

3.6.2 Cell Processing for Subsequent Assays

1. At t_0 and t_{final}, trypsinize cells in T25 flasks (*see* Subheading 3.4.3) using 300 μL of trypsin-EDTA and add 1 mL of complete cell-culture medium to block trypsin activity.

2. Collect cells in 1.5 mL polypropylene microcentrifuge tubes (*see* **Note 33**).

3. Divide t_{final} samples (transfected cells) into two aliquots.

4. Centrifuge cells for 5 min at 4 °C at $1000 \times g$ and wash the obtained pellets with 500 μL of PBS.

5. Fix cells in half the aliquots of t_{final} samples in fixation buffer as described in Subheading 3.4.3 and store samples at 4 °C for the following cytofluorimetric analysis.

6. For t_0 samples and the remaining aliquots of t_{final}, resuspend the obtained cell pellets in 150 μL 5% SSA.

7. Freeze-thaw twice using liquid nitrogen and incubate for 5 min at 4 °C (*see* **Note 34**).

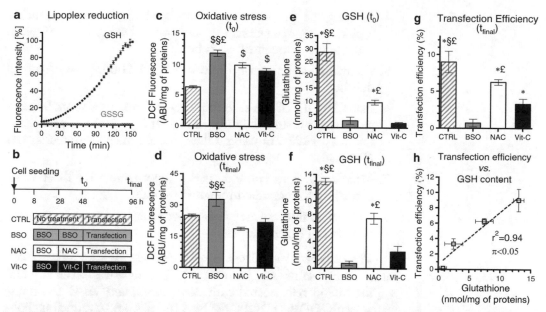

Fig. 2 (a) Disassembly of 16.7:33.3:50 (molar ratio) DOPC/DOPE/SS14 lipoplexes at CR 5 in the presence of GSH or GSSG. Results are presented as fluorescence % with respect to uncomplexed DNA. **(b)** Outline of the experimental procedure of glutathione depletion/repletion studies. Four groups were analyzed: untreated CTRL, BSO-, NAC-, and Vit-C-treated cells. Following pharmacological treatment (t_0), cells were transfected for 48 h (t_{final}) with 16.7:33.3:50 (molar ratio) DOPC/DOPE/SS14 lipoplexes at CR 5. Oxidative stress and GSH content were measured at t_0 ((**c**) and (**d**), respectively) and after transfection ((**e**) and (**f**), respectively). **(g)** Transfection efficiency, expressed as % of positive (*green fluorescent*) cells. **(h)** A linear correlation between GSH content and transfection efficiency was observed. Results are expressed as mean ± SEM ($n=3$). \$ $p<0.05$ vs. CTRL; *$p<0.05$ vs. BSO; § $p<0.05$ vs. NAC; £ $p<0.05$ vs. Vit-C. From [3]

8. Centrifuge the extracts for 10 min at 4 °C at $10,000 \times g$ to pellet precipitated proteins.

9. Keeping samples on ice, collect the supernatants in new polypropylene microcentrifuge tubes and measure their volume (*see* **Note 35**). Supernatants can now be stored at −80 °C.

10. Add to the protein pellets a volume of 25 mM NaOH equal to the corresponding measured volume of supernatant and resuspend them (*see* **Note 36**).

11. Evaluate transfection efficiency of the PFA-fixed samples by cytofluorimetry as described in Subheading 3.4.4.

3.6.3 Evaluation of Oxidative Stress

1. At t_0 and t_{final} wash cells cultured in 24-well plates with 500 μL of PBS and incubate with 10 μM DCFH-DA in PBS (500 μL/ well) for 15 min at 37 °C (*see* **Note 37**).

2. Wash cells twice with 500 μL of PBS.

3. Lyse cells by adding 300 μL of 0.5 % (v/v) Tween 20 in 50 mM Tris–HCl, pH 7.5, and incubate for 15 min on ice.

4. Keeping the samples on ice, detach cells from the well surface with the help of a cell scraper and collect lysate in 1.5 mL polypropylene microcentrifuge tubes.

5. Centrifuge samples for 5 min at 4 °C at $1000 \times g$ to pellet cell debris.

6. Place 200 µL of the resulting supernatants in a black 96-well plate and measure the fluorescence at $\lambda_{em} = 530$ nm and exciting at $\lambda_{ex} = 485$ nm using a fluorescence microplate reader (*see* **Note 38**).

7. Measure protein content of the supernatants by BCA assay, according to manufacturer's instructions.

8. Normalize fluorescence results over the total protein content of each cell lysate sample.

The obtained normalized sample fluorescence is an index of cellular oxidative stress (*see* **Note 37**) [8]. Oxidative stress levels at t_0 and t_{final} for MG63 cells treated with BSO, NAC, and Vit-C and transfected with DOPC/DOPE/SS14 (16.7:33.3:50) reducible lipoplexes (*see* Subheading 3.6.1) are shown in Fig. 2c, d, respectively. Results show that, at t_0, oxidative stress levels of BSO-treated cells increased by almost two-fold with respect to untreated cells (CTRL) while the antioxidant treatment with NAC and Vit-C equally alleviated BSO effects. At t_{final}, 48 h post-transfection, oxidative stress levels in NAC- and Vit-C-treated groups were equal to CTRL while those of BSO-treated cells were still higher ($p < 0.05$).

3.6.4 GSH Quantification

1. Add in duplicate 10 µL of known concentrations of GSH in 5 % SSA (GSH standards, 3.125–100 µM) and of unknown samples (supernatants collected in Subheading 3.6.2, **step 9**) in a transparent 96-well plate (*see* **Note 39**).

2. Add in duplicate 10 µL of 5 % SSA as reagent blanks.

3. Add 150 µL of working solution (without GSH Reductase) to each well and incubate for 15 min at RT. Measure absorbance at $\lambda = 412$ nm (OD_{412}), using an absorbance microplate reader (*see* **Note 40**).

4. Add 50 µL of GSH Reductase-NADPH solution to each well with a multichannel pipette and mix by pipetting.

5. Measure OD_{412} for 10 min at 1 min intervals.

Calculation of Reduced GSH Content

1. Subtract the average OD_{412} of the reagent blank replicates from the OD_{412} of all standards and unknown samples recorded at Subheading 3.6.4, **step 3**.

2. Plot the average blank-corrected OD_{412} for each GSH standard against its concentration and fit a linear standard curve.

3. Calculate the reduced GSH concentration of each unknown sample using the standard curve.

4. Measure protein content of the samples obtained at Subheading 3.6.2, **step 10** by BCA assay, according to manufacturer's instructions (*see* **Note 41**).

5. Normalize the measured reduced GSH concentrations of each sample with the corresponding protein concentrations; reduced GSH content will be expressed as mmol of GSH/mg of proteins.

Calculation of Total Glutathione (GSH and GSSG)

1. Subtract the average OD_{412} of the reagent blank replicates from the OD_{412} of all the measurements recorded at Subheading 3.6.4, **step 5**.

2. For each standard and sample, calculate the $\Delta OD_{412}/min$ (*see* **Note 42**) by fitting a linear trend line (OD_{412} vs. time). $\Delta OD_{412}/min$ is represented by the slope (angular coefficient) of the fitted linear trendline.

3. Plot the average $\Delta OD_{412}/min$ for each GSH standard against its concentration and fit a standard curve.

4. Calculate the total glutathione concentration of each unknown sample using the standard curve.

5. Normalize the measured total glutathione concentrations of each sample with the corresponding protein concentrations (*see* Subheading 3.6.4.1, **step 4**); total glutathione content will be expressed as mmol of (GSH+GSSG)/mg of proteins (*see* **Note 43**).

Reduced GSH levels at t_0 and t_{final} for MG63 cells treated with BSO, NAC, and Vit-C and transfected with DOPC/DOPE/SS14 (16.7:33.3:50) reducible lipoplexes (*see* Subheading 3.6.1) are shown in Fig. 2e, f, respectively. As expected, results show that only incubation of GSH-depleted cells with NAC significantly restored GSH levels at t_{final} (57% repletion in GSH content compared to BSO-untreated CTRL). Taking into account the transfection results in the four groups (Fig. 2g), a linear correlation between GSH content and transfection efficiency ($r^2 = 0.94$) could be observed (Fig. 2h). Inversely, oxidative stress levels and transfection efficiency did not correlate at all ($r^2 = 0.35$), demonstrating the pivotal role of intracellular GSH levels in the transfection process of 16.7:33.3:50 (molar ratio) DOPC/DOPE/SS14 reducible lipoplexes.

4 Notes

1. LiposoFast™ is a manually powered extruder designed for researchers who use only small amounts of liposomes. Vesicles (lipid emulsions) prepared with LiposoFast™ are repeatedly extruded through a porous polycarbonate membrane forced back and forth by specially modified gas-tight syringes [9]. The apparatus can be autoclaved in order to produce sterile liposomes.

2. Transfection experiments in antibiotic-free medium are recommended since the increase in cell membrane permeability by cationic liposomes during transfection could lead to higher antibiotic uptake and consequently increase the cytotoxicity.

3. The use of glass or stainless steel in the presence of organic solutions is recommended; the use of vials made of polymeric materials should be avoided as impurities could leach out of the container.

4. The preparation of 16.7:33.3:50 (molar ratio) formulation is here reported as an example, but desired molar ratios can be easily obtained by changing the volume ratio of the starting lipid solutions.

5. The final physicochemical and transfection properties of the obtained liposomes can be strongly influenced by the aqueous solution where they are prepared; other buffers such as PBS and 10 mM Hepes buffer, pH 7, can be used. The use of buffers containing EDTA is not recommended as it could cause liposome aggregation.

6. If vortexing is ineffective, bath sonicate the lipid dispersion for 2–5 min, until clarity is obtained.

7. The use of two stacked polycarbonate membranes helps yielding monodisperse, nanometric-sized liposomes. Liposomes of different dimensions can be obtained by simply using polycarbonate membranes with different pore sizes (e.g., 50, 100, 200, 400 nm; available from Avestin).

8. An odd number of passages is recommended (at least 21) to finally have extruded liposomes in the, initially empty, receiving syringe, thus avoiding contamination with unextruded vesicles which might remain inside the loading syringe.

9. Usually liposomes are stable up to 1 year at 4 °C. However it is recommended to periodically verify liposome stability by measuring their mean size (hydrodynamic diameter) and ζ-potential (*see* Subheading 3.2).

10. For both characterization experiments and lipoplex formation, the dilution of liposome formulations in the same aqueous solution where they were prepared, is recommended.

11. PDI is a dimensionless parameter that evaluates the width of the particle size distribution. A high PDI indicates a large variability in the particle size. If PDI is higher than 0.2 or mean size is much higher than membrane pore size, it may be necessary to extrude liposomes again. In these cases, lipid concentration during extrusion should be reduced.

12. A positive ζ-potential is expected for cationic liposomes in dH_2O.

13. DNA phosphate density (and then negative charge density) is 3.03 nmol of PO_4/µg of DNA.

14. SS14 is assumed to carry 4 positive charges per molecule while DOPC and DOPE are neutral in dH_2O at pH 7.

15. In these works, lipoplexes were always prepared at RT.

16. SYBR® Green I is the DNA stain of choice for these experiments because it has been shown to be much less mutagenic and much more sensitive than ethidium bromide [10].

17. It is recommended to prepare a triplicate of each sample to take into account experimental and instrumental variability. The use of black polystyrene microplates is also suggested for fluorescence analysis as they minimize light scattering and well-to-well crosstalk and have low background fluorescence.

18. Maximum DNA condensation is often necessary to obtain efficient lipoplexes; if a plateau is not observed, test higher CRs.

19. Size (hydrodynamic diameter) and ζ-potential measurements of polyplexes are recommended: to assure DNA complexation and lipoplex interaction with negatively charged cell surfaces, positively charged lipoplexes are necessary (when using cationic liposomes as transfection reagents).

20. Transfection efficiency and cytotoxicity of lipoplexes are strongly cell-dependent. If high cytotoxicity or poor transfection results are observed, optimal cell seeding density and/or lipoplex dose should be identified [11].

21. If using other cell lines or primary cells, the appropriate culture medium should be chosen, according to existing literature. Presence of serum in the culture medium may affect the transfection efficiency of nonviral gene delivery vectors, therefore sometimes it could be preferable to carry out transfection experiments in serum-free transfection medium.

22. Washing step can be avoided to reduce cell detachment if culture medium is the same before and during transfection.

23. Medium change after 4 h can be carried out to reduce cytotoxicity and is often necessary in case of transfection in serum-free medium.

24. GFP expression usually peaks at 24–48 h post-transfection, even though longer incubation times could be necessary for some liposomal formulations.

25. AlamarBlue® is a nontoxic, nondestructive cell growth indicator. The use of AlamarBlue® as cell viability assay allows to test the same samples in the following cytofluorimetric analysis.

26. Increase/decrease incubation time if too low/too high (saturated) signal is observed.

27. To facilitate cell detachment gently tap the plate, then check by optical microscope. Put the plate again at 37 °C for 1–2 more min, if necessary.

28. Mock transfected cells are a negative control used to determine any nonspecific effects that may be caused by the transfection reagent or processes such as background fluorescence and autofluorescence of transfected cells.

29. In some cases the simple presence of a reducing agent such as GSH is not sufficient to lead to lipoplex disassembly and nucleic acid release. In these cases, in order to demonstrate the reducibility of the complexes, it is necessary to add a counter ion such as heparin in the reducing solution. If DNA is released in the presence of heparin and GSH but not of heparin and GSSG, nucleic acid release from lipoplexes in reducing environment can be considered effective. A DNA/heparin w/w ratio of 1 is often appropriate for this purpose, but it should be optimized specifically for each transfectant.

30. 6-well culture plates can also be used; smaller size wells are not recommended since a high number of cells is necessary for the following assays. Cells are also seeded in 24-well plates to allow the evaluation of the oxidative stress levels by DCFH-DA assay.

31. Prepare enough samples considering the number of treatments investigated and the fact that cells will be analyzed at two different time points, t_0 (immediately before transfection) and t_{final} (48 h after transfection).

32. BSO is a glutathione depletor, NAC is a glutathione repletor and Vit-C is an antioxidant. The concentrations of BSO, NAC, and Vit-C to be used for these experiments are cell-dependent. It is recommended to optimize concentrations for each cell type used in order to obtain adequate levels of GSH depletion/repletion together with low cytotoxicity.

33. Approximately $0.5–1.0 \times 10^6$ and $2.0–3.0 \times 10^6$ cells should be obtained from a T25 flask at t_0 and t_{final}, respectively.

34. A sonication step could be added to facilitate cell rupture but usually the freeze-thaw step in 5 % SSA is enough to efficiently lyse cells and release GSH.

35. The volume should be around 140–145 µL.

36. The addition of 25 mM NaOH is necessary to guarantee complete protein resuspension. Samples can be now stored at –80 °C.

37. The nonfluorescent fluorescein derivative DCFH-DA is relatively resistant to oxidation, but upon cellular uptake, it is deacetylated to form DCFH whose oxidization by intracellular oxidants lead to the formation of highly fluorescent compound 2′,7′-dichlorofluorescein (DCF) [8].

38. Supernatants can be now stored at –80 °C directly in the 96-well plate.

39. Do not exceed 10 μL volume.

40. Measuring the absorbance at 412 nm before the addition of GSH Reductase and NADPH allows to quantify the intracellular levels of reduced GSH and not of the redox couple GSH-GSSG.

41. 25 mM NaOH is compatible with BCA assay. In case of using different assays for protein quantification, check the compatibility.

42. Since the signal of samples with high concentrations of glutathione could saturate within the 10 min of reading, it is important to exclude saturated values when fitting the linear curve.

43. Both reduced and total glutathione should be measured. If it is not possible to adequately quantify reduced GSH owing to low signal, total glutathione can be taken into account. The technique for the quantification of total glutathione is in fact more sensitive since it exploits a kinetic assay in which GSH causes a continuous reduction of DTNB and the GSSG formed in the process is recycled by glutathione reductase, thus strongly increasing the absorbance signal.

References

1. Pezzoli D, Chiesa R, De Nardo L, Candiani G (2012) We still have a long way to go to effectively deliver genes! J Appl Biomater Funct Mater 10(2):e82–e91

2. Pezzoli D, Candiani G (2013) Non-viral gene delivery strategies for gene therapy: a "menage a trois" among nucleic acids, materials, and the biological environment. J Nanopart Res 15(3):1523

3. Candiani G, Pezzoli D, Ciani L, Chiesa R, Ristori S (2010) Bioreducible liposomes for gene delivery: from the formulation to the mechanism of action. PLoS One 5(10), e13430

4. Pezzoli D, Zanda M, Chiesa R, Candiani G (2013) The yin of exofacial protein sulfhydryls and the yang of intracellular glutathione in in vitro transfection with SS14 bioreducible lipoplexes. J Control Release 165(1):44–53

5. Kumar VV, Chaudhuri A (2004) On the disulfide-linker strategy for designing efficacious cationic transfection lipids: an unexpected transfection profile. FEBS Lett 571(1-3):205–211

6. Candiani G, Frigerio M, Viani F, Verpelli C, Sala C, Chiamenti L, Zaffaroni N, Folini M, Sani M, Panzeri W, Zanda M (2007) Dimerizable redox-sensitive triazine-based cationic lipids for in vitro gene delivery. ChemMedChem 2(3):292–296

7. Candiani G, Pezzoli D, Cabras M, Ristori S, Pellegrini C, Kajaste-Rudnitski A, Vicenzi E, Sala C, Zanda M (2008) A dimerizable cationic lipid with potential for gene delivery. J Gene Med 10(6):637–645

8. Wang H, Joseph JA (1999) Quantifying cellular oxidative stress by dichlorofluorescein assay using microplate reader. Free Radic Biol Med 27(5-6):612–616

9. Macdonald RC, Macdonald RI, Menco BPM, Takeshita K, Subbarao NK, Hu LR (1991) Small-volume extrusion apparatus for preparation of large, unilamellar vesicles. Biochim Biophys Acta 1061(2):297–303

10. D'Andrea C, Pezzoli D, Malloggi C, Candeo A, Capelli G, Bassi A, Volonterio A, Taroni P, Candiani G (2014) The study of polyplex formation and stability by time-resolved fluorescence spectroscopy of SYBR Green I-stained DNA. Photochem Photobiol Sci 13(12):1680–1689

11. Malloggi C, Pezzoli D, Magagnin L, De Nardo L, Mantovani D, Tallarita E, Candiani G (2015) Comparative evaluation and optimization of off-the-shelf cationic polymers for gene delivery purposes. Polymer Chem 6:6325–6339

Chapter 15

From Artificial Amino Acids to Sequence-Defined Targeted Oligoaminoamides

Stephan Morys, Ernst Wagner, and Ulrich Lächelt

Abstract

Artificial oligoamino acids with appropriate protecting groups can be used for the sequential assembly of oligoaminoamides on solid-phase. With the help of these oligoamino acids multifunctional nucleic acid (NA) carriers can be designed and produced in highly defined topologies. Here we describe the synthesis of the artificial oligoamino acid Fmoc-Stp(Boc$_3$)-OH, the subsequent assembly into sequence-defined oligomers and the formulation of tumor-targeted plasmid DNA (pDNA) polyplexes.

Key words Proton-sponge, Sequence-defined, Polyplex, Oligoaminoamides, Gene transfer, Tumor targeting, cMet

1 Introduction

Gene therapy is a very attractive but also challenging approach for curing diseases caused by genetic disorders. Before the ultimate goal of clinical application can be reached, researchers designing artificial nonviral vectors are struggling with different requirements for a successful gene delivery. Starting with a sufficient nucleic acid (NA) packaging, protection and shielding against the immune system, specific, cellular uptake into the intended target cells, and finally escape from endolysosomes into the cytoplasm are most critical prerequisites for a therapeutic utilization [1–3].

Linear polyethylenimine (lPEI) is considered to be an effective polymeric gene delivery agent, since it fulfills several of the mentioned requirements as a result of its chemical structure. The repeating diaminoethane motif of lPEI causes a characteristic sequential protonation [4] guaranteeing both sufficient charge density for NA binding and condensation at neutral pH and a buffer capacity in the lower endosomal pH range for a vesicular escape via the hypothesized proton sponge effect [2, 5, 6]. Unfortunately lPEI also exhibits concentration dependent toxicity in vitro [7, 8] and in vivo [9]. In addition,

Gabriele Candiani (ed.), *Non-Viral Gene Delivery Vectors: Methods and Protocols*, Methods in Molecular Biology, vol. 1445, DOI 10.1007/978-1-4939-3718-9_15, © Springer Science+Business Media New York 2016

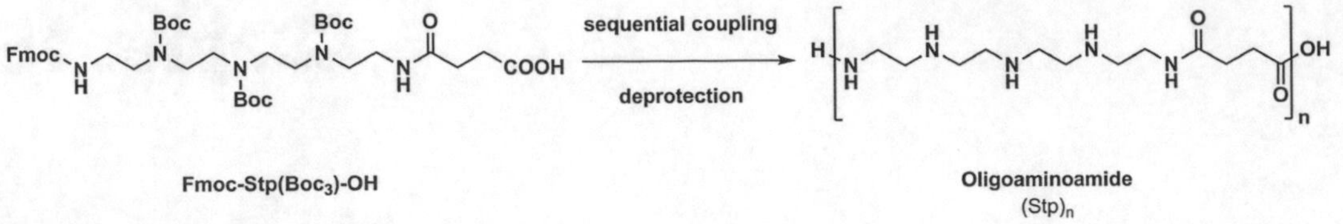

Fmoc-Stp(Boc₃)-OH   Oligoaminoamide (Stp)n

Fig. 1 The artificial amino acid Fmoc-Stp(Boc₃)-OH and the sequential assembly into oligoaminoamides

lPEI generally possesses certain polydispersity, and extensive, site-specific modification to meet additional demands is sophisticated.

For this reason, Schaffert et al. developed artificial amino acids containing defined oligoamine segments mimicking the chemical structure of lPEI, a conjugated diacid as molecular connector and suitable protecting groups for complete compatibility with classical solid phase peptide synthesis (Fig. 1) [10, 11]. By this means, the synthesis of sequence-defined oligoaminoamides with precise topology and site-specific functionalization could be realized [10, 12–15]. Long linear structures solely containing the artificial oligoamino acid succinyl-tetraethylene pentamine (Stp) [16] as well as branched topologies with additional cysteines, for supramolecular assembly via reducible cross-linkings, showed high efficiency while maintaining cell viability [10, 14, 17]. The intrinsic buffer capacity of the artificial amino acids in the oligomer was enhanced by the integration of buffering histidines (His) with a pK_a around 6 which additionally boosted endosomal escape [2], like it had been observed also in context of other polycationic delivery systems before [18–20]. The combination of alternating Stp and His turned out to be an efficient pH responsive motif both ensuring NA binding at neutral pH and proton-sponge activity.

Another issue about artificial gene vehicles is preventing innate immune responses. Hereby polyethylene glycol (PEG) is a current state of the art, as it represents a generally well-tolerated hydrophilic polymer which can circumvent unspecific interactions like immunogenicity and toxicity by sterical hindrance [21]. This so-called "shielding agent" prevents opsonization and thereby prolongs circulation time in vivo [22]. However also intended interactions, such as the uptake and endosomolysis in target cells, are affected by the particle shielding. To circumvent this so-called "PEG-Dilemma," and especially to achieve tissue specificity, targeting peptides, antibodies, or proteins can be conjugated to the PEG.

This methodical chapter focuses on tumor specific targeting; so an approach of coupling a novel targeting peptide onto two-arm structures containing His as well as Stp is described. For tumor targeting, HGFR (Hepatocyte Growth Factor Receptor) also called c-Met, was chosen as a target receptor. c-Met is a proto-oncogene and is usually occurring in stem cells or progenitor cells [23].

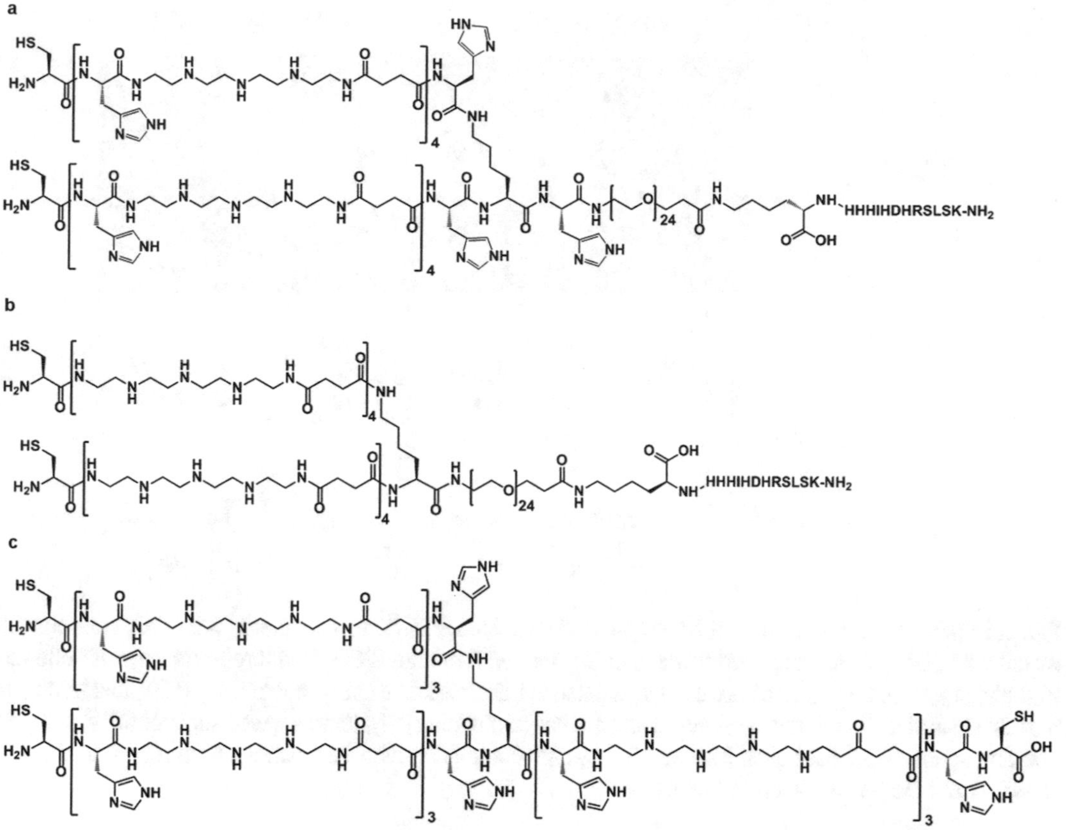

Fig. 2 Sequence defined oligomers for pDNA delivery. cMBP2 targeted, PEGylated structures (**a**) *442* with histidines and (**b**) *443* without histidines. (**c**) His and polycation rich co-oligomer *689*

Upregulated activation of c-Met's gene product Met can lead to tumorigenesis and metastasis. It is found in many kinds of solid tumors like brain, breast, pancreas and prostate as well as hepatocellular carcinoma [24, 25].

cMBP2 (c-met binding peptide 2), a phage display derived peptide (KSLSRHDHIHHH) [25] has been shown to mediate sequence-specific binding of model nanoparticles and pDNA polyplexes to HGFR expressing cells and remarkably increased gene transfer activity [26, 27].

Briefly, Kos et al. showed that the PEG shielded, His-rich, Stp oligomer *442* (Fig. 2a) performed equally well as untargeted 22 kDa lPEI in in vitro transfections, but with higher specificity and no observable toxicity [26]. At higher N/P (protonatable nitrogens of the oligomer–phosphates of used NA) ratio it even outperformed lPEI (unpublished data). Comparing the transfection results with the His-free conjugate *443* (Fig. 2b) demonstrated that His are crucial for the high gene transfer activity. Although the best performer *442* could also mediate ligand-dependent transgene

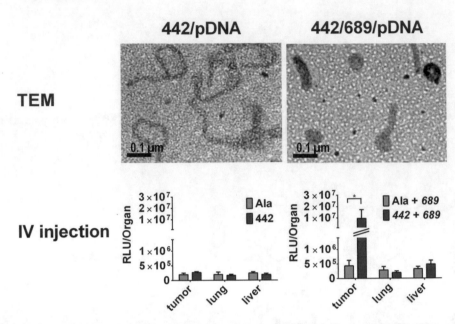

Fig. 3 Single- and dual-oligomer/pDNA polyplex formulations. PEGylated oligomers (*442* or Ala control) were mixed with pDNA alone (single formulation) or together with the non-PEGylated three-arm oligomer 689 (co-formulation). Resulting polyplexes were investigated in transmission electron microscopy (TEM) and transgene expression in vivo after intravenous (IV) injection. Dual-formulation polyplexes showed superior pDNA compaction and ligand-dependent gene transfer after systemic administration. Reproduced from ref. [26] with permission from the Royal Society of Chemistry

expression in the tumor after local injection, it was inactive after systemic administration in mice (Fig. 3).

As a consequence of the high PEG content, the plasmid DNA (pDNA) condensation in *442* polyplexes is poor, leading to rather loose worm-like structures and a hampered passive accumulation in the tumor. Therefore, the polycation–PEG ratio in the polyplexes was increased by mixing with an untargeted, non-PEGylated, His-rich Stp oligomer *689* (Fig. 2c). Due to previous work, a more rod- or toroid-like structure of the then formed polyplexes was expected, as the cation density compared to PEG was increased [15]. This co-formulation at the optimal ratio of 7:3 (*442–689*, normalized to nitrogen content) improved pDNA condensation into more compact round-shaped nanoparticles, as determined by transmission electron microscopy (Fig. 3).

In vitro stability size measurements validated a prolonged serum stability of the co-formulation polyplexes compared to the single *442* formulation. Consequently this combination at N/P 12 was applied again intravenously in tumor bearing mice. Here a ligand-dependent gene transfer in the tumor was found.

In sum, the different requirements for a successful targeted gene delivery in vivo were demonstrated. The combination of cMBP2 as a targeting ligand for solid tumors, pDNA binding Stp,

His improving the pH-responsiveness of oligomers as well as good pDNA compaction of the co-formulation polyplexes resulted in a promising nonviral gene delivery system.

In this methodical chapter the synthesis of the building block Fmoc-Stp(Boc₃)-OH as well as the oligomers *442*, *443*, and *689* is described.

2   Materials

Use solvents and reagents of high quality for all synthesis steps and experiments.

2.1 Building Block Synthesis

1. Laboratory glassware. 500 mL round-bottom flasks, 1 L round-bottom flasks, beakers, dropping funnels, separatory funnels, filter funnels, Büchner flask and funnel.

2. Reflux condenser.

3. Filter paper.

4. Vacuum pump.

5. Vacuum line.

6. Rotary evaporator.

7. Heating plate with magnetic stirrer.

8. Polystyrene box for ice bath.

9. Dewar for acetone–dry ice cooling bath.

10. Dry column vacuum chromatography (DCVC) apparatus (Büchner funnel with sintered glass disk, approximately 10 cm in diameter and 18 cm height, adapter with side-arm for vacuum connection, separatory funnel, fraction collection tubes).

11. Thin layer chromatography (TLC) chamber.

12. TLC spotting capillaries.

13. TLC plates, silica gel 60 F_{254} (Merck Millipore, Darmstadt, Germany).

14. UV lamp ($\lambda = 254$ nm).

2.1.1 Synthesis of bis-tfa-Tp(Boc₃)

1. Technical grade dichloromethane (DCM), distilled before use.

2. Analytical grade methanol (MeOH).

3. n-hexane, purissimum.

4. Tetraethylene pentamine pentahydrochloride (TEPA × 5 HCl).

5. Triethylamine (TEA).

6. Ethyl trifluoroacetate (TFAEt).

7. Di-tert-butyl dicarbonate (Boc anhydride).

8. Sodium hydrogen carbonate ($NaHCO_3$).

9. Sodium sulfate (Na_2SO_4) anhydrous.

*2.1.2 Synthesis
of Tp(Boc₃)*

1. Analytical grade absolute ethanol (EtOH).
2. Deionized water (dH$_2$O), in house purification.
3. bis-tfa-Tp(Boc$_3$).
4. Sodium hydroxide (NaOH).
5. Na$_2$SO$_4$ anhydrous.

*2.1.3 Synthesis
of Fmoc-Stp(Boc₃)-OH*

1. Technical grade acetone.
2. Analytical grade tetrahydrofuran (THF).
3. HPLC grade acetonitrile (ACN).
4. Dry ice.
5. Tp(Boc$_3$).
6. Succinic anhydride.
7. *N,N*-Diisopropylethylamine (DIPEA) (Iris Biotech, Marktredewitz, Germany).
8. Fmoc *N*-hydroxysuccinimide ester (Fmoc-OSu) (Iris Biotech, Marktredewitz, Germany).
9. Trisodium citrate dihydrate.
10. Na$_2$SO$_4$ anhydrous.
11. Celite S (Sigma-Aldrich, Munich, Germany).
12. Ninhydrin.

*2.1.4 Purification
of Fmoc-Stp(Boc₃)-OH
by DCVC*

1. Analytical grade n-heptane.
2. Ethyl acetate (EtOAc), distilled before use.
3. Analytical grade MeOH.
4. Analytical grade chloroform (CHCl$_3$).

2.1.5 Solutions

1. 5 % (w/v) NaHCO$_3$ solution: 50 g of NaHCO$_3$ in 1 L of dH$_2$O.
2. Trisodium citrate buffer: 0.1 M of trisodium citrate dihydrate, adjusted to pH 5.5.
3. TLC staining solution: 0.4 g of ninhydrin dissolved in 200 mL of 100:4.5:0.5 (v/v/v) n-butanol–dH$_2$O–acetic acid (CH$_3$COOH).

**2.2 Solid-Phase
Synthesis (SPS)**

Use solvents and reagents of high quality for all experiments (*see* **Note 1**). The SPS can be carried out manually on a laboratory vacuum manifold (Promega Corporation, Madison, WI, USA) or an overhead shaker using microreactors (*see* **Note 2**) with polyethylene filters (Multisyntech GmbH, Witten Germany) for vacuum filtration. As solid phase 2-chlorotrityl chloride resin (Iris Biotech, Marktredewitz, Germany) is used.

2.2.1 Amino Acids

1. Fmoc and Boc-protected α-amino acids (Iris Biotech, Marktredwitz, Germany).

2. Fmoc-Stp(Boc$_3$)-OH synthesis is described in Subheading 3.1.

3. Fmoc-N-amido-dPEG$_{24}$-OH (Quanta Biodesign, Powell, Ohio, USA).

2.2.2 Reagents and Solvents

1. DCM.

2. N,N-dimethylformamide (DMF).

3. DIPEA.

4. 1-hydroxybenzotriazole (HOBt).

5. Benzotriazol-1-yl-oxy tripyrrolidinophosphonium hexafluoro-phosphate (Pybop®) (Multisyntech GmbH, Witten, Germany).

6. Fmoc-deprotection solution: 20% (v/v) piperidine–DMF.

7. Capping solution: 80:15:5 (v/v/v) DCM–MeOH–DIPEA.

8. Kaiser's test solutions: 80% (w/v) phenol in EtOH; 5% (w/v) ninhydrin in EtOH; 20 μM KCN in pyridine (2 mL of 1 mM KCN (aq) in 98 mL of pyridine).

9. ivDde-deprotection solution: 4% (v/v) hydrazine monohydrate in DMF.

10. Cleavage cocktail: 95:2.5:2.5 (v/v/v) trifluoro acetic acid (TFA)–triisopropylsilane (TIS)–dH$_2$O.

11. Precipitating solution: 1:1 (v/v) methyl *tert*-butyl ether (MTBE)–n-hexane.

12. Sephadex G10 size exclusion chromatography (SEC) medium (GE Healthcare, Freiburg, Germany).

2.3 Polyplex Formation

1. pCMV Luc pDNA (Plasmidfactory, Bielefeld, Germany).

2.4 Biophysical Polyplex Characterization

1. Agarose powder.

2. GelRed (VWR, Darmstadt, Germany).

3. UV transilluminator.

4. Zetasizer Nano ZS with backscattering detection and folded capillary cells (Malvern Instruments, Worcestershire, UK).

2.5 Buffers

1. TBE Buffer: 89 mM TRIS, 89 mM boric acid, 2 mM ethylene-diaminetetraacetic acid disodium salt (EDTA-Na$_2$), pH 8.0.

2. HBG: 5% (w/v) glucose in 20 mM HEPES, pH 7.4.

3. Electrophoresis 6× loading buffer: 6 mL of glycerine, 1.2 mL of 0.5 M EDTA-Na$_2$ solution, pH 8.0, 2.8 mL of dH$_2$O, 20 mg of bromophenol blue.

4. Size exclusion running buffer: 70:30 (v/v) 10 mM HCl in dH$_2$O/ACN.

3 Methods

3.1 Building Block Synthesis

The artificial oligoamino acid Stp is based on TEPA which constitutes a structure analog of lPEI with precise length. The succinic acid at one terminal primary amine serves as molecular adapter to connect one oligoamine segment to the other during oligoaminoamide assembly. The remaining primary amine is protected with a base-labile Fmoc group to avoid random polymerization; the secondary amines are blocked by acid-labile Boc protecting groups. The particular structure and protecting groups were designed and selected for complete compatibility with Fmoc chemistry peptide synthesis and qualify for the use on solid phase. The synthesis of Stp is carried out in three steps (Fig. 4).

1. The primary amines of TEPA are transiently protected as trifluoroacetamides using TFAEt to allow site-specific Boc-protection of the secondary amines by Boc anhydride in a one-pot-reaction. The intermediate product bis-tfa-Tp(Boc$_3$) can be obtained in good yields as white crystals after recrystallization.

2. Alkaline hydrolysis of the trifluoroacetamide groups quantitatively results in the oily intermediate Tp(Boc$_3$).

3. The asymmetrical substitution of the primary amines with succinic acid and Fmoc by reaction with succinic anhydride and Fmoc-OSu gives the final building block Fmoc-Stp(Boc$_3$)-OH ready for subsequent solid-phase synthesis, which can be isolated by DCVC.

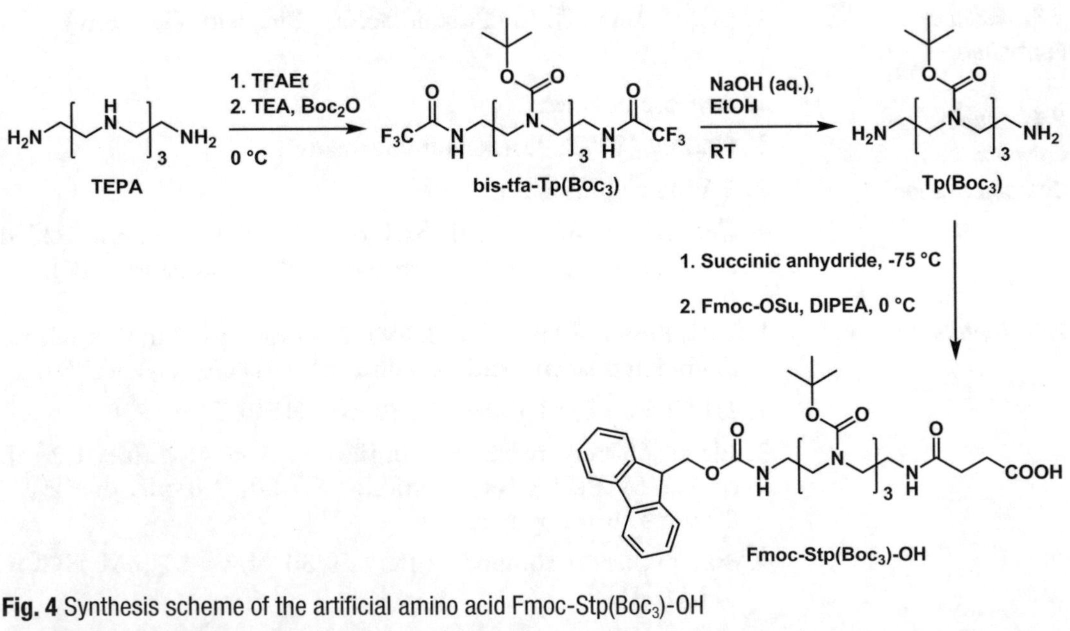

Fig. 4 Synthesis scheme of the artificial amino acid Fmoc-Stp(Boc$_3$)-OH

3.1.1 Synthesis
of bis-tfa-Tp(Boc₃)

1. Weigh 20 g of TEPA×5 HCl (53.8 mmol, 1 eq.) in a 500 mL round-bottom flask (*see* **Note 3**).

2. Put a magnetic stir bar into the flask.

3. Add 60 mL of DCM and 60 mL of MeOH.

4. Stir the mixture on a magnetic stirrer.

5. Slowly add 37.3 mL of TEA (269.1 mmol, 5 eq.) and keep stirring until a clear solution is formed (*see* **Note 3**).

6. Put an ice bath in a polystyrene box on the magnetic stirrer and cool the round-bottom flask to 0 °C.

7. Weigh 16.1 g of TFAEt (113.3 mmol, 2.1 eq.) into a beaker and dissolve it with 50 mL of DCM.

8. Put a dropping funnel on the round-bottom flask, close the stopcock and poor the TFAEt solution in the funnel.

9. Add the solution dropwise to the reaction mixture over 2 h.

10. After complete addition, the reaction mixture is allowed to warm up to room temperature (RT) and stirred for 2 h more.

11. Weigh 47.0 g of Boc anhydride (215.5 mmol, 4 eq.) into a beaker and dissolve it in 50 mL of DCM.

12. Slowly add 29.8 mL of TEA (215.3 mmol, 4 eq.) to the reaction mixture in the round-bottom flask under stirring.

13. Poor the Boc anhydride solution into the dropping funnel and add it to the reaction mixture dropwise over a period of 2 h. Continue stirring overnight.

14. Concentrate the reaction mixture to a volume of approximately 100 mL using a rotary evaporator.

15. Poor the reaction mixture into a separatory funnel and wash it three times with 50 mL of 5% $NaHCO_3$ solution and three times with dH_2O.

16. Collect the organic phase in a beaker and add Na_2SO_4 portion wise under slight shaking until the solution is dry (*see* **Note 4**).

17. Filter the solution directly into a 1 L round-bottom flask using a filter paper and filter funnel.

18. Evaporate the organic solvent using first the rotary evaporator and second a vacuum line.

19. Set up a reflux apparatus consisting of a magnetic stirrer, heated bath and reflux condenser.

20. Put a magnetic stir bar into the round-bottom flask and fit it in the reflux apparatus.

21. Add 20 mL of DCM and start heating under stirring.

22. Add DCM portion wise through the condenser under reflux until bis-tfa-Tp(Boc₃) is dissolved completely.

23. Slowly add n-hexane portion-wise through the condenser until considerable clouding occurs at the drop-in point.

24. Remove the heating bath and let the mixture cool down to RT, then put the mixture into the fridge overnight.

25. Isolate the crystals by filtration and wash them with n-hexane.

26. Dry the bis-tfa-Tp(Boc$_3$) in vacuo.

3.1.2 Synthesis of Tp(Boc₃)

1. Weigh 20 g of bis-tfa-Tp(Boc$_3$) (29.3 mmol, 1 eq.) in a 500 mL round-bottom flask.

2. Put a magnetic stir bar into the flask and add 175 mL of EtOH and 200 mL of 3 M NaOH solution (600 mmol, 20.5 eq.).

3. Stir the mixture using a magnetic stirrer overnight.

4. Remove the EtOH of the reaction mixture using a rotary evaporator.

5. Fill the mixture into a separatory funnel and extract the organic compound four times with 100 mL of DCM.

6. Combine the organic phases in a beaker and add Na$_2$SO$_4$ portion wise under slight shaking until the solution is dry (*see* **Note 4**).

7. Weigh an empty 1 L round-bottom flask and note the tare.

8. Filter the solution directly into the round-bottom flask using a filter paper and filter funnel.

9. Evaporate the organic solvent using first the rotary evaporator and second a vacuum line to obtain Tp(Boc$_3$) as a highly viscous compound.

3.1.3 Synthesis of Fmoc-Stp(Boc₃)-OH

1. Determine the mass of isolated Tp(Boc$_3$) by weighing the round-bottom-flask and subtracting the tare.

2. Calculate the required amounts of succinic anhydride, DIPEA and Fmoc-OSu according to the determined amount of Tp(Boc$_3$). Table 1 shows an exemplary calculation for the synthesis using 10 g of Tp(Boc$_3$).

3. Add 50 mL of THF and a magnetic stir bar into the round-bottom flask and dissolve Tp(Boc$_3$).

4. Fill acetone into a dewar and add dry ice in small portions from time to time. The optimal temperature has been reached when some dry ice stays solid in the bath after addition (*see* **Note 5**).

5. Install the round-bottom flask with dropping funnel in the acetone–dry ice cooling bath on a magnetic stirrer.

6. Weigh half of the calculated amount of required succinic anhydride into a beaker and dissolve it in 200 mL of THF.

7. Close the stopcock of the dropping funnel and poor the succinic anhydride solution in.

Table 1
Exemplary calculation of reagents for the synthesis of Fmoc-Stp(Boc₃)-OH

	Tp(Boc₃)	Succinic anhydride	DIPEA	Fmoc-Osu
eq.	1	1.25	3	1.5
MW	489.7	100.7	129.3	337.3
m [g]	10.0	2.6	7.9	10.3
n [mmol]	20.4	25.5	61.2	30.6
V [mL]	–	–	10.7	–

8. Add the solution slowly dropwise to the reaction mixture under stirring. Add some dry ice into the cooling bath from time to time.

9. After complete addition prepare the second half of succinic anhydride and proceed the same way as described in Subheading 3.1.3, **steps 6–8**.

10. After complete addition, the mixture is stirred in the cooling bath for 1 h and subsequently for another h without cooling bath.

11. Add the DIPEA slowly to the reaction mixture under stirring.

12. Weigh the calculated amount of Fmoc-OSu into a beaker and dissolve it in a mixture of 60 mL of ACN and 30 mL of THF.

13. Put an ice bath in a polystyrene box on the magnetic stirrer and cool the reaction mixture to 0 °C.

14. Poor the Fmoc-OSu solution into the dropping funnel and add it dropwise to the cooled reaction mixture.

15. Stir the reaction mixture.

16. The next day, concentrate the solution to approximately 50 mL using a rotary evaporator.

17. Add 100 mL of DCM and transfer the solution to a separatory funnel. Wash the organic phase five times with 100 mL of trisodium citrate buffer.

18. Collect the organic phase in a beaker and add Na_2SO_4 portion wise under slight shaking until the solution is dry (*see* **Note 4**).

19. Filter the solution directly into a 1 L round-bottom flask using a filter paper and filter funnel.

20. Add 32 g of Celite into the flask and evaporate the organic solvent using first the rotary evaporator and second a vacuum line.

21. Purify Fmoc-Stp(Boc₃)-OH by DCVC.

*3.1.4 Purification
of Fmoc-Stp(Boc₃)-OH
by DCVC*

1. Set up a DCVC apparatus (Fig. 5).

2. Pack the column by stepwise addition of silica gel into the Büchner funnel. After each portion being added, apply vacuum to produce a compact silica gel bed of finally approximately 10 cm height.

3. Put a filter paper on top of the silica gel bed.

4. Precondition the column by pouring n-heptane in portions of 100 mL on the filter paper and applying vacuum after each addition. Continue until a straight solvent front runs through the whole column and reaches the collection funnel of the apparatus.

5. Disintegrate the crude Fmoc-Stp(Boc₃)-OH into a fine powder using mortar and pestle.

6. Distribute the powder evenly on the filter paper of the column and put a second filter paper on top.

7. Purify the crude product by adding 100 mL fractions of solvent mixture (*see* **Notes 6** and **7**), applying vacuum and collecting the individual eluates. Remove Fmoc by-products by using a solvent gradient of n-heptane–EtOAc from 50:50 to 5:95 (*see* **Note 6**), and elute the product Fmoc-Stp(Boc₃)-OH with a gradient of EtOAc–MeOH from 100:0 to 80:20 (*see* **Note 7**).

8. Analyze samples of each fraction by TLC using a solvent mixture of 7:3 CHCl₃–MeOH and investigate fluorescence quenching under a UV lamp.

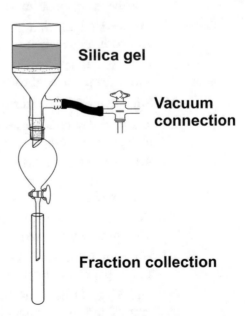

Fig. 5 Schematic illustration of a dry column vacuum chromatography (DCVC) apparatus

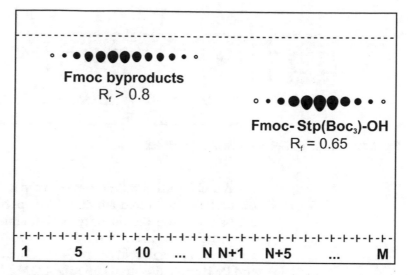

Fig. 6 Exemplary TLC of the DCVC purification. *Numbers* and *letters* at the bottom indicate the individual fractions. The fluorescence quenching spots with R_f values > 0.8 are caused by Fmoc by-products. The product Fmoc-Stp(Boc$_3$)-OH has an R_f of 0.65

9. Maintain the composition of fraction 10 (5:95 n-heptane–EtOAc) until no Fmoc by-products ($R_f > 0.8$) can be observed any longer (Fraction N, Fig. 6).

10. Maintain the composition of fraction N + 5 (80:20 EtOAc–MeOH) until no more product Fmoc-Stp(Boc$_3$)-OH ($R_f = 0.65$) can be observed (Fraction M, Fig. 6) (*see* **Note 8**).

11. Pool all fractions containing the Fmoc-Stp(Boc$_3$)-OH and no by-products in a tared round-bottom flask and evaporate the organic solvent using first the rotary evaporator and second a vacuum line to obtain the product as a foamy solid.

12. Analyze the product Fmoc-Stp(Boc$_3$)-OH by ^{1}H-NMR (*see* **Note 9**) and ESI-MS (*see* **Note 10**).

3.2 Solid-Phase Synthesis (SPS)

SPS offers a way to synthesize precisely defined oligomer structures. Depending on the desired topology a targeting domain can be inserted into these structures. Targeted oligomers *442* and *443* as well as the untargeted oligomer *689* are generated by standard Fmoc-SPS always following a repetitive synthesis cycle (Fig. 7):

1. Coupling (60 min).

2. Washing (3× DMF, 3× DCM).

3. Kaiser's test.

4. Deprotection (10 min with 20% (v/v) piperidine/DMF for four times).

5. Washing (3× DMF, 3× DCM).

6. Kaiser's test.

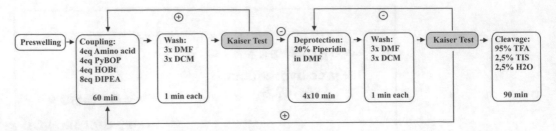

Fig. 7 Standard procedure of a solid phase synthesis cycle

A 2-chlorotrityl chloride resin is used as solid support. Coupling of the Fmoc protected amino acids is performed with a fourfold excess (based on the quantity of free amines) whilst an identical excess of HOBt and PyBOP is used for preactivation. DIPEA is added with an eightfold excess (also related to free amines). HOBt and PyBOP are dissolved in 5 mL of DMF/g of resin and the (artificial) amino acids are dissolved in 5 mL of DCM/g of resin. The corresponding amount of DIPEA is added, the solutions are mixed for preactivation and added to the resin. Routinely coupling time is chosen as 1 h (*see* **Note 11**).

After each coupling step (as well as after each step of deprotection), three washes with DMF as well as with DCM (10 mL/g of resin) are carried out.

20% (v/v) piperidine/DMF is applied for Fmoc-removal four times per 10 min by default (10 mL/g resin).

Coupling, as well as deprotection are verified by testing for free amines qualitatively using Kaiser's test [28]. If the result is unsatisfying the previous coupling or deprotection step is repeated.

3.2.1   Resin Loading

1. Place 0.5 g of 2-chlorotrityl chloride resin in a 10 mL syringe reactor.

2. Swell the resin for approximately 20 min in 5 mL of dry DCM in the closed reactor while shaking (*see* **Note 12**).

3. Discard the DCM.

4. Dissolve 0.25 mmol of the intended Fmoc-amino acid, either 143.7 mg Fmoc-Lys(ivDde)-OH in case of *442* and *443*, or 146.3 mg Fmoc-Cys(Trt)-OH in case of 689 in 5 mL of dry DCM and 130.8 µL of DIPEA (0.75 mmol).

5. Add the solution to the resin and incubate in the closed reactor for 60 min under shaking.

6. Discard the solution and add 5 mL of the capping solution for at least 30 min to cap remaining active chloride groups on the resin.

7. Discard the solution and wash three times with DMF as well as with DCM (5 mL each).

8. Dry the resin under high vacuum and weight triplicate samples (between 5 and 10 mg each) into polypropylene microcentrifuge tubes subsequently.

9. Add 1 mL of Fmoc-deprotection solution to the samples and incubate for 90 min at RT under gentle shaking.

10. Take 25 μL of the supernatant and dilute it 1:40 by adding 975 μL of DMF.

11. Vortex and calculate resin loading based on the absorbance at λ = 301 nm against an equally prepared blank of deprotection solution (*see* **Notes 13** and **14**). While determining the resin loading, add 5 mL of Fmoc-deprotection solution to the resin four times for 10 min.

12. Wash the resin three times with both DMF and DCM 10 mL/g of resin, then perform a Kaiser's test.

13. When receiving a positive result, dry the resin at high vacuum and store under exclusion of air and moisture.

3.2.2 Kaiser's Test

1. Transfer a few beads of resin into a polypropylene microcentrifuge tube, and add one drop of each Kaiser's test solution.

2. Vortex and spin down quickly.

3. Incubate at 100 °C for 4 min, although a positive reaction should occur within the first 2 min, usually. Free amines are indicated by blue color.

3.2.3 Synthesis of 442 and 443

1. Here the synthesis of His rich *442* oligomer will be described. *443* is synthesized analogously, but leaving out the His coupling steps (*see* **Note 15**). Considering resin loading and desired synthesis scale size, take the required amount of preloaded Lys(ivDde)-OH resin and transfer into the corresponding reactor (*see* **Note 2**).

2. Swell the resin for 30 min with 10 mL/g of DCM.

3. Synthesize the cMBP2 ligand (KSLSRHDHIHHH) by sequential coupling and deprotection of 3 Fmoc-L-His(Trt)-OH amino acids. Continue with Fmoc-L-Ile-OH, Fmoc-L-His(Trt)-OH, Fmoc-L-Asp(tBu)-OH, Fmoc-L-His(Trt)-OH, Fmoc-L-Arg(Pbf)-OH, Fmoc-L-Ser(tBu)-OH, Fmoc-L-Leu-OH, Fmoc-L-Ser(tBu)-OH and end with a Fmoc-Lys(Boc)-OH.

4. To end this arm, use Boc anhydride in an 8 fold excess dissolved in DCM with 16-fold excess of DIPEA (*see* **Note 16**).

5. For ivDde deprotection, freshly prepare a 4% (v/v) hydrazine hydroxide solution in DMF and apply 5 mL/g of resin for 10 min while shaking, and exchange the solution every 10 min.

6. After the first and every 10 cycles of deprotection, take the solution and measure the absorbance against a blank of unused

hydrazine deprotection solution at $\lambda = 290$ nm. Deprotection is finished when absorbance is below 0.02 for at least 10 cycles.

7. Continue with the synthesis at the freed amine by coupling Fmoc-dPEG$_{24}$-OH using the standard coupling conditions (*see* Subheading 3.2 and Fig. 7).

8. Couple the amino acid of the backbone Fmoc-L-His(Trt)-OH at the free amine of the dPEG$_{24}$.

9. After deprotection and Kaiser's test (*see* Subheading 3.2.2), attach a branching Fmoc-L-Lys-(Fmoc)-OH. From this step on, the number of resin attached amines is doubled (*see* **Note 17**).

10. Under the standard coupling and deprotection conditions (*see* Subheading 3.2 and Fig. 7), alternatingly attach Fmoc-L-His(Trt)-OH and Fmoc-Stp(Boc$_3$)-OH to the growing oligomer chain. It results in the alternating sequence containing 5 His and 4 Stp (*see* Fig. 2). Then couple Boc-L-Cys(Trt)-OH without subsequent Fmoc deprotection (*see* **Note 18**).

11. Dry *442* on high vacuum for approximately 30 min.

12. Prepare a cleavage cocktail for cleaving the resin from the acid labile linker (*see* Subheading 2.2.2).

13. Apply 10 mL/g of cleavage solution to resin for 90 min at RT while shaking and collect it afterwards.

14. Wash the resin three times with 10 mL TFA per g resin (*see* **Note 19**).

15. Allow the combined solutions to evaporate under nitrogen (N$_2$) stream to 1 mL and precipitate in a dropwise manner into 50 mL of ice-cold precipitating solution.

16. Centrifuge for 20 min ($4000 \times g$, 4 °C), discard the supernatant and dry the precipitate under nitrogen (N$_2$) stream.

17. Dissolve the obtained product in size exclusion running buffer and purify it by SEC.

18. Take the product containing fractions, and pool them into a tared 15 mL tube, then snap-freeze and lyophilize.

19. Determine the product yield by balancing and analyze the oligomer by ^{1}H-NMR and RP-HPLC (*see* **Notes 20** and **21**).

20. Store the obtained yellow HCl salt of the oligomer (*see* **Note 22**) at −20 °C, preferably sealed (*see* **Notes 23** and **24**).

3.2.4 Synthesis of 689

1. Considering resin loading and desired synthesis scale size, take the required amount of preloaded and deprotected L-Cys(Trt) resin and transfer into the corresponding reactor (*see* **Note 2**).

2. Swell the resin for 30 min with 10 mL/g of DCM.

3. Couple a Fmoc-L-His(Trt)-OH onto the resin.

4. Couple the artificial building block Fmoc-Stp(Boc$_3$)-OH three times altering with three times Fmoc-L-His(Trt)-OH.

5. Deprotect the resin after each coupling step using the standard deprotection conditions (*see* Subheading 3.2 and Fig. 7).

6. After deprotection, couple Fmoc-L-Lys(Fmoc)-OH as a branching point resulting in doubled amount of free amines after successful deprotection (*see* **Note 17**).

7. Continue the synthesis by coupling another Fmoc-L-His(Trt) and Fmoc-Stp(Boc$_3$)-OH.

8. After repeating the coupling of these 2 amino acids twice, attach 1 final Fmoc-L-His(Trt) to the sequence on the resin and end synthesis by coupling the Boc-L-Cys(Trt).

9. After the synthesis, dry the resin on high vacuum for cleavage. In the meanwhile, prepare the cleavage solution as described before (*see* Subheading 2.2.2).

10. Apply 10 mL/g of cleavage solution to resin for 90 min while shaking (*see* **Note 19**).

11. Collect the cleavage solution and wash the resin three times with 10 mL/g of resin with pure TFA.

12. After evaporating the solvent to approximately 1 mL, precipitate the remaining solution in 50 mL of ice-cold precipitating solution.

13. Centrifuge for 20 min ($4000 \times g$, 4 °C), discard the supernatant and dry the precipitate under N$_2$ stream.

14. Dissolve the obtained product in SEC running buffer and purify it by SEC.

15. Pool the product containing fractions in a tared 15 mL tube, snap-freeze and lyophilize overnight.

16. Determine the product yield by balancing and analyze the oligomer by ^{1}H-NMR and RP-HPLC (*see* **Notes 25** and **21**).

17. Store the white or yellow HCl salt of the oligomer (*see* **Note 22**), preferably sealed (*see* **Notes 23** and **24**) at −20 °C.

3.3 Polyplex Formation

Successful formulation of polyplexes is occurring if positively charged oligomers complex negatively charged nucleic acid. Stability of these polyplexes is highly depending on the ratio between polymer and nucleic acid. In our case basic oligomers with protonatable nitrogens are used, so the N/P is very frequently used to describe the oligomer to NA proportions within the formulated polyplex.

To determine the optimal N/P guaranteeing a stable polyplex, several ratios need to be evaluated (*see* **Note 26**).

The most favored N/P for in vivo experiments is determined as 12. This means 70 % of N/P 12 are covered by *442* and 30 % by *689* in the mixture. For calculations this implies an amount of *442* calculated as N/P 8.4 and *689* matching N/P 3.6 (*see* **Note 27**). Polyplex formation is described for in vitro transfections. For other experiments preparation is done the same way with adjusted amounts of oligomer and pDNA.

1. Dilute 0.2 µg of pDNA in 10 µL of HBG for each desired N/P.

2. Dilute the calculated amount of oligomer in 10 µL of HBG for each desired N/P.

3. Add the oligomer solution to the pDNA solution and mix by vigorous pipetting up and down ten times.

4. Incubate the solution for 40 min at RT to complete polyplex formation by disulfide bonding. Experiments should be carried out immediately after incubation time is completed.

3.4 Biophysical Polyplex Characterization

Two methods are very common to determine and characterize polyplexes.

On the one hand, polyplex formulations can be screened by agarose gel retardation assay. This method takes advantage of the fact that negatively charged (free) pDNA migrates in the electrical field. As soon as all NA is complexed by oligomer, electrophoretic mobility is inhibited due to loss of negative charge and increased size. So this assay's output is the general ability of the oligomer to bind pDNA (compared to others) as well as the minimal required fraction of oligomer for total binding (according to N/P).

On the other hand, dynamic light scattering (DLS) is a very common way to determine particle size and ζ-potential, this gives further information about polyplex consistency.

3.4.1 Gel Migration Assay for pDNA Polyplexes

1. Fix a 15 cm × 15 cm UV-transparent gel tray in a gel casting unit.

2. For pDNA polyplexes, weigh 1.8 g of agarose powder (1 % gel, w/v) into a beaker and add 180 mL of TBE buffer.

3. Dissolve agarose by heating up to boiling until a clear solution is obtained (*see* **Note 28**).

4. Allow the solution to cool down to 50 °C, then add 18 µL of 10,000× concentrate GelRed for the subsequent NA staining.

5. Pour the Gel into the gel casting unit. Eliminate air bubbles with a pipette tip before a well comb is fixed and the gel is solidified (usually within at least 30 min).

6. Prepare polyplexes containing 0.2 µg of pDNA at different N/Ps as described in Subheading 3.3 (*see* **Note 26**).

7. After completed polyplex incubation for 40 min, add 4 µL of 6× loading buffer.

8. Remove the well comb of the set gel to expose sample pockets, and transfer the gel into the electrophoresis unit.

9. Fill the chamber with TBE buffer until the gel is totally covered and all sample pockets are filled.

10. Load the samples into the sample pockets and apply a voltage of 120 V for 80 min.

11. Observe the gel under UV light exposure (*see* **Note 29**).

3.4.2 Size Measurement via DLS and Measurement of ζ-Potential

1. Prepare oligomer solution of the desired N/P in 400 µL of HBG.

2. Prepare a solution by adding 8 µg of pDNA to 400 µL of HBG.

3. Prepare polyplexes as described in Subheading 3.3 (*see* **Note 30**).

4. After 40 min of incubation, transfer the polyplex solution into a folded capillary cell.

5. For the size measurements, set the method of the zetasizer to three measurements with 15 subruns of 10 s at 25 °C.

6. For the determination of the ζ-potential, measure each sample three times with 10–30 subruns of 10 s at 25 °C (*see* **Note 31**).

4   Notes

1. Especially care is required with DMF as it tends to hydrolyze to formic acid and dimethylamine when exposed for a longer time to air and moisture. This can reduce coupling efficiency during synthesis and cause false positive results in Kaiser tests. Therefore, always use peptide grade quality DMF and store it with caution.

2. Syringe micro reactors are available in different sizes (2–100 mL) and have to be chosen according to the resin amount. The amount of resin depends on the determined resin loading and of the scale size (scale size[mmol]/L[mmol/g] = resin amount[g]). Approximately 10 µmol of resin correlate with approximately 20 mg of yield in case of *442* and *443* as well as *689*.

3. Technical grade free base TEPA with a purity of $\geq 80\%$ can also be used for the synthesis. In this case the reagent amounts have to be adjusted to the lower molecular weight (MW). Moreover, the initial addition of 5 eq. of TEA (*see* Subheading 3.1.1, **step 5**) can be skipped, since this step is only required for the transformation of TEPA×5 HCl into the free base form.

4. As soon as portions of Na_2SO_4 float freely in the solvent without clotting after addition and shaking, the drying can be terminated.

5. Be aware that during the first additions of dry ice a strong gas development can cause bubbling and splashing of the cooling bath. For this reason, the portions should be added carefully.

Table 2
Solvent composition of the first part of the purification

Fraction	1	2	3	4	5	6	7	8	9	10-N
n-heptane [mL]	50	45	40	35	30	25	20	15	10	5
EtOAc [mL]	50	55	60	65	70	75	80	85	90	95

Table 3
Solvent composition of the second part of the purification

Fraction	N+1	N+2	N+3	N+4	N+5	...	M
EtOAc [mL]	100	95	90	85	80	80	80
MeOH [mL]	0	5	10	15	20	20	20

6. During the first part of the purification (Fractions 1 to N, removal of Fmoc by-products) the solvent mixtures are composed of n-heptane and EtOAc according to the gradient protocol described in Table 2.

7. During the second part of the purification (Fractions N+1 to M, elution of Fmoc-Stp(Boc$_3$)-OH) the solvent composition is switched to a EtOAc/MeOH gradient according to Table 3.

8. Some by-products lacking Fmoc can elute with lower R_f value than Fmoc-Stp(Boc$_3$)-OH. Ninhydrin staining is required to detect the spots without fluorescence quenching on the TLC plate and to ensure purity of the collected product fractions.

9. ^{1}H-NMR (500 MHz, CDCl$_3$): $\delta = 7.77$ (d, $J=7.6$ Hz, 2H), 7.60 (d, $J=8.2$ Hz, 2H), 7.41 (t, $J=7.5$ Hz, 2H), 7.32 (t, $J=7.8$ Hz, 2H), 4.30–4.52 (m, 2H), 4.21 (t, $J=7.0$ Hz, 1H), 3.63–3.06 (m, 16H), 2.80–2.39 (m, 4H), 1.47 (m, 27H).

10. The chemical formula of Fmoc-Stp(Boc$_3$)-OH is C$_{42}$H$_{61}$N$_5$O$_{11}$, exact mass 811.4368, MW 811.9740.

11. In our case a Heidolph Reax 2 overhead shaker is used, but any stirring mechanism guaranteeing steady mixing of the solution can be accepted.

12. Dry DCM is required as otherwise H$_2$O can react with the resin's linker and become reactive positions in further couplings. Therefore, always store the DCM over calcium chloride (CaCl$_2$) and keep it away from moisture.

13. Calculate resin load by the following formula:

$$\text{Loading}\left[\frac{\text{mmol}}{\text{g}}\right] = \frac{1000 v A_{301}}{D v 7800 v m [\text{mg}]}$$

with D as dilution factor (0.025) and 7800 as molar extinction coefficient

[$Lvmol^{-1}vcm^{-1}$] of Fmoc. Calculate the arithmetic mean of the triplicate values as final resin loading.

14. The determined loading should be approx. 0.3 mmol/g of resin.

15. *442*: K-$_\alpha$[cMBP2]-$_\varepsilon$[PEG$_{24}$-H-K$_{\alpha,\varepsilon}$[H-(Stp-H) $_4$-C]$_2$]
    443: K-$_\alpha$[cMBP2]-$_\varepsilon$[PEG$_{24}$-K$_{\alpha,\varepsilon}$[(Stp) $_4$-C]$_2$]
    689: C-H-(Stp-H)$_3$- K$_{\alpha,\varepsilon}$[H-(Stp-H) $_3$-C]$_2$]

16. Successful bocylation should also be proven by a negative Kaiser's test, otherwise further coupling will abrogate ligand specificity.

    At this point a "mini cleavage" is suggested for mass spectrometry as well as a HPLC run. Therefore, 15–20 mg of the vacuum-dried resin is incubated with 1 mL of cleavage solution and proceeded as described in Subheading 3.2.3, **steps 13–16**. The retrieved product is dissolved in 0.1% formic acid in H$_2$O and analyzed by mass spectrometry (MW: 1631 Da) and RP-HPLC.

17. After a branching lysine, the molar amounts of coupling reagents (amino acid, PyBOP, HOBt, and DIPEA) have to be doubled since the number of resin attached amines is doubled.

18. By using the bocylated L-Cys(Trt) no further deprotection is required as the acid labile boc group will be removed during TFA cleavage (*see* Subheading 3.2.3, **step 13** and Subheading 3.2.4, **step 10**).

19. TFA is a very aggressive acid, so wear protective clothes and protective goggles.

20. ^{1}H-NMR spectrum of *442* in D$_2$O. δ (ppm)=1.0–2.0 (comp, 40 H, βγH arginine, βγδH isoleucine, βγδH leucine, βγδH lysine), 2.4–2.6 (comp, 34 H, -CO-CH$_2$-CH$_2$-CO- succinic acid, -CO-CH$_2$-dPEG$_{24}$), 2.8–3.5 (comp, 176 H, -CH$_2$- tepa, δH arginine, βH aspartate, βH cysteine, βH His, εH lysine, βH serine), 3.67 (s, 98 H, -CH$_2$-O- dPEG$_{24}$, -CH$_2$-N- dPEG$_{24}$), 4.0–4.6 (comp, 27 H, αH amino acids), 4.79 (s, HDO), 7.1–7.3 (m, 16 H, aromatic H His), 8.48–8.58 (m, 16 H, aromatic H His).

    ^{1H}-NMR spectrum of *443* in D$_{2O}$. δ (ppm) = 1.0–2.0 (comp, 40 H, βγH arginine, βγδH isoleucine, βγδH leucine, βγδH lysine), 2.4–2.6 (comp, 34 H, -CO-CH$_2$-CH$_2$-CO- succinic acid, -CO-CH$_2$- dPEG$_{24}$), 2.8–3.6 (comp, 156 H, -CH$_2$- tepa, δH arginine, βH aspartate, βH cysteine, βH His, εH lysine, βH serine), 3.66 (s, 98 H, -CH$_2$-O- dPEG$_{24}$, -CH$_2$-N- dPEG$_{24}$), 3.9–4.6 (comp, 16 H, αH amino acids), 4.80(s, HDO), 7.24–7.25 (m, 5 H, aromatic H His), 8.61 (s, 5 H, aromatic H His). comp indicates a group of overlaid protons.

21. For the analysis by RP-HPLC the use of a C18 column and a water/acetonitrile gradient containing 0.1% (v/v) TFA are recommended. The compounds can be detected photometrically at $\lambda = 214$ nm.

22. After SEC the quantitative HCl salt of the multiple protonatable amines of the oligomers is obtained. This has to be considered in the calculation of the MW. MW(*442*) = 8412.25 g/mol; MW(*443*) = 6506.47 g/mol; MW(*689*) = 6037.97 g/mol.

23. The generated salts tend to be hygroscopic, and therefore, seal the containers well and preserve them from air and moisture to prevent it from oxidation.

24. Stock solutions should be prepared in high concentrations in H_2O and frozen in aliquots. This hampers oxidation of the stock solution as it can be kept frozen.

25. ¹H-NMR spectrum of *689* in D_2O. δ (ppm) = 1.1–1.4 (comp, 6H, βγδH lysine), 2.3–2.7 (comp, 36 H, -CO-CH_2-CH_2-CO-succinic acid), 2.9–3.8 (comp, 176 H, -CH_2- tepa, βH cysteine, βH His, εH lysine), 4.1–4.7 (comp, 16 H, αH cysteine, lysine, His), 4.79 (s, HDO), 7.2–7.4 (m, 12 H, aromatic H His), 8.5–8.7 (m, 12 H, aromatic H His). comp indicates a group of overlaid protons.

26. By standard N/P 3, 6, 12, and 20 are tested.

27. n(phosphate) = m(pDNA)/av. MW of nucleotides

$$n(\text{nitrogen}) = n(\text{phosphate}) \times \text{desired} \, N / P$$

$$v(\text{Sample}) = \frac{n(\text{nitrogen})}{c(\text{polymer}) \times \text{number of protonatable amines}}$$

Av. MW of nucleotides is 327 g/mol. Number of protonatable amines are calculated by counting all available secondary (Stp) amines as well as N-terminal primary amines. Neither His amines nor amines within the targeting peptide are considered in the calculations. The unit of c(oligomer) is mol/L.

28. Boiling the agarose gel in a microwave reduces risk of superheating, but once in a while shake in between.

29. Always wear gloves and lab coat and never look directly into the UV light as it can cause serious eye damage. Usually, total binding of pDNA is already achieved at low N/P 3 in case of the described oligomers *442*, *443*, and *689*.

30. Since N/P 12 is used for in vivo experiments, size determination at this N/P is considered important.

31. Due to positive charge in the targeting peptide, *442* and *443* containing polyplexes exhibit a ζ-potential of 15 mV +/– 2 and a size of approximately 200 nm.

Acknowledgements

This work was supported by the German Research Foundation (DFG) Excellence Cluster "Nanosystems Initiative Munich" and DFG Collaborative Research Center SFB824. We thank Wolfgang Rödl and Miriam Höhn for technical support, and Olga Brück for skillful assistance.

References

1. Schaffert D, Wagner E (2008) Gene therapy progress and prospects: synthetic polymer-based systems. Gene Ther 15(16):1131–1138

2. Lächelt U, Kos P, Mickler FM et al (2014) Fine-tuning of proton sponges by precise diaminoethanes and histidines in pDNA polyplexes. Nanomed NBM 1:35–44. doi:10.1016/j.nano.2013.07.008

3. Lächelt U, Wagner E (2015) Nucleic acid therapeutics using polyplexes: a journey of 50 years (and beyond). Chem Rev. 115(19):11043–11078. doi:10.1021/cr5006793

4. Ziebarth JD, Wang Y (2010) Understanding the protonation behavior of linear polyethylenimine in solutions through Monte Carlo simulations. Biomacromolecules 11(1):29–38. doi:10.1021/bm900842d

5. Boussif O, Lezoualc'h F, Zanta MA et al (1995) A versatile vector for gene and oligonucleotide transfer into cells in culture and in vivo: polyethylenimine. Proc Natl Acad Sci U S A 92(16):7297–7301

6. Behr JP (1997) The proton sponge: a trick to enter cells the viruses did not exploit. Chimia 51(1-2):34–36

7. Fischer D, Li Y, Ahlemeyer B et al (2003) In vitro cytotoxicity testing of polycations: influence of polymer structure on cell viability and hemolysis. Biomaterials 24(7):1121–1131

8. Breunig M, Lungwitz U et al (2007) Breaking up the correlation between efficacy and toxicity for nonviral gene delivery. Proc Natl Acad Sci U S A 104(36):14454–14459. doi:10.1073/pnas.0703882104

9. Chollet P, Favrot MC et al (2002) Side-effects of a systemic injection of linear polyethylenimine-DNA complexes. J Gene Med 4(1):84–91

10. Schaffert D, Badgujar N, Wagner E (2011) Novel Fmoc-polyamino acids for solid-phase synthesis of defined polyamidoamines. Org Lett 13(7):1586–1589. doi:10.1021/ol200381z

11. Schaffert D, Troiber C, Salcher EE et al (2011) Solid-phase synthesis of sequence-defined T-, i-, and U-shape polymers for pDNA and siRNA delivery. Angew Chem Int Ed Engl 50(38):8986–8989. doi:10.1002/anie.201102165

12. Schaffert D, Troiber C, Wagner E (2012) New sequence-defined polyaminoamides with tailored endosomolytic properties for plasmid DNA delivery. Bioconjug Chem 23(6):1157–1165. doi:10.1021/bc200614x

13. Scholz C, Kos P, Wagner E (2014) Comb-like oligoaminoethane carriers: change in topology improves pDNA delivery. Bioconjug Chem 25(2):251–261. doi:10.1021/bc400392y

14. Salcher EE, Kos P, Fröhlich T et al (2012) Sequence-defined four-arm oligo(ethanamino) amides for pDNA and siRNA delivery: Impact of building blocks on efficacy. J Control Release 164(3):380–386. doi:10.1016/j.jconrel.2012.06.023

15. Martin I, Dohmen C, Mas-Moruno C et al (2012) Solid-phase-assisted synthesis of targeting peptide-PEG-oligo(ethane amino)amides for receptor-mediated gene delivery. Org Biomol Chem 10(16):3258–3268. doi:10.1039/c2ob06907e

16. Scholz C, Kos P, Leclercq L et al (2014) Correlation of length of linear oligo(ethanamino) amides with gene transfer and cytotoxicity. ChemMedChem 9(9):2104–2110. doi:10.1002/cmdc.201300483

17. Klein PM, Müller K, Gutmann C et al (2015) Twin disulfides as opportunity for improving stability and transfection efficiency of oligoaminoethane polyplexes. J Control Release 205:109–119. doi:10.1016/j.jconrel.2014.12.035

18. Leng QX, Mixson AJ (2005) Modified branched peptides with a histidine-rich tail enhance in vitro gene transfection. Nucleic Acids Res 33(4):e40. doi:10.1039/nar/gni040

19. Midoux P, Monsigny M (1999) Efficient gene transfer by histidylated polylysine/pDNA complexes. Bioconjug Chem 10(3):406–411. doi:10.1021/bc9801070

20. Hashemi M, Parhiz BH et al (2011) Modified polyethyleneimine with histidine-lysine short

peptides as gene carrier. Cancer Gene Ther 18(1):12–19. doi:10.1038/cgt.2010.57

21. Knop K, Hoogenboom R et al (2010) Poly(ethylene glycol) in drug delivery: pros and cons as well as potential alternatives. Angew Chem Int Ed Engl 49(36):6288–6308. doi:10.1002/anie.200902672

22. Hatakeyama H, Akita H, Harashima H (2013) The polyethyleneglycol dilemma: advantage and disadvantage of PEGylation of liposomes for systemic genes and nucleic acids delivery to tumors. Biol Pharm Bull 36(6):892–899

23. Boccaccio C, Comoglio PM (2006) Invasive growth: a MET-driven genetic programme for cancer and stem cells. Nat Rev Cancer 6(8):637–645. doi:10.1038/nrc1912

24. Zhao P, Grabinski T, Gao C et al (2007) Identification of a met-binding peptide from a phage display library. Clin Cancer Res 13(20):6049–6055. doi:10.1158/1078-0432.CCR-07-0035

25. Kim EM, Park EH, Cheong SJ et al (2009) In vivo imaging of mesenchymal-epithelial transition factor (c-Met) expression using an optical imaging system. Bioconjug Chem 20(7):1299–1306. doi:10.1021/bc8005539

26. Kos P, Lächelt U, Herrmann A et al (2015) Histidine-rich stabilized polyplexes for cMet-directed tumor-targeted gene transfer. Nanoscale 7(12):5350–5362. doi:10.1039/c4nr06556e

27. Broda E, Mickler FM, Lächelt U et al (2015) Assessing potential peptide targeting ligands by quantification of cellular adhesion of model nanoparticles under flow conditions. J Control Release 213:79–85. doi:10.1016/j.jconrel.2015.06.030

28. Kaiser E, Colescott RL et al (1970) Color test for detection of free terminal amino groups in the solid-phase synthesis of peptides. Anal Biochem 34(2):595–598

Chapter 16

Gene Delivery Method Using Photo-Responsive Poly(β-Amino Ester) as Vectors

Nan Zheng, Yang Liu, and Jianjun Cheng

Abstract

Nonviral vectors show great potential in delivering nucleic acids (NA) into many mammalian cells to achieve efficient gene transfection. Among these, cationic polymer is one of the most widely used nonviral gene delivery vectors, forming the polymer/NA complexes for the intracellular transportation and release of the genetic materials into the target mammalian cells. Here we describe the poly(β-amino ester) (PBAE) with the photo-responsive domain built in the polymers, as a UV-light-responsive nonviral gene delivery vector to deliver and release plasmid DNA (pDNA) into HeLa cells and achieve enhanced transfection efficiency.

Key words Nonviral gene delivery, Poly (β-amino ester)s, Photo-responsive, Transfection efficiency

1 Introduction

Gene therapy has emerged as a promising approach in treating various genetic diseases [1]. Compared with viral vectors, nonviral vectors have received growing attention and have been developed as safer alternatives to the viral vectors due to their limited immunogenicity and oncogenicity effect [2, 3]. Cationic polymer is one of the major class of nonviral vectors, which is capable of condensing negatively charged nucleic acids (NA) to form stable complexes (polyplexes) for intracellular delivery [4–6]. Among all cationic polymers being developed and studied, poly(β-amino ester) (PBAE) has attracted particular interest because of its ease of synthesis and high efficiency of gene delivery capability [7–9].

PBAE typically degrades through the hydrolysis of the backbone ester linkages. To enable controlled degradation of PBAE, we recently developed photo-responsive PBAEs by incorporating nitrobenzyl esters into the PBAE backbone [10, 11]. The photo-responsive PBAEs were synthesized through the poly-addition of (2-nitro-1, 3-phenylene)bis(methylene) diacrylate and a bisfunctional amine. Upon external UV-triggering, the nitrobenzyl ester

Gabriele Candiani (ed.), *Non-Viral Gene Delivery Vectors: Methods and Protocols*, Methods in Molecular Biology, vol. 1445,
DOI 10.1007/978-1-4939-3718-9_16, © Springer Science+Business Media New York 2016

bonds can be almost instantaneously cleaved and the PBAEs were degraded, releasing the complexed NA [12].

Here we describe the method of using the photo-responsive PBAEs as nonviral gene delivery vectors to deliver plasmid DNA (pDNA) encoded with enhanced green fluorescence protein (EGFP) (pEGFP) into HeLa cells. Upon UV irradiation, the release of DNA was demonstrated and the enhanced gene transfection efficiency was observed.

---

2   Materials

2.1   pDNA and Delivery Vectors (PBAEs)

1. pDNA encoding enhanced green fluorescence protein (EGFP) (pEGFP) (Elim Biopharm, Hayward, CA, USA) (*see* **Note 1**).

2. PBAEs were synthesized via Michael addition reaction (*see* **Note 2**).

2.2   Reagents for In Vitro Experiments

1. YOYO-1 (Life Technologies, Carlsbad, CA, USA) (*see* **Note 3**).

2. Ethidium bromide (EtBr).

3. RIPA lysis buffer. 250 mL of 0.1 M Tris, 210 mL of 0.1 M hydrochloric acid (HCl), and 40 mL of dH$_2$O to get the Tris–HCl buffer, pH 7.4. Add 5 g of NP40, 0.5 g of sodium dodecyl sulfate (SDS), and 4.383 g of sodium chloride (NaCl) into the freshly prepared Tris–HCl buffer and stir overnight.

4. 25 mM sodium acetate buffer (CH$_3$COONa), pH 5.2.

5. Human cervix adenocarcinoma cells (HeLa) (American Type Culture Collection, Rockville, MD, USA).

6. Complete cell-culture medium: Dulbecco's Modified Eagle Medium (DMEM) containing 10 % (v/v) fetal bovine serum (FBS) and 1 % (v/v) penicillin-streptomycin (*see* **Note 4**).

7. Opti-MEM.

8. 3-(4, 5-dimethylthiahiazol-2-yl)-2, 5-diphenyl-2H-tetrazolium bromide (MTT).

9. Bicinchoninic acid (BCA) assay.

10. Dimethyl sulfoxide (DMSO).

11. 20 mg/mL of heparin in deionized water (dH$_2$O).

12. Polypropylene microcentrifuge tubes.

13. Vortex.

14. Spectrophotometer-spectrofluorimeter (e.g., SpectraMax® M2 Multi-detection reader).

15. Flow cytometer.

3   Methods

3.1   Preparation of PBAE/DNA Complexes

1. Dissolve the PBAEs in DMSO to a final concentration of 100 mg/mL in a glass vial.

2. Dilute the polymers using 25 mM CH_3COONa buffer, pH 5.2, to the final concentration of 1 mg/mL in a 1.5 mL polypropylene microcentrifuge tube.

3. Determine the initial DNA concentration by measuring the absorbance (optical density, OD) at $\lambda = 260$ using the following calculation:

$$\text{DNA concentration} = 50\ \mu g\,/\,mL \times OD_{260} \times \text{dilution factor}$$
$$(\text{dilute the sample to give OD readings between 0.1 and 1.0}).$$

4. Dilute pEGFP in dH_2O to the final concentration of 0.2 mg/mL in a 1.5 mL polypropylene microcentrifuge tube.

5. Add 10 μL of 0.2 mg/mL polymer solution (*see* **Note 5**) to 2 μL of 0.2 mg/mL pEGFP solution (*see* **Note 6**) in a 1.5 mL polypropylene microcentrifuge tube, then vortex for 30 s and incubate for 20 min at room temperature (RT) to allow the formation of PBAE/DNA polyplexes with the polymer/DNA weight ratio of 5. Instead, add 20 μL of 0.2 mg/mL polymer solution to 2 μL of 0.2 mg/mL pEGFP solution to allow the formation of PBAE/DNA polyplexes with the polymer/DNA weight ratio of 10 (*see* **Note 7**).

3.2   UV-Triggered Polyplex Dissociation and DNA Release

1. Add 999 μL of dH_2O to 1 μL of 10 mg/mL EtBr to get a final 10 μg/mL EtBr solution.

2. Add 1 μL of 1 mg/mL pEGFP solution to 10 μL of 10 μg/mL EtBr solution in a 1.5 mL polypropylene microcentrifuge tube, vortex, and incubate the mixture for 1 h at RT to get 11 μL of EtBr-stained DNA solution.

3. Mix 50 μL of 0.2 mg/mL polymer solution with 11 μL of EtBr-stained DNA solution, vortex the mixture and incubate for 20 min at RT to allow the formation of polyplexes (polymer/DNA weight ratio of 10) (*see* **Note 8**). Add 39 μL of dH_2O to make the final volume of 100 μL.

4. UV-irradiate polyplex at $\lambda = 365$ nm, 20 mW/cm^2, for 5 min (*see* **Note 9**).

5. Add 0.5, 1, 2.5, 5, 25, and 100 μL of 20 mg/mL heparin to polyplexes solutions to make the final heparin concentrations of 0.1, 0.2, 0.5, 1, 2, 5, and 10 mg/mL, respectively.

6. Incubate the mixtures for 1 h at 37 °C.

7. Read the fluorescence intensity on a spectrofluorimeter at $\lambda_{ex} = 510$ nm and $\lambda_{em} = 590$ nm.

8. Calculate the DNA condensation efficiency (%) according to the following equation:

$$\text{DNA condensation efficiency} \left(\%\right) = \left(1 - \frac{F - F_{\text{EtBr}}}{F_0 - F_{\text{EtBr}}}\right) \times 100$$

Where F_{EtBr}, F, and F_0 denote the fluorescence intensity of pure EtBr solution, DNA/EtBr solution with polymer, and DNA/EtBr solution without any polymer, respectively (Fig. 1).

3.3 Intracellular Delivery of DNA

1. Seed HeLa cells onto 24-well plates at 2.5×10^4 cells/cm^2 in 0.5 mL/well of complete cell-culture medium.

2. When cells reach confluency, replace the complete cell-culture medium from each well with 0.2 mL/well of Opti-MEM.

3. Label DNA using YOYO-1 dye by mixing 2 μL of 1 mg/mL DNA solution, 3 μL of 5 mM/mL YOYO-1, and 5 μL of dH$_2$O to obtain a final concentration of 0.2 mg/mL YOYO-1-DNA. Determine the DNA concentration as described in Subheading 3.1, **step 3** (*see* **Note 10**).

4. Incubate the mixture for 20 min at RT in the dark.

5. Add 25 μL of 0.2 mg/mL polymers to 2.5 μL of 0.2 mg/mL YOYO-1-DNA solution in a polypropylene microcentrifuge tube (*see* **Note 11**).

6. Vortex the mixture, and incubate for 20 min at RT to allow the formation of polyplexes with the polymer/DNA weight ratio of 10 (*see* Subheading 3.1, **step 5**).

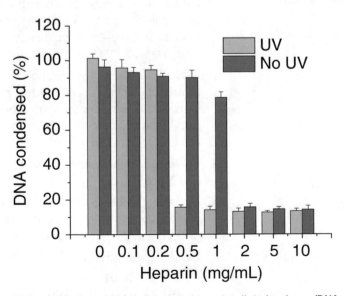

Fig. 1 DNA release from UV-irradiated and non-irradiated polymer/DNA polyplexes in the presence of heparin at various concentrations (*n* = 3)

7. Add 100 µL of polyplexes containing 0.5 µg of YOYO-1-DNA to each well seeded with cells (*see* **Note 12**).

8. After incubation for 4 h at 37 °C, wash the cells thrice with 1 mL of PBS (*see* **Note 13**).

9. Add 500 µL of RIPA lysis buffer to each well to lyse the cells and mix vigorously.

10. Rock the plate for 20 min at RT.

11. Monitor the YOYO-1-DNA content of 50 µL/well lysates in a 96-well plate by means of a spectrofluorimeter at $\lambda_{ex} = 485$ nm and $\lambda em = 530$ nm.

12. Prepare a set of 50 µL/well YOYO-1 DNA standards by diluting the 0.2 mg/mL YOYO-1 DNA into RIPA lysis buffer with 1, 0.5, 0.2, 0.1, 0.05, 0.02, and 0.01 µg/mL concentrations and read the fluorescence (*see* Subheading 3.3, **step 11**).

13. Prepare BCA working solution based on the BCA kit protocol (*see* **Note 14**), add 200 µL to each well containing 20 µL/well of cell lysates and the standards and then incubate for 30 min at 37 °C in a 96-well plate.

14. Read the absorbance at $\lambda = 562$ nm by means of a spectrophotometer.

15. Express the YOYO-1-DNA uptake level as ng of DNA/mg of cellular proteins (Fig. 2).

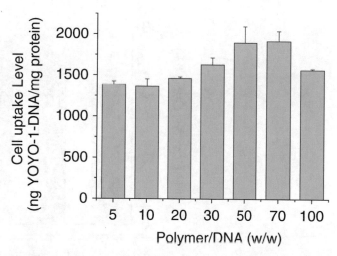

Fig. 2 Uptake level of polymer/DNA polyplexes with various weight ratios following incubation at 37 °C for 4 h ($n=3$)

3.4 In Vitro Transfection

1. Seed HeLa cells in 24-well plates at 2.5×10^4 cells/cm^2 in 0.5 mL of complete culture medium and culture cells until they reach 70 % confluence.

2. When cells reach confluence, replace the complete culture medium from each well with 0.2 mL/well fresh aliquots of Opti-MEM.

3. Add 125 µL of 0.2 mg/mL polymers to 2.5 µL of 0.2 mg/mL DNA solutions in a polypropylene microcentrifuge tube, vortex the mixture and incubate for 20 min at RT to allow the formation of polyplex with the polymer/DNA weight ratio of 10 (*see* **Note 11**).

4. Add 127.5 µL of polyplexes containing 0.5 µg of DNA/well to each well seeded with cells (*see* **Note 12**).

5. After incubation for 4 h at 37 °C, replace the culture medium from each well with 500 µL/well of complete cell-culture medium.

6. UV-irradiate the cells at $\lambda = 365$ nm, 20 mW/cm^2 for 0.5, 1, 2, 3, and 10 min (*see* **Note 9**).

7. Incubate the cells for further 44 h.

8. Evaluate the EGFP expression levels by flow cytometry and express the results as percentage of EGFP positive cells (Fig. 3).

3.5 Cytotoxicity

1. Seed HeLa cells at 3×10^4 cells/cm^2 on 96-well plates and cultured in 100 µL/ well of complete cell-culture medium.

2. After 24 h, remove the complete cell-culture medium from each well and add 100 µL/well of Opti-MEM.

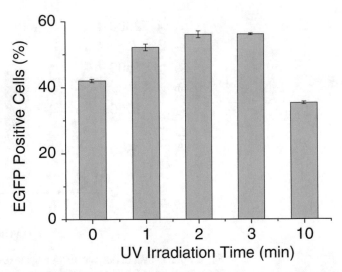

Fig. 3 Transfection efficiencies (TE) of polymer/DNA polyplexes at weight ratio of 50 in HeLa cells in response to UV irradiation ($\lambda = 365$ nm, 20 mW/cm^2) for various time

3. Add 25 μL of 0.2 mg/mL polymers to 0.5 μL of 0.2 mg/mL DNA solutions in a polypropylene microcentrifuge tube. Vortex the mixture and incubate for 20 min at RT to allow the formation of polyplex with the polymer/DNA weight ratio of 10.

4. Add 25.5 μL of polyplexes containing 0.1 μg of DNA/well to each well containing cells (*see* **Note 12**).

5. After incubation for 4 h at 37 °C, replace the old culture medium from each well with 500 μL/well of complete cell-culture medium.

6. UV-irradiate the cells at $\lambda = 365$ nm, 20 mW/cm^2 for 3, 5, or 10 min, and culture them for further 44 h (*see* **Note 9**).

7. Prepare 500 mg/mL of MTT solution by dissolving the 3-(4, 5-dimethylthiazol-2-yl)-2, 5-diphenyltetrazolium bromide into DMSO, then dilute it in PBS to the final concentration of 5 mg/mL.

8. Add 20 μL of MTT solution to each well and incubate for 4 h at 37 °C (*see* **Note 15**).

9. Read the absorbance at $\lambda = 570$ nm, with a reference $\lambda = 650$ nm using a microplate reader.

9. Calculate cell viability as percentage viability of control cells (%) according to the following equation:

$$\text{Cell viability}\,(\%) = \frac{A_{\text{p}}}{A_{\text{c}}} \times 100$$

Where A_{p}, and A_{c} denote the absorbance values of cells with the treatment of polyplexes and the cells without any treatment, respectively (Fig. 4).

4 Notes

1. For in vitro assays, pDNA was first dissolved at 1 mg/mL in dH$_2$O and stored at -20 °C and then diluted in dH$_2$O to the final concentration of 0.2 mg/mL.

2. Polymers were dissolved at 100 mg/mL in DMSO and stored at -20 °C avoiding light. For in vitro assays, polymers were further diluted in 25 mM sodium acetate buffer (pH = 5.2) to the final concentration of 1 mg/mL.

3. YOYO-1 was stored at -20 °C avoiding light.

4. HeLa cells were passaged at a subcultivation ratio of 1.4 and the cell-culture medium was renewed from twice to thrice per week.

5. The amount of polymer was based on the designated polymer/DNA weight ratio and the amount of DNA in each well. For example, in a 96-well plate and the weight ratio is 10, the formulation should

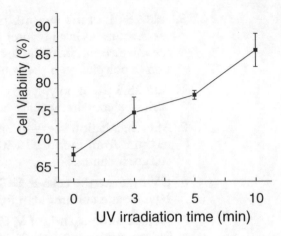

Fig. 4 Viabilities of HeLa cells transfected with polyplexes at polymer/DNA weight ratio of 50 and irradiated with UV light ($\lambda = 365$ nm, 20 mW/cm^2) for various time ($n = 3$)

    be the addition of 5 μL of 0.2 mg/mL polymer solution to 0.5 μL of 0.2 mg/mL pDNA solution.

6. The amount of DNA was based on the number of seeded cells and experiments. For a 96-well plate, the dose of pDNA in each well is 0.1 μg/well, while for a 24-well plate, the dose of pDNA is 0.5 μg/well.

7. Slightly pipette the mixture and vortex it before doing experiments since the polyplexes may aggregate in the bottom of the tube.

8. The diluted EtBr was incubated in the dark environment. Prepare as control pure EtBr solution by mixing 1 μL of dH$_2$O and 10 μL of 10 μg/mL EtBr solutions.

9. Use non UV-irradiated polyplexes as controls.

10. The labeling process is by mixing YOYO-1 and DNA together. YOYO-1 is a "turn-on" dye. Free YOYO-1 doesn't have fluoresce. No purification step is needed according to the manual protocol of YOYO-1.

11. Prepare polyplexes with various polymer/DNA weight ratios tuning the volume of the polymers (*see* Subheading 3.1, **step 5**).

12. Use cells without any polyplexes treatment as controls. The uptake, transfection, and toxicity experiments were designed at least in triplicates.

13. Add PBS into each well and shake the plate slightly to remove the polymers and DNA bound to the cell membranes.

14. Prepare working solutions by mixing 50 parts of BCA Reagent A with 1 part of BCA Reagent B (50:1 (v/v) Reagent A:B) based on the description in the protocol.

15. Time could be between 2 and 4 h depending on the density of cells.

References

1. Candolfi M, Xiong WD, Yagiz K, Liu CY, Muhammad AKMG, Puntel M et al (2010) Gene therapy-mediated delivery of targeted cytotoxins for glioma therapeutics. Proc Natl Acad Sci U S A 107:20021–20026

2. Mintzer MA, Simanek EE (2009) Nonviral vectors for gene delivery. Chem Rev 109:259–302

3. Nishikawa M, Huang L (2001) Nonviral vectors in the new millennium: delivery barriers in gene transfer. Hum Gene Ther 12:861–870

4. Hunter AC (2006) Molecular hurdles in polyfectin design and mechanistic background to polycation induced cytotoxicity. Adv Drug Deliv Rev 58:1523–1531

5. Ko IK, Ziady A, Lu S, Kwon YJ (2008) Acid-degradable cationic methacrylamide polymerized in the presence of plasmid DNA as tunable non-viral gene carrier. Biomaterials 29:3872–3881

6. Barua S, Joshi A, Banerjee A, Matthews D, Sharfstein ST, Cramer SM, Kane RS, Rege K (2009) Parallel synthesis and screening of polymers for nonviral gene delivery. Mol Pharm 6:86–97

7. Lynn DM, Langer R (2000) Degradable poly(β-amino esters): synthesis, characterization, and self-assembly with plasmid DNA. J Am Chem Soc 122:10761–10768

8. Akinc A, Anderson DG, Lynn DM, Langer R (2003) Synthesis of poly(β-amino ester)s optimized for highly effective gene delivery. Bioconjug Chem 14(5):979–988

9. Berry D, Lynn DM, Sasisekharan R, Langer R (2004) Poly(beta-amino ester)s promote cellular uptake of heparin and cancer cell death. Chem Biol 11:487–498

10. Lee HI, Wu W, Oh JK, Mueller L, Sherwood G, Peteanu L, Kowalewski T, Matyjaszewski K (2007) Light-induced reversible formation of polymeric micelles. Angew Chem Int Ed Engl 46:2453–2457

11. Schumers JM, Fustin CA, Gohy JF (2010) Light-responsive block copolymers. Macromol Rapid Commun 31:1588–1607

12. Deng X, Zheng N, Song Z, Yin L, Cheng J (2014) Trigger-responsive, fast-degradable poly(beta-amino ester)s for enhanced DNA unpackaging and reduced toxicity. Biomaterials 35:5006–5015

Chapter 17

Thermo-Responsive Polyplex Micelles with PEG Shells and PNIPAM Layer to Protect DNA Cores for Systemic Gene Therapy

Junjie Li, Zengshi Zha, and Zhishen Ge

Abstract

Simultaneous achievement of prolonged retention in blood circulation and efficient gene transfection activity in target tissues has always been a major challenge hindering in vivo applications of nonviral gene vectors via systemic administration. The engineered strategies for efficient systemic gene delivery are under wide investigation. These approaches include the thermo-responsive formation of a hydrophobic intermediate layer on PEG-shielded polyplex micelles. Herein, we constructed novel rod-shaped ternary polyplex micelles (TPMs) via complexation between the mixed block copolymers of poly(ethylene glycol)-b-poly{N'-[N-(2-aminoethyl)-2-aminoethyl]aspartamide} (PEG-b-PAsp(DET)) and poly(N-isopropylacrylamide)-b-PAsp(DET) (PNIPAM-b-PAsp(DET)) and plasmid DNA (pDNA) at room temperature (RT), exhibiting distinct temperature-responsive formation of a hydrophobic intermediate layer between PEG shells and pDNA cores through facile temperature increase from RT to body temperature (~37 °C).

Key words Polyplex micelle, Nonviral gene delivery system, Cancer gene therapy, Prolonged blood circulation, Temperature-responsive

1 Introduction

Poly(ethylene glycol) (PEG)-block-polycation block copolymers can form polyplex micelles via complexation with plasmid DNA (pDNA). The PEG-shielded polyplex micelles were recognized as promising nonviral in vivo gene vectors, especially for applications of systemic administration [1–4].

However, the polyplex micelles based on sole electrostatic interaction still suffered from unstable systemic circulation. In addition to the nuclease attack, which abundantly presents in blood, strong polyanions, particularly, heparan sulfate existing abundantly in the glomerular basement membrane (GBM) in kidney, is suggested as a major cause that induce dissociation of the electrostatic-formulated

Gabriele Candiani (ed.), *Non-Viral Gene Delivery Vectors: Methods and Protocols*, Methods in Molecular Biology, vol. 1445, DOI 10.1007/978-1-4939-3718-9_17, © Springer Science+Business Media New York 2016

structures [5]. Therefore, tolerability against these obstacles was considered to be critical challenge in developing polyplex micelles towards successful systemic gene delivery.

We have designed a ternary polyplex micelle system (TPM) characterized with hybrid shells via complexation between pDNA and the mixture of block copolymers, PEG-b-poly{N'-[N-(2-aminoethyl)-2-aminoethyl]aspartamide} (PEG-b-PAsp(DET)) and poly(N-isopropylacrylamide)-b-PAsp(DET) (PNIPAM-b-PAsp(DET)) [6]. The polyplex micelles were constructed through electrostatic interactions at 25 °C which is lower than lower critical solution temperature (LCST) (~32 °C), where both PEG and PNIPAM segments were water-soluble (see Fig. 1). Upon heating up to 37 °C, PNIPAM blocks turn out to be insoluble, and collapsed onto the core of polyplex micelles representing a hydrophobic intermediate layer between PEG shells and complexed pDNA cores [7]. The hydrophobic PNIPAM layer was expected to work as another barrier to the complexed pDNA cores in addition to PEG shells for restricting accessibilities of nuclease and strong counter polyanion. Accordingly, prolonged blood circulation and enhanced gene transfection efficacy in tumor tissue can be anticipated after intravenous injection of TPMs.

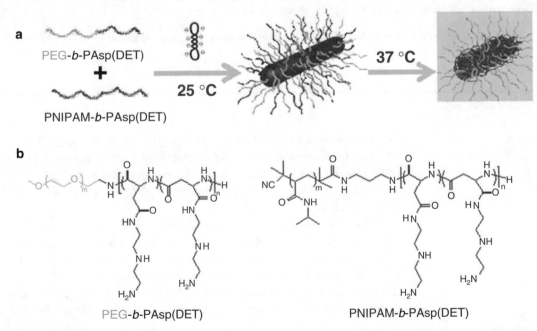

Fig. 1 (a) Schematic illustration of preparation of rod-like ternary polyplex micelles (TPMs) with thermo-responsive formation of hydrophobic intermediate barrier between PEG shells and complexed pDNA. (b) Structures of diblock copolymers, PEG-b-PAsp(DET) and PNIPAM-b-PAsp(DET)

2   Materials

2.1   Preparation of Ternary Polyplex Micelles

1. Anhydrous *N*-methyl-2-pyrrolidone (NMP).
2. Anhydrous *N,N*-dimethylformamide (DMF).
3. Anhydrous diethylenetriamine (DET).
4. Anhydrous dichloromethane (DCM).
5. Anhydrous hexane.
6. *N*-isopropylacrylamide (NIPAM).
7. Azobis(isobutyronitrile) (AIBN).
8. β-Benzyl-L-aspartate *N*-carboxyanhydride (BLA-NCA).
9. Nuclease-free ultrapure water (18 MΩ-cm at 25 °C).
10. 10 mM HEPES buffer, pH 7.4.
11. pDNA encoding luciferase (Luc), or soluble fms-like tyrosine kinase 1 (sFlt-1) with a CAG promoter was amplified in competent DH5α *Escherichia coli* and purified with a QIAGEN HiSpeed Plasmid MaxiKit (Germantown, Maryland, USA).

2.2   Tolerability of Polyplex Micelles Against Nuclease Digestion

1. TPMs(1:1), TPMs (1:3), and TPMs(3:1) at 33.3 μg/mL of DNA (*see* **Note 1**).
2. 1 U/μL of RNase-free DNase I.
3. Magnesium sulfonate.

2.3   Stability of Polyplex Micelles Against Counter Polyanion Exchange Reaction

1. TPMs(1:1), TPMs (1:3), and TPMs(3:1) at 33.3 μg/mL of DNA (*see* **Note 1**).
2. 20 μM of sodium dextran sulfate solution in 10 mM HEPES buffer, pH 7.4.
3. 1 μg/mL of ethidium bromide (EtBr) solution in deionized water (dH$_2$O).

2.4   Circulation of Polyplex Micelles in Bloodstream

1. pDNA labeled with Cy5 (Cy5-pDNA) using a Label IT Nucleic Acid Labeling Kit (Mirus Bio Corporation, Madison, WI), according to the manufacturer's protocol.
2. 1:1 (w/w) TPMs at 100 μg/mL of DNA.
3. 7-weeks-old female BALB/c mice (Charles River Laboratories, Yokohama, Japan).
4. 2.0–3.0% (w/w) isofurane in air.

2.5   Antitumor Activity Evaluation

1. 1:1 (w/w) TPMs at 100 μg/mL of sFlt-1 pDNA.
2. 150 mM sodium chloride (NaCl) in dH$_2$O.
3. Male 7-weeks-old CD-1(ICR) mice (Vital River Laboratory Animal Technology Co. Ltd., Beijing, China).

4. The murine hepatic cancer cell line, H22 (Shanghai Institute of Cell Biology, Shanghai, China).

5. Digital vernier caliper.

3 Methods

3.1 Preparation of Ternary Polyplex Micelles

1. Synthesize the block copolymers of $PNIPAM_{80}$-b-$PAsp(DET)_{34}$ and PEG_{272}-b-$PAsp(DET)_{64}$ according to the literature method [6].

2. Dissolve the block copolymers, $PNIPAM_{80}$-b-$PAsp(DET)_{34}$ and PEG_{272}-b-$PAsp(DET)_{64}$, as well as pDNA in 1 mL of 10 mM HEPES buffer, pH 7.4, as stock solutions.

3. Add the mixture of $PNIPAM_{80}$-b-$PAsp(DET)_{34}$ and PEG_{272}-b-$PAsp(DET)_{64}$ solutions with different PNIPAM/PEG weight ratios into a two-fold excess volume of pDNA solution for complexation at varying N/P ratios (residual molar ratio of amino groups in block copolymer to phosphate groups in pDNA) at 25 °C (see Note 1).

4. Adjust the final pDNA concentrations in all the polyplex micelles to 33.3 μg/mL in 10 mM HEPES buffer, pH 7.4 for in vitro experiments and 100 μg/mL in 10 mM HEPES buffer, pH 7.4 with 150 mM NaCl for in vivo experiments (see Note 2).

5. Incubate overnight at 4 °C followed by TEM and DLS charaterization at varying temperatures (see Note 3).

3.2 Tolerability of Polyplex Micelles Against Nuclease Digestion

1. Incubate the TPMs (1/3), TPMs (1/1), TPMs (3/1), or BPMs (1 mL) in 10 mM HEPES buffer, pH 7.4 with 5 mM magnesium sulfonate at 33.3 μg/mL of DNA for 30 min.

2. Add 10 μL of 1 U/μL DNase I into the above solutions.

3. Incubate for a predetermined time continually.

4. Monitor the absorbance change at λ_{260} nm by means of a microplate reader (ELX-800, BioTek, USA). Naked pDNA was subjected to immediate degradation as evidenced by the dramatic increase in absorbance of the reaction solution at $\lambda = 260$ nm.

3.3 Stability of Polyplex Micelles Against Counter-Polyanion Exchange Reaction

1. Incubate the TPMs (1/3), TPMs (1/1), TPMs (3/1), or BPMs (1 mL) in 10 mM HEPES buffer, pH 7.4 at 33.3 μg/mL DNA at 37 °C or 25 °C for 30 min.

2. Add 10 μL sodium dextran sulfate solutions in 10 mM HEPES buffer, pH 7.4, at various concentrations (see Notes 4 and 5).

3. Incubate for 3 h.

4. Mix the above solutions with 100 μL of 1 μg/mL EtBr solution.

5. Incubate for 10 min.

6. Measure the fluorescence at $\lambda_{em} = 590$ nm and $\lambda_{ex} = 310$ nm by means of a spectrofluorimeter (Hitachi F-4500, Japan).

3.4 Circulation of Polyplex Micelles in Bloodstream

1. Anesthetize 7-week-old female BALB/c mice with 2.0–3.0 % isofurane by intraveneous injection.

2. Place the mice on a temperature-controlled pad at 37 °C.

3. Fix the ear lobe dermis beneath a coverslip.

4. Inject 200 µL of polyplex micelle solution in 10 mM HEPES with 150 mM NaCl loading Cy5-labeled pDNA at 100 µg/mL pDNA via the tail vein.

5. Acquire video capture at snapshots every min (*see* **Note 6**).

3.5 Antitumor Activity Evaluation

1. Inoculate CD-1 (ICR) mice subcutaneously with murine H22 cells (4×10^6 cells per mouse).

2. Inject polyplex micelles containing 100 µg/mL of sFlt-1 pDNA in 10 mM HEPES buffer, pH 7.4, with 150 mM NaCl from tail vein on d 0 and 4 when the tumor size reached ~50 mm^3.

3. Measure tumor size every 2 or 3 days with a digital vernier caliper across its longest (*a*) and shortest diameters (*b*) (*see* **Note 7**).

4 Notes

1. The polyplex micelles prepared from the mixture of block copolymers, PNIPAM$_{80}$-*b*-PAsp(DET)$_{34}$ and PEG$_{272}$-*b*-PAsp(DET)$_{64}$ with various PNIPAM/PEG weight ratios of 1:3, 1:1, 3:1, and 0:1 were denoted as TPMs (1:3), TPMs (1:1), TPMs (3:1), and BPMs, respectively.

2. Prepare a fresh polyplex micelle solution each time.

3. Morphology observation of the polyplex micelles loading pBR322 pDNA at N/P 4 was conducted by an H-7000 electron microscope (Hitachi, Tokyo, Japan) operated at 75 kV acceleration voltage. Copper TEM grids with carbon-coated collodion film were glow-discharged for 10 s using an Eiko IB-3 ion coater (Eiko Engineering Co. Ltd., Japan). The grids were then dipped into desired polyplex micelle solution which has been treated by uranyl acetate (UA) solution (2 % (w/v)) for 30 s for DNA staining. The sample grids were blotted by filter paper to remove excess complex solution, followed by drying for 10 min (*see* Fig. 2).

4. The S/Ps (sulfate groups on dextran sulfate/phosphate groups on pDNA) of sodium dextran sulfate to DNA were set to 0, 0.5, 1.0, 2.0, 4.0, 10, and 20, respectively.

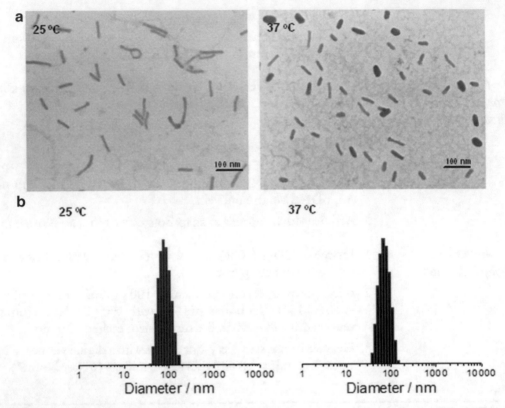

Fig. 2 Characterization of the polyplex micelles. (**a**) TEM images and (**b**) size distribution by DLS of TPMs (1/1) prepared at 25 °C followed by 20 min incubation at 37 °C

5. Calculate decomplexation degree of polyplex micelles against sodium dextran sulfate according to the literature Equation (*see* Fig. 3) [6, 8].

6. The circulation of polyplex micelles in bloodstream was investigated using IVRTCLSM in live mice. All pictures were acquired using a Nikon A1R confocal laser scanning microscope system connected to an upright ECLIPSE FN1 (Nikon Corp., Tokyo, Japan) with a 20× objective, 640 nm diode laser, and a band-pass emission filter of 700/75 nm. The pinhole diameter was set with a 10 μm optical slice. The average fluorescence intensity at each time point was determined by comparing the selected regions of interest in the veins and interstitial space of ear lobe. The retention half-life of the polyplex micelles in blood circulation was defined as the time when the remaining fluorescence intensity in the vein was half of the maximum (*see* Fig. 4).

7. Tumor size was measured every 2 or 3 days with a digital vernier caliper across its longest (*a*) and shortest diameters (*b*). Calculate volume of tumor (*V*) according to the formula $V = a \times b^2/2$. Tumor progression was evaluated in terms of relative tumor volume to day 1, $n = 5$ (*see* Fig. 5).

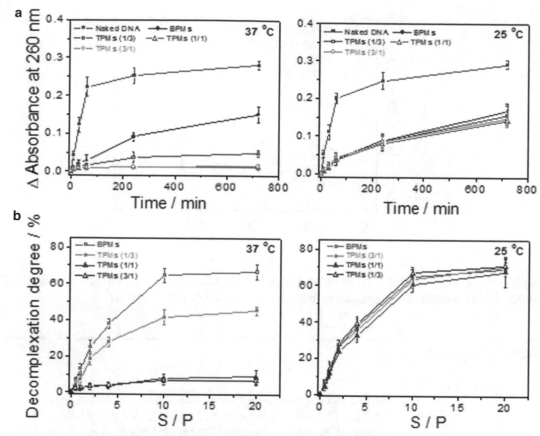

Fig. 3 (**a**) Degradation profiles of pDNA loaded into polyplex micelles (BPMs, TPMs (1/3), TPMs (1/1), and TPMs (3/1)) at 37 °C and 25 °C in the presence of 10 U DNase I. (**b**) Decomplexation degrees of polyplex micelles at 37 and 25 °C against an exchange reaction with dextran sulfate at various S/P ratios (the molar ratio of sulfate groups of dextran sulfate to phosphate groups of pDNA) after 3 h incubation. The results are expressed as mean ± s.d. ($n = 3$)

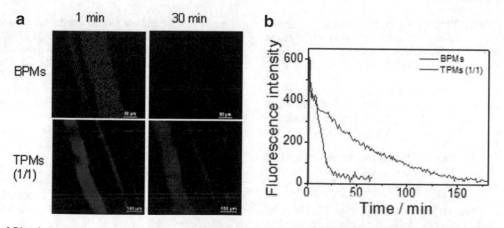

Fig. 4 Blood circulation and tumor accumulation of the polyplex micelles (BPMs and TPMs (1/1)). (**a**) IVRTCLSM images of the polyplex micelles (BPMs and TPMs (1/1)) loading Cy5-labeled pDNA in mouse earlobe blood vessels after intravenous injection for 1 and 30 min. (**b**) Time-dependent in vivo fluorescence intensity of polyplex micelles by comparing the selected regions of vein (*square*) and interstitial space (*dotted square*)

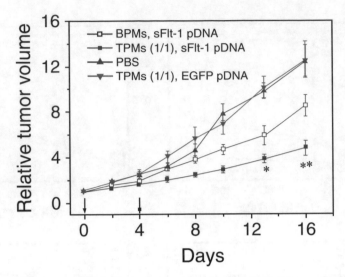

Fig. 5 Antitumor effects of TPMs (1/1) and BPMs loading sFlt-1 pDNA. TPMs (1/1) loading EGFP pDNA and PBS as the negative controls. Data are expressed as mean ± s.d. ($n=5$). *$P < 0.05$, **$P < 0.01$

Acknowledgment

The financial support from the National Natural Scientific Foundation of China (NNSFC) (Projects 51273188), the Foundation for the Author of National Excellent Doctoral Dissertation of PR China (FANEDD) (201224), and the Fundamental Research Funds for the Central Universities (WK3450000002, WK2060200012) is gratefully acknowledged.

References

1. Miyata K, Nishiyama N, Kataoka K (2012) Rational design of smart supramolecular assemblies for gene delivery: chemical challenges in the creation of artificial viruses. Chem Soc Rev 41:2562–2574

2. Mintzer MA, Simanek EE (2009) Nonviral vectors for gene delivery. Chem Rev 109:259–302

3. Guo X, Huang L (2012) Recent advances in nonviral vectors for gene delivery. Acc Chem Res 45:971–979

4. Yin H, Kanasty RL, Eltoukhy AA, Vegas AJ, Dorkin JR, Anderson DG (2014) Non-viral vectors for gene-based therapy. Nat Rev Genet 15:541–555

5. Zuckerman JE, Choi CHJ, Han H, Davis ME (2012) Polycation-siRNA nanoparticles can disassemble at the kidney glomerular basement membrane. Proc Natl Acad Sci U S A 109:3137–3142

6. Li J, Chen Q, Zha Z, Li H, Toh K, Dirisala A, Matsumoto Y, Osada K, Kataoka K, Ge Z (2015) Ternary polyplex micelles with PEG shells and intermediate barrier to complexed DNA cores for efficient systemic gene delivery. J Control Release 209:77–87

7. Schild HG (1992) Poly(N-isopropylacrylamide)-experiment, theory and application. Prog Polym Sci 17:163–249

8. Jiang XA, Zheng YR, Chen HH, Leong KW, Wang TH, Mao HQ (2010) Dual-sensitive micellar nanoparticles regulate DNA unpacking and enhance gene-delivery efficiency. Adv Mater 22:2556–2560

Part III

Substrate-Mediated Gene Delivery

Application of Polyethylenimine-Grafted Silicon Nanowire Arrays for Gene Transfection

Hongwei Wang, Jingjing Pan, Hong Chen, and Lin Yuan

Abstract

Polyplexes are one of the most important and promising approaches to deliver exogenous DNA into cells. However, it is severely restricted by the aggregation of polyplexes. Surface-tethered polyplexes can inhibit the aggregation effect and increase the local concentrations of DNA, exhibiting an excellent potential in gene transfection. Since silicon nanowires have the ability to penetrate the cell membrane, branched polyethylenimine (bPEI)-grafted silicon nanowire arrays (SiNWAs) can stimulate gene transfection to a great extent. Herein, the method for the preparation of bPEI-grafted SiNWAs, as an example of surface-tethered polyplexes, is introduced in detail.

Key words Surface, Polyplexes, DNA, Polycation, Gene transfection

1 Introduction

Polyplexes, the polyelectrolyte complexes of polycations and DNA, can deliver heterogenous genetic materials into cells, playing an important role in gene transfection as nonviral vectors. However, there are some limitations for the application of polyplexes as pharmaceutical products. The major problem is their poor stability in aqueous solutions, including in the circulatory system in vivo. In these environments, polyplexes tend to form aggregates, which decrease their concentration during transfection and may cause some trouble in the storage [1, 2]. Therefore, one of the crucial issues is to develop new methods for maintaining the dispersity of polyplexes and keeping as high as possible their local concentration.

Several strategies based on biomaterials have been used to improve the stability of polyplexes, such as formation of micro- or nano-particles [3, 4], encapsulation in hydrogels [5, 6], loading into porous scaffolds [7, 8], and tethering onto material surfaces [9, 10]. These methods may not only inhibit the aggregation of polyplexes due to the isolation from close contact, but also increase the local

Gabriele Candiani (ed.), *Non-Viral Gene Delivery Vectors: Methods and Protocols*, Methods in Molecular Biology, vol. 1445,
DOI 10.1007/978-1-4939-3718-9_18, © Springer Science+Business Media New York 2016

concentrations of DNA due to its release from the material. Among them, surface-tethered polyplexes have received great attention since they can be well controlled on the surface coverage and can make use of the physical properties of material surfaces.

In the application to form surface-tethered polyplexes, polyethylenimine (PEI), poly-L-(lysine) (PLL), poly (2-(dimethylamino) ethylmethacrylate) (PDMAEMA), and chitosan are the most widely used polycations due to their ability to achieve high transfection efficiencies. Segura et al. tethered DNA-containing polyplexes with biotin-functionalized PEI and PLL through specific binding with avidin on the surfaces [11, 12]. Park et al. reported another strategy to load DNA on gold surfaces modified by adamantine groups via the host-guest recognition with β-cyclodextrin-functionalized PEI [13]. Li et al. prepared polycaprolactone (PCL) surfaces functionalized with (PDMAEMA)/gelatin complexes and adsorbed DNA on the surfaces [14]. Instead, Holmes et al. studied polyelectrolyte multilayers composed of glycol-chitosan and hyaluronic acid able to carry DNA to NIH3T3 fibroblasts and HEK293 kidney cells in vitro [15]. Interestingly, all of these surface-tethered polyplexes exhibited enhanced gene transfection efficiencies.

In order to further increase DNA delivery into cells, we developed a new method by forming polyplexes on branched PEI (bPEI)-grafted silicon nanowire arrays (SiNWAs) [10]. Since this method takes advantage of surface-tethered polyplexes in carrying DNA and direct penetration of nanowires into cells, a great promotion of transfection efficiency was observed. Herein, the procedure for fabrication of SiNWAs, modification of bPEI on the surfaces and formation of polyplexes are introduced as an example of surface-tethered polyplexes for in vitro DNA transfection.

2 Materials

All reagents are purchased from Shanghai Chemical Reagent Co. and stored at room temperature (RT) (unless otherwise indicated). Organic reagents are purified before use. All the solutions are prepared by using ultrapure water (dH$_2$O, purifying deionized water to attain a sensitivity of 18.2 MΩ-cm at 25 °C) (*see* **Note 1**). Use high purity nitrogen gas (N$_2$, 99.999 %) in this method. Waste materials are disposed according to all waste disposal regulations.

2.1 Substrate Components

1. Silicon wafers [n-doped, (100)-oriented] (Guangzhou Semiconductor Materials Research Institute, Guangzhou, China).

2. Nitric acid (HNO$_3$) cleaning solution: 100 mL of concentrated HNO$_3$ in 200 mL of dH$_2$O (*see* **Note 2**).

3. Etching solution: dissolve 1.53 g of AgNO$_3$ in 135 mL of dH$_2$O, and add 45 mL HF (*see* **Note 3**).

4. "Piranha" solution (*see* **Note 4**).

5. Acetone.

6. Absolute ethanol (EtOH).

7. Anhydrous toluene solution.

8. 3-Aminopropyltriethoxysilane (APTES).

9. Acetonitrile (CH_3CN).

10. NPC activation solution: anhydrous CH_3CN solution containing 51 g/L of 4-nitrophenyl chloroformate (NPC) and 3.6 % (v/v) of triethylamine (TEA).

11. Teflon autoclaves (with diameter of 10 cm and height of 2 cm).

12. Incubator.

13. Ultrasonic cleaner.

2.2 Polyplex Components

1. Plasmid DNA (pDNA), pRL-CMV (Promega, Madison, WI) (*see* **Note 5**).

2. DNA solution: 0.1 µg/µL of pDNA in dH_2O (*see* **Note 6**).

3. DNA salt solution: 75 ng/µL of DNA in 150 mM sodium chloride (NaCl) in dH_2O (*see* **Note 7**).

4. bPEI solution: disperse 50 mg of bPEI (molecular weight, MW, 25 kDa, Sigma-Aldrich, Saint Louis, MO) in 10 mL of dH_2O (*see* **Note 8**).

5. 75 % (v/v) EtOH in dH_2O.

6. Toluene.

7. Dichloromethane (CH_2Cl_2).

8. Methanol (MeOH).

9. 48-well polystyrene plate.

2.3 Cell Culture and Gene Transfection

1. HeLa cells, human adenocarcinoma cell line (ATCC, Manassas, VA).

2. Serum-free cell culture medium: Dulbecco's Modified Eagle Medium (DMEM) supplemented with 100 U/mL of penicillin and 100 µg/mL of streptomycin.

3. Complete cell culture medium: serum-free cell culture medium with 10 % (v/v) fetal bovine serum (FBS).

4. Sterile phosphate-buffered saline (PBS).

5. Cell lysis reagent (Promega).

6. Renilla Luciferase Assay (Promega).

7. Bradford Protein Assay Kit (Beyotime, Shanghai, China).

8. 48-well polystyrene cell culture plates.

9. Incubator.

10. Microplate luminometer.

3   Methods

3.1   Chip Preparation

The cleaning and etching of silicon chips are conducted in the Teflon autoclaves. Clean and dry these autoclaves before use (*see* **Note 9**).

1. Polish silicon wafers on one side and cut into square chips before use (*see* **Note 10**).

2. Clean the chips by ultrasound with acetone for 2 min, with EtOH for 2 min, and with dH_2O for 2 min, sequentially and for at least thrice.

3. Immerse the chips in "piranha" solution for further cleaning for 10 min.

4. Remove the "piranha" solution, rinse the chips extensively with dH_2O, and dry under N_2 stream (*see* **Note 11**).

3.2   Fabrication of Silicon Nanowire Arrays (SiNWAs)

1. Separate the cleaned silicon chips evenly in the Teflon autoclave and put into the incubator for 10 min at 50 °C (*see* **Note 12**).

2. Preheat 30 mL of etching solution at 50 °C and pour into each Teflon autoclave until all the chips are immersed (*see* **Note 13**).

3. After 10 min, remove the etching solution from the autoclaves and carefully rinse the chips with dH_2O. SiNWs will form on the surfaces of silicon chips, covered by a layer of silver dendrites (*see* **Note 14**).

4. Carefully add HNO_3 cleaning solution into each autoclave until all the chips are immersed. Wait for 1 min until silver dendrites are dissolved by HNO_3 solution.

5. Remove the cleaning solution and rinse extensively the resulting materials with dH_2O (*see* **Note 15**).

3.3   Preparation of PEI-Grafted SiNWAs (SiNWAs-PEI)

The procedure for surface modification is performed as shown in Fig. 1. During the preparation, SiNWAs should be forced facing upwards without any contact with the containers.

1. Prepare hydroxyl-terminated SiNWAs (SiNWAs-OH) by adding SiNWAs to 20 mL of "piranha" solution and incubate for 2 h at 90 °C. Hydroxyl groups will be generated on the surface of SiNWAs with the chemical bonds as Si-OH.

2. Rinse extensively the SiNWAs-OH with dH_2O and acetone, then dry the cleaned materials under N_2 stream.

3. Functionalize SiNWAs with amino groups (SiNWAs-NH_2) by immersing the freshly prepared hydroxyl-terminated SiNWAs in 20 mL of anhydrous toluene solution.

4. Add dropwise 0.4 mL of APTES to the solution under the protection of N_2 gas.

5. Incubate for 18 h at 80 °C to allow the amino groups to chemically bond on the surface of SiNWAs.

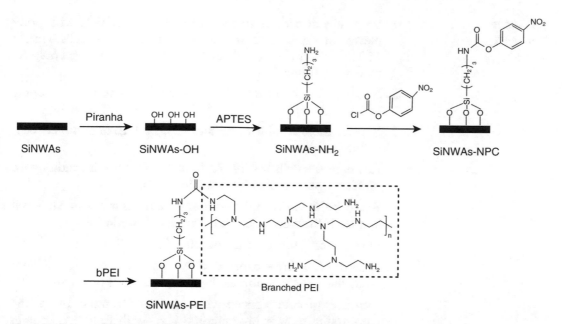

Fig. 1 Surface modification of silicon nanowire arrays (SiNWAs)

6. Rinse extensively the SiNWAs-NH$_2$ with toluene, CH$_2$Cl$_2$, MeOH, dH$_2$O, and acetone.

7. Dry the cleaned materials under N$_2$ stream.

8. Activate SiNWAs-NH$_2$ with NPC (NPC-activated SiNWAs-NH$_2$) by immersing SiNWAs-NH$_2$ in 10 mL of NPC activation solution (*see* **Note 16**).

9. Clean the NPC-activated SiNWAs-NH$_2$ with CH$_3$CN, dH$_2$O, and acetone.

10. Dry the cleaned materials under N$_2$ stream.

11. Prepare bPEI-grafted SiNWAs by immersing the freshly prepared NPC-activated SiNWAs-NH$_2$ into 6 mL of PEI solution for 18 h at 30 °C.

12. Wash the bPEI-grafted surfaces with abundant dH$_2$O and acetone to remove the unreacted bPEI and then dry under N$_2$ stream (*see* **Note 17**).

3.4 Polyplex Formation on PEI-Grafted Surfaces

1. Immerse bPEI-grafted SiNWAs in 75% EtOH for 20 min at RT, at least twice, for sterilization.

2. Rinse extensively the bPEI-grafted SiNWAs with dH$_2$O and dry in air.

3. Place the sterilized bPEI-grafted SiNWAs into the wells of a 48-well plate.

4. Add 20 μL of DNA solution onto the surface of bPEI-grafted SiNWAs for 30 min to ensure maximum loading of the DNA (*see* **Note 18**).

3.5 Gene Transfection on Surfaces

1. Seed cells directly onto the bPEI-grafted SiNWAs with polyplexes on the surface at a density of 6.25×10^4 cells/cm^2 in 250 μL of serum-free cell culture medium in a 48-well polystyrene cell culture plate.

2. Incubate for 3 h at 37 °C, 99% humidity with regular supply of 5% CO_2.

3. Replace the old culture medium with 250 μL of complete cell-culture medium.

4. Incubate the cells for 24–72 h at 37 °C, 99% humidity with regular supply of 5% CO_2 (*see* **Note 19**).

5. Remove the old complete cell-culture medium from each well and wash the cells twice with 250 μL of sterile PBS.

6. Lyse the cells using 65 μL of cell-culture lysis reagent.

7. Quantify Luciferase expression by using the Renilla Luciferase Assay System according to the manufacturer's protocol.

8. Evaluate protein concentration in each sample using the Coomassie brilliant blue method [16] with Bradford Protein Assay Kit.

9. Calculate the transfection efficiency by means of the expression products from the heterogenous genes and standardize over the quantity of cellular proteins (*see* **Note 20**).

4   Notes

1. Since sodium azide affects cell growth, it is not added in the reagents.

2. HNO_3 is a strong acid and a powerful oxidizing agent. The dilution of HNO_3 in dH_2O will release heat. It is dangerous to contact with HNO_3 vapor. The handling of HNO_3 should be performed under the fume hood to avoid violent reactions. To avoid acids splash out of the containers, the cleaning solution is prepared by dropwise addition of HNO_3 in dH_2O at low temperature.

3. HF is highly corrosive which does dissolve glass. The experiments using HF have to be performed in Teflon containers. HF solutions should be freshly prepared before use. $AgNO_3$ is light sensitive and can undergo decomposition when exposed to light. The etching solution should be kept away from light.

4. Before preparation, both concentrated sulfuric acid (H_2SO_4) and 30% (v/v) hydrogen peroxide (H_2O_2) should be laid in the ice bath. Add 9 mL of ice-cold H_2O_2 slowly into 21 mL of concentrated H_2SO_4. At the same time mix them carefully and prevent high temperature while mixing. Concentrated H_2SO_4 is a strong acid and a powerful oxidizing agent. The handling

of H_2SO_4 should be performed under the fume hood and require a full face shield, heavy duty rubber gloves. In order to avoid violent reactions and explosion, always add the H_2O_2 to H_2SO_4 very slowly in the conditions with low temperature when preparing the "piranha" solution. "Piranha" solution is very likely to become hot and explosive. It cannot be stored in a closed container and for a long time.

5. DNA can be the commercial pDNA or constructed ones by different labs. For example, pRL-CMV encoding the Renilla luciferase reporter gene, is used for gene transfection in this study. In order to amplify the pDNA, it is suggested to transform DNA into *Escherichia coli* (*E. coli*).

6. Since the purity of pDNA will affect the gene transfection, purify the DNA with the pDNA purification kit (TIANprep Midi, TIANGEN Biotech., Beijing, China) following the manufacturer's protocol. Measure the purity and concentration of DNA by the absorbance at $\lambda = 260$ nm and $\lambda = 280$ nm. An appropriate ratio of A260/280 around 1.8 (at 1.7–1.9) can reflect high purity of DNA.

7. Prepare fresh DNA salt solution before use. The volumes of NaCl solution, DNA solution, and dH_2O are changed according to pDNA concentration in DNA solution. For example, if DNA concentration in DNA solution is 0.1 g/L, the volumes of NaCl solution, DNA solution, and dH_2O should be 30 μL, 150 μL, and 20 μL, respectively.

8. Since the application of bPEI with large MW result in a high transfection rate, 25 kDa bPEI is suggested in this method.

9. The etching of silicon chips can be affected by some other ions. Be sure that there are no contaminant ions remaining in the autoclave.

10. SiNWAs are all formed on the polished side. The size of chips is chosen according to the requirement of transfection experiments. For convenient operation, the suggested size is 0.5 cm × 0.5 cm.

11. For characterization of the properties of the materials, at least 150 similar chips are selected for the following steps.

12. We suggest to put 20–30 chips in each autoclaves.

13. During the reaction, keep the Teflon autoclaves closed by the caps and stayed still at 50 °C. Any movement during the etching of silicon chips may result in the failure to form SiNWAs.

14. Generally, SiNWAs with the length of ~10 μm and the diameter ~60 nm will generate on the top surface of silicon chips (*see* Fig. 2a).

15. Silicon nanowires are all vertically aligned. They should be faced upwards. Otherwise, the touch or friction of nanowires

with the containers may break the nanowires, causing the defect of SiNWAs' structure.

16. Perform the reaction for 18 h at 30 °C under protection of N_2 to generate NPC-activated SiNWAs.

17. The morphology of SiNWAs-PEI is similar to that of SiNWAs (*see* Fig. 2).

18. The volume of DNA salt solution used to form polyplexes is dependent on the amino density of PEI- grafted SiNWAs. Generally, the N/P ratio (molar ratio of nitrogen to phosphate) is suggested to be around 8.0 for achieving high transfection efficiency. The amino density of the surfaces can be measured by 4-nitrobenzaldehyde. Briefly, several chips of PEI-grafted SiNWAs are immersed in 20 mL of anhydrous EtOH containing 20 mg of 4-nitrobenzaldehyde and 16 μL of acetic acid (CH_3COOH) for 3 h at 50 °C. After rinsing in absolute EtOH for 2 min and drying under a N_2 stream, the samples are immersed in 3.5 mL of dH_2O containing 7 μL of CH_3COOH, and the solution is incubated for 3 h at 40 °C. The amount of 4-nitrobenzaldehyde liberated, which is equivalent to the surface amine content, is determined by measuring the absorbance at $\lambda = 268.5$ nm. The content of phosphor (P) in DNA is 3 nmol P/μg DNA.

19. Additional PEI-DNA polyplexes will increase the transfection efficiency. Specifically, according to a previous study [10], polyplexes formed by using 2 kDa PEI with DNA at N/P ~80.

20. The transfection efficiency could be expressed as relative light units per milligram of the cellular protein (RLU/mg protein).

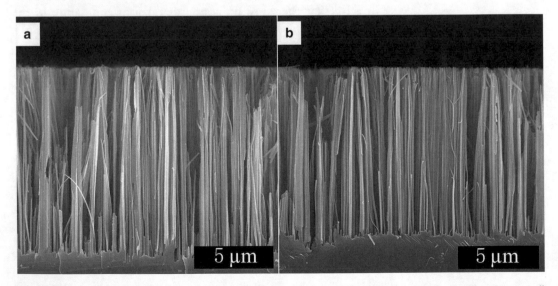

Fig. 2 SEM images of silicon nanowire arrays. (**a**) Freshly prepared silicon nanowire arrays without any modification and (**b**) PEI-grafted silicon nanowire arrays (PEI-grafted SiNWAs)

Acknowledgement

This work was supported by the National Natural Science Foundation of China (21334004, 21374070 and 21474072), and the Natural Science Foundation of the Jiangsu Higher Education Institutions of China (13KJA430006).

References

1. Bengali Z, Shea LD (2005) Gene delivery by immobilization to cell-adhesive substrates. MRS Bull 30:659–662

2. Gersbach CA, Coyer SR, Le Doux JM, Garcia AJ (2007) Biomaterial-mediated retroviral gene transfer using self-assembled monolayers. Biomaterials 28:5121–5127

3. Blum JS, Saltzman WM (2008) High loading efficiency and tunable release of plasmid DNA encapsulated in submicron particles fabricated from PLGA conjugated with poly-L-lysine. J Control Release 129:66–72

4. Bowman K, Sarkar R, Raut S, Leong KW (2008) Gene transfer to hemophilia A mice via oral delivery of FVIII-chitosan nanoparticles. J Control Release 132:252–259

5. Wieland JA, Houchin-Ray TL, Shea LD (2007) Non-viral vector delivery from PEG-hyaluronic acid hydrogels. J Control Release 120:233–241

6. Kong HJ, Kim ES, Huang YC, Mooney DJ (2008) Design of biodegradable hydrogel for the local and sustained delivery of angiogenic plasmid DNA. Pharm Res 25:1230–1238

7. Jang JH, Shea LD (2003) Controllable delivery of non-viral DNA from porous scaffolds. J Control Release 86:157–168

8. Guo T, Zhao J, Chang J, Ding Z, Hong H, Chen J, Zhang J (2006) Porous chitosan-gelatin scaffold containing plasmid DNA encoding transforming growth factor-β1 for chondrocytes proliferation. Biomaterials 27:1095–1103

9. Bielinska AU, Yen A, Wu HL, Zahos KM, Sun R, Weiner ND, Baker JR, Roessler BJ (2000) Application of membrane-based dendrimer/DNA complexes for solid phase transfection in vitro and in vivo. Biomaterials 21:877–887

10. Pan J, Lyu Z, Jiang W, Wang H, Liu Q, Tan M, Yuan L, Chen H (2014) Stimulation of gene transfection by silicon nanowire arrays modified with polyethylenimine. ACS Appl Mater Interfaces 6:14391–14398

11. Segura T, Shea LD (2002) Surface-tethered DNA complexes for enhanced gene delivery. Bioconjug Chem 13:621–629

12. Segura T, Volk MJ, Shea LD (2003) Substrate-mediated DNA delivery: role of the cationic polymer structure and extent of modification. J Control Release 93:69–84

13. Park IK, Von Recum HA, Jiang SY, Pun SH (2006) Supramolecular assembly of cyclodextrin-based nanoparticles on solid surfaces for gene delivery. Langmuir 22:8478–8484

14. Li CY, Yuan W, Jiang H, Li JS, Xu FJ, Yang WT, Ma J (2011) PCL film surfaces conjugated with P(DMAEMA)/gelatin complexes for improving cell immobilization and gene transfection. Bioconjug Chem 22:1842–1851

15. Holmes CA, Tabrizian M (2013) Substrate-mediated gene delivery from glycol-chitosan/hyaluronic acid polyelectrolyte multilayer films. ACS Appl Mater Interfaces 5:524–531

16. Bradford MMA (1976) Rapid and sensitive method for the quantitation of microgram quantities of protein utilizing the principle of protein-dye binding. Anal Biochem 72:248–254

INDEX

Gabriele Candiani (ed.), *Non-Viral Gene Delivery Vectors: Methods and Protocols*, Methods in Molecular Biology, vol. 1445,
DOI 10.1007/978-1-4939-3718-9, © Springer Science+Business Media New York 2016

Printed in the United States
By Bookmasters